Introduction to
Medical Immunology

IMMUNOLOGY SERIES

Editor-in-Chief
NOEL R. ROSE
Professor and Chairman
Department of Immunology and
Infectious Diseases
The Johns Hopkins University
School of Hygiene and Public Health
Baltimore, Maryland

European Editor
ZDENEK TRNKA
Basel Institute for
Immunology
Basel, Switzerland

1. Mechanisms in Allergy: Reagin-Mediated Hypersensitivity
   Edited by Lawrence Goodfriend, Alec Sehon and Robert P. Orange

2. Immunopathology: Methods and Techniques
   Edited by Theodore P. Zacharia and Sidney S. Breese, Jr.

3. Immunity and Cancer in Man: An Introduction
   Edited by Arnold E. Reif

4. *Bordetella pertussis:* Immunological and Other Biological Activities
   J.J. Munoz and R.K. Bergman

5. The Lymphocyte: Structure and Function (in two parts)
   Edited by John J. Marchalonis

6. Immunology of Receptors
   Edited by B. Cinader

7. Immediate Hypersensitivity: Modern Concepts and Development
   Edited by Michael K. Bach

8. Theoretical Immunology
   Edited by George I. Bell, Alan S. Perelson, and George H. Pimbley, Jr.

9. Immunodiagnosis of Cancer (in two parts)
   Edited by Ronald B. Herberman and K. Robert McIntire

10. Immunologically Mediated Renal Diseases: Criteria for Diagnosis and Treatment
    Edited by Robert T. McCluskey and Giuseppe A. Andres

11. Clinical Immunotherapy
    Edited by Albert F. LoBuglio

12. Mechanisms of Immunity to Virus-Induced Tumors
    Edited by John W. Blasecki

13. Manual of Macrophage Methodology: Collection, Characterization, and Function
    Edited by Herbert B. Herscowitz, Howard T. Holden, Joseph A. Bellanti, and Abdul Ghaffar

14. Suppressor Cells in Human Disease
    Edited by James S. Goodwin

15. Immunological Aspects of Aging
    Edited by Diego Segre and Lester Smith

16. Cellular and Molecular Mechanisms of Immunologic Tolerance
    Edited by Tomáš Hraba and Milan Hašek

Introduction to
Medical Immunology
Second Edition

edited by

Gabriel Virella
Jean-Michel Goust
H. Hugh Fudenberg

Medical University of South Carolina
Charleston, South Carolina

MARCEL DEKKER, INC.   New York and Basel

Library of Congress Cataloging-in-Publication Data

Introduction to medical immunology / edited by Gabriel Virella, Jean-Michel
Goust, H. Hugh Fudenberg. -- 2nd ed.
   p. cm. -- (Immunology series ; 50)
   Includes bibliographical references.
   ISBN 0-8247-8229-1
   1. Immunology. 2. Immunologic diseases. I. Virella, Gabriel,
II. Goust, Jean-Michel, III. Fudenberg, H. Hugh, IV. Series: Immunology
series ; v. 50
   [DNLM: 1. Immunity. 2. Immunologic Diseases. W1 IM53K v.50 /
QW 504 I6226]
QR181.I516   1990
616.079--dc20
DNLM/DLC
for Library of Congress   89-71546
                                                 CIP

This book is printed on acid-free paper.

MARCEL DEKKER INC.
270 Madison Avenue, New York, New York 10016

Current printing (last digit):
10 9 8 7 6 5 4 3 2 1

PRINTED IN THE UNITED STATES OF AMERICA

Series Introduction

The teaching of immunology to students of medicine and other health professions presents a major challenge to the educator. Immunology has emerged relatively recently as a distinct scientific discipline; for most of its century-long existence it was considered a junior partner of microbiology. Separate courses in immunology are still a rarity in the medical curriculum. Students, therefore, have in the past encountered immunology in a number of guises. Often their study of immunology dealt only with defense against infectious diseases. These limited slices of immunology conveyed to students a biased view suggesting that immunology was only an applied discipline. Students failed to perceive the full scope and import of this science of biological recognition. They did not appreciate the critical importance of self versus non-self discrimination in multicellular, metazoan life. The result is that the immune system was not seen in its proper perspective—as a primary physiological regulatory system. The student, in turn, did not grasp the central function of the immune system in health maintenance as well as in the protection from disease.

This historical anomaly relegated immunology to a subsidiary position in medical education and must be corrected by including unified courses in the medical curriculum that present immunology as a distinct biological discipline. Well-written, comprehensive, and authoritative textbooks are required for such courses. We are fortunate that a few such texts are now available. The present textbook, edited by Drs. Virella, Goust, and Fudenberg, is an outstanding example of such a book. Written by a group of active investigators and experienced teachers, it combines the best features of a multiauthored and a tightly edited volume. Its widespread acceptance is evident from the need to prepare a second edition so soon after the first one. I believe that health science educators will find this new edition even more useful than the first.

Noel R. Rose

Foreword

The original edition of this textbook was developed over a number of years, predominantly by the immunology faculty at the Medical University of South Carolina. The editors' purpose was to compile a textbook, primarily aimed at medical students, that covered both the essential basic concepts of immunology and aspects relevant to medical practice that are usually not well developed in introductory textbooks. The general outline of the book is based on a course that has been taught for over 12 years and obviously has been extensively field-tried. In keeping with those goals, the original text was lucid and well organized and contained a variety of features (diagrams, question-and-answer sections, detailed index, etc.) that resulted in good acceptance among the intended readership. The rapid progress and expansion of knowledge in immunology over the past four years has prompted the authors to produce a significantly revised second edition. Two additional contributors, Drs. Henry C. Stevenson (National Institutes of Health) and Domingos Silveira Machado (University of Lisbon), have joined the team of authors participating in the second edition.

The valuable organizational and self-evaluation features of the original text have been carried forward into the second edition. Following a revised introductory chapter that provides an expanded overview of the field and introduces the reader to a series of important concepts that are detailed subsequently, the major revisions in the Basic Immunology section are in the following chapters: "Tissues and Cells in the Immune Response," "Major Histocompatibility Complex," "Antigenicity and Immune Recognition," "Lymphocyte Ontogeny and Membrane Markers," "Cell-Mediated Immunity," and "Humoral Immune Response." In the Diagnostic Immunology section, the chapters on immunoserology and diagnostic immunochemistry as well as on the diagnostic evaluation of cell-mediated immunity have been significantly updated. In the Clinical Immunology section, the chapters covering tolerance and autoimmunity, immunosuppression and immunomodulation, transplantation immunology, tumor immunology, and immunodeficiency diseases have been revised. In addition, it is important to note that new information on vaccines ("Humoral Immune Response") and AIDS ("Immunodeficiency Diseases") has been incorporated into the second edition. Along with the new and revised information, the authors have also updated the selected bibliographies of the revised chapters, which will continue to allow interested readers to obtain further information and ultimately access the classical literature.

The second edition of this text is a major asset for medical students. Further, the authors have provided appropriate updates that will keep the text useful to beginning graduate students in immunology and continue to make it an important reference for physicians requiring a concise review of the ever evolving field of immunology.

Paul C. Montgomery, Ph.D.
Professor and Chair
Department of Immunology and Microbiology
Wayne State University Medical School
Detroit, Michigan

Preface to the Second Edition

Four years ago the first edition of *Introduction to Medical Immunology* was published, introducing a new textbook written specifically for medical students, in an attempt to achieve a very difficult balance between basic information and significant clinical concepts. In this we succeeded, at least in part, judging from the response of our students and of students from other schools in the United States and overseas. But soon it was apparent to us that the publication of an updated and revised second edition was necessary. In the first place, immunology is progressing at an astounding pace; hence the need to introduce new concepts and to revise old dogmas soon became clear. On the other hand, some chapters in the first edition fell short of our expectation, as was obvious from students' feedback. We hope to have corrected both problems in this second edition, while retaining the features that made this book so valuable for medical students. Most chapters have been carefully and extensively revised—some have been virtually rewritten—and we feel that we have significantly improved the quality of this textbook.

In preparing the second edition we were assisted by Ms. Sherry Lorenz, who helped us prepare the original manuscript, by Mr. Brooks Hart, who was responsible for all new artwork, and by our production editor, Ms. Barbara Dunleavy. The feedback and criticisms of our students had a significant impact in our revision, and we wish to recognize their collective collaboration, past and future. We also want to express our gratitude to our families, who have been patient and supportive throughout the many years of gestation of this textbook. Dr. Noel R. Rose, as Editor-in-Chief of the Immunology Series in which this textbook has been included, has supported our undertaking since the first day; we thank him and also our publishers, Marcel Dekker, Inc., for having accepted the risk of publishing *another* immunology textbook.

Gabriel Virella, M.D., Ph.D.
Jean-Michel Goust, M.D.
H. Hugh Fudenberg, M.D.

Preface to the First Edition

The first question that will cross any immunologist's mind at this time is "Do we need another textbook of immunology?" The answer is clear to us, and it has been obvious to us for the last decade: otherwise we would not have undertaken the task of putting this together. During this period many immunology textbooks have been published, but none achieved what we believed were the ideal goals for a medically oriented textbook to be used as an introduction to the field. In our minds such a textbook should be clear, concise, and up-to-date and should present a balanced perspective of basic, clinical, and diagnostic immunology. Many textbooks achieved some of these goals, but we were unable to find one that would satisfy the needs of our medical students, residents, and interns. A successful textbook for such readers cannot be over-detailed or too research-oriented; the reader should be able to get at the major concepts without dealing with all the related details; it needs to be current, but not too controversial; it also must be written in such a way that readers perceive the relevance of the concepts for their future professional activity. We hope that through several years of collaboration, in which most of these chapters were developed as part of a syllabus for medical students, we have achieved our goal of producing a textbook which our readers will find helpful to the pursuit of their educational goals. Thinking specifically about medical students, we have added ten board-type questions with answers, explained when necessary, to each chapter. Also, the bibliographies for each chapter are intended as sources of relevant additional readings for advanced medical students, residents, and interns.

In preparing this textbook we were assisted by many, in a variety of ways: Linda Paddock, Nancy Butler, and Michelle Dopson spent long hours on word processors, typing and revising the manuscript; Kevin McPhillips was responsible for most of the drawings and diagrams; Gail Hull and Cathy Moore assisted us with various secretarial tasks; and Carolyn King and Greg Hardigree helped us immensely with the proofs. To all of them we owe a great deal. We are also indebted to a wide array of reviewers and friends who helped us with friendly (and not so friendly) criticism in the painstaking process of polishing the manuscript to its final form. Finally, we would like to acknowledge the support of Professor Noel R. Rose, and the trust reposed in us by Marcel Dekker and Dr. Maurits Dekker, who dared to go ahead with this immense undertaking.

Gabriel Virella, M.D., Ph.D.
Jean-Michel Goust, M.D.
H. Hugh Fudenberg, M.D.
Christian C. Patrick, M.D., Ph.D.

Contents

Contents

Contributors

Robert J. Boackle, Ph.D. Department of Basic and Clinical Immunology and Microbiology, Medical University of South Carolina, Charleston, South Carolina

H. Hugh Fudenberg, M.D. Department of Basic and Clinical Immunology and Microbiology, Medical University of South Carolina, Charleston, South Carolina

Robert M. Galbraith, M.D. Department of Basic and Clinical Immunology and Microbiology, Medical University of South Carolina, Charleston, South Carolina

Jean-Michel Goust, M.D. Department of Basic and Clinical Immunology and Microbiology, Medical University of South Carolina, Charleston, South Carolina

Domingos Silveira Machado, M.D. Department of Nephrology, Hospital de Santa Cruz and University of Lisbon, Lisbon, Portugal

Janardan P. Pandey, Ph.D. Department of Basic and Clinical Immunology and Microbiology, Medical University of South Carolina, Charleston, South Carolina

Christian C. Patrick, M.D., Ph.D. Department of Infectious Diseases, St. Jude Children's Research Hospital, Memphis, Tennessee

Mary Ann Spivey, M.T. (A.S.C.P.) S.B.B. Department of Pathology and Laboratory Medicine, Medical University of South Carolina, Charleston, South Carolina

Henry C. Stevenson, M.D.   Division of Cancer Treatment, National Cancer Institute, National Institutes of Health, Bethesda, Maryland

Kwong-Y. Tsang, Ph.D.   Department of Basic and Clinical Immunology and Microbiology, Medical University of South Carolina, Charleston, South Carolina

Gabriel Virella, M.D., Ph.D.   Department of Basic and Clinical Immunology and Microbiology, Medical University of South Carolina, Charleston, South Carolina

I
Basic Immunology

1

Introduction

GABRIEL VIRELLA

The fundamental observation that led to the development of immunology as a
scientific discipline was that an individual can become resistant for life to a certain disease after having contracted it only one single time. The term *immunity*
derived from the Latin *immunis* (exempt from taxation, military service, public
duty in general) was adopted to designate this naturally acquired protection
against diseases such as measles or smallpox.

Even before the infectious theory was properly formulated, the notion that
some diseases were transmitted from person to person was widespread in the
East and eventually in the West. For example, the inoculation of healthy individuals with the contents of skin pustules of patients with mild cases of smallpox was witnessed by Lady Montagu in Turkey in the mid-1700s, and this practice was introduced into England soon thereafter. It was known as *variolation*
and was supposed to induce a mild form of smallpox that would result in immunity, but this did not always happen. Edward Jenner, a physician and natur-
alist and a friend of the great John Hunter, made the brilliant observation that
milkmaids contracted a benign disease, usually in their hands, from cows suffering a poxlike disease. This disease, known as cowpox, was characterized by a
rash, localized on the hands, that healed spontaneously; the milkmaids who
contracted it became immune to smallpox. This was the basis of vaccination
(from the Latin *vacca*, cow), which two centuries later led to the extinction of
the disease. In retrospect, one cannot but admire Jenner's intuition and ingen-

uity in developing an animal-derived viral vaccine when no one had the slightest idea about the nature of viruses.

The emergence of immunology as a discipline was closely tied to the development of microbiology. The work of *Pasteur, Koch, Metchnikov,* and all the other pioneers of the golden age was fundamental in giving impulse to the two areas. One has to understand that the motivation of these brilliant scientists was the desire to solve problems for mankind. Infectious diseases ranked as the most common causes of death at the time, and the discovery of new infectious agents was closely followed by attempts to prevent or cure the diseases caused by them. A modern parallel has been provided by the emergence of AIDS. An unprecedented, massive effort has been applied to the investigation of the biological characteristics of the causative virus and, simultaneously, to the development of therapies and preventive measures. The motivation of Louis Pasteur and his contemporaries was equally straightforward: to identify the agent of a disease and find the best way to cure it or prevent its spread. The impact of vaccination against infectious diseases such as tetanus, diphtheria, and smallpox, to name just a few examples, is difficult to grasp today when small pox has disappeared and tetanus and diphtheria are seen only sporadically. It is fair to state that the impact of vaccination and sanitation on the welfare and life expectancy of humans has had no parallel in any other development of medical science.

Because the major concern of the early immunologists was the prevention and control of infectious diseases, it is natural that immunology acquired its working definition as a discipline designed to study the mechanisms of defense against infectious agents. Only in the second part of this century did immunology transcend its early boundaries and become a more general discipline. Today, the study of immunological defense mechanisms is still an important area of research, but immunologists are involved in a much wider array of problems, such as self-nonself discrimination, control of cell and tissue differentiation, cancer immunotherapy, etc. The focus of interest has shifted toward the basic understanding of how the immune system works, in hopes that this insight will allow novel approaches to its manipulation. In this introduction we shall attempt to give a general (though simplified) overview of our current knowledge hoping to facilitate the understanding of the following chapters.

I. ANTIGENS, ANTIBODIES, AND THE IMMUNE RESPONSE

The specific protective responses developed by the immune system, also known as *immune responses*, are usually directed against nonself substances (cells, proteins, polysaccharides) that can be generally designated as *antigens*. The recognition systems of the immune system are activated by the interaction with small portions of these foreign cells or proteins, designated as *antigenic determinants* or *epitopes*.

An adult human being has the capacity to recognize millions of different antigens, some of microbial origin, others present in the environment, and even some artificially synthesized. The ensuing state of immunity is exquisitely specific. For example, small modifications in the side groups of a simple chemical compound may induce specific immunity for each different spatial configuration. Besides *specificity*, the second major characteristic of immunity is *memory*, i.e., the ability that the organism has to react faster and more intensely when repeatedly exposed to the same antigen.

Ehrlich, Landsteiner, and other scientists were greatly interested in the understanding of what substances or compounds mediated the immune response, and they eventually designated as *antibodies* the proteins that appear in circulation after immunization and that have the ability to react specifically with the antigen used to immunize. Because antibodies are soluble and present in virtually all body fluids ("humors"), the term *humoral immunity* was introduced to designate the response to antigens mediated by antibody production.

Great progress has been made in the last 30 to 40 years in our knowledge about the nature of antibodies. In the 1950s it was first discovered that most animals have two major populations of antibody molecules (also designated as *immunoglobulins*) differing in their size, and in the 1960s it was demonstrated that antibodies could be classified into several different families (immunoglobulin isotypes). With the determination of the amino acid sequence of immunoglobulin molecules it became clear that two major *functional regions* could be distinguished in the molecule. The one involved with antigen binding was highly variable from molecule to molecule, while the region determining other biological properties of the antibody molecule is relatively constant, at least within the major classes of immunoglobulins. This structural duality corresponds to a complex multigenic control of immunoglobulin synthesis, and it is known that the genes determining the synthesis of the variable region are highly diversified as a result of the existence of multiple germ line genes that undergo recombinations and mutations mainly during embryonic differentiation. As a result of this diversity, the wide array of different antibody combining sites necessary to react with millions of different antigens is generated.

II. ANTIGEN-ANTIBODY REACTIONS, COMPLEMENT, AND PHAGOCYTOSIS

The knowledge that the serum of an immunized animal contained protein molecules able to bind specifically to the antigen led to exhaustive investigations of the characteristics and consequences of the *antigen-antibody reactions*. Some consequences are detectable by simple observation. If the antigen is soluble, the reaction with specific antibody under appropriate conditions results in precipitation of large antigen-antibody aggregates. If the antigen is present on a cell membrane, the cells will be cross-linked by antibody and form visible clumps (agglutination). But more interesting are the studies concerning the physiological effects of the reaction between antigen and antibody. For example, soluble toxins released by bacteria lose their pathogenic properties after reaction with the corresponding antibodies (neutralization reaction). However, the reaction of an antibody molecule with a live microorganism does not directly result in the destruction of the latter. Other humoral factors can assist antibodies in their purpose of eliminating an infectious agent, the most important being the *complement system*. This system is constituted by nine major proteins that are sequentially activated. Among different mechanisms of complement activation, the most efficient are antigen-antibody reactions involving antibody molecules with specific structural characteristics that lead to interaction with the complement system. Complement activation will trigger a cascade of enzymes that, in the end, is able to disrupt cell membranes; such disruption leads to the destruction of the microbial agent.

The other major mechanism by which antibodies indirectly lead to the destruction of a microorganism is by promoting its ingestion by *phagocytic cells*. The importance of phagocytic cells in the protection against infectious agents was first stressed in the late 1800s by Metchnikov, and it is now clear that the ingestion and intracellular destruction of infectious agents, termed phagocytosis, can be mediated by both immunological and nonimmunological recognition mechanisms. The induction of phagocytosis by immunological mechanisms involves the binding of antibodies and complement to the outer surface of the infectious agent (*opsonization*) and the recognition of the bound antibody and/ or complement as a signal for ingestion by the phagocytic cell.

III. CELL-MEDIATED IMMUNITY

Many different types of cells play important roles in the immune system, chiefly the *lymphocytes*. These cells were first found to be responsible for skin reactions triggered by the exposure to infections of chemical agents, which are considered as manifestations of *cutaneous hypersensitivity*. Indeed, the intradermal injection of bacterial products or chemical substances often results in the acquisition of immunity expressed by skin reactions (redness and induration) when the antigen is reintroduced by the same route. This reactivity expresses itself 24 to 48 hours after reintroduction of the antigen (for which reason it can also be designated as *delayed hypersensitivity*), and it is not mediated by antibodies but rather by lymphocytes. From these observations emerged the concept of *cell-mediated immunity* as the type of immune response in which lymphocytes play the major role as effector cells.

Cell-mediated immune mechanisms also play a very important role in rejection of foreign organs or tissues (graft rejection). The interest in organ transplantation has led to detailed studies of the mechanisms by which an individual will reject an organ from an unrelated donor. After a period in which the recipient is sensitized to cellular antigens present in the grafted organ, termed *transplantation* or *histocompatibility antigens*, a population of *cytotoxic lymphocytes* of the recipient becomes activated and able to destroy specifically the cells of the graft. This antigenic system allows discrimination of self versus nonself. However, teleologically this system could not have evolved as a barrier against organ transplantation. Its origin appears to be related to the need that an organism has to recognize *self* (against which immune responses are suppressed) and, perhaps, to recognize *altered-self*. Studies on how the immune system fights viral infections have revealed that cytotoxic lymphocytes specifically directed against infected cells play a most important role in promoting the elimination of the infective virus. Since virus-infected cells are originally self, the question of how they are recognized as undesirable and destroyed after viral infection was a fundamental point in need of clarification. It is known that once a virus starts multiplying in a cell, it codes for viral proteins that are inserted in the cell membrane. At first it would appear that the elimination of infected cells could be mediated simply by recognition of these newly expressed viral proteins. However, experimental studies demonstrated that the cytotoxic lymphocytes destroy virus-infected cells only when they share identical histocompatibility antigens. The most popular interpreation for this observation is that the reaction of cytotoxic lymphocytes against virus-infected cells is triggered by the recognition of virally modified histocompatibility antigens on the membrane of infected cells, or in other words, by the recognition of altered-self.

IV. LYMPHOCYTE SUBPOPULATIONS

Although lymphocytes appear as a fairly monotonous population in a peripheral blood film, a remarkable functional heterogeneity exists in these cells. Two large groups of lymphocytes were initially defined: the *T lymphocytes*, designated as T because the thymus plays a key role in their differentiation, and the *B lymphocytes*, designated as B because in birds a peri-intestinal lymphoid organ known as the bursa of Fabricus plays a major role in their differentiation, whereas in man they appear to arise in the bone marrow. B lymphocytes are identified by the presence of immunoglobulin molecules on their cell membrane, whereas T lymphocytes carry a variety of membrane antigens not expressed by B lymphocytes. Functionally, T lymphocytes are responsible for cell-mediated immunity, whereas B lymphocytes differentiate into antibody-producing cells (plasma cells), antibodies being the basis for humoral immunity.

The *T lymphocyte* population has been found to be constituted by three main subpopulations. One is constituted by cells that assist the triggering of humoral and cellular immune responses and are designated as *helper* cells. A second subpopulation turns down unnecessary responses, such as those directed against self or those directed against an antigen that has already been eliminated. This is known as the T *suppressor* cell subpopulation. Finally, a third subpopulation is constituted by the *cytotoxic* T lymphocytes, able to destroy cells expressing nonself or altered cell antigens. Other cells, such as the *monocytes, macrophages* and specialized macrophage-derived cells found in many tissues, play important roles by modifying and presenting antigens to lymphocytes and releasing soluble factors (*interleukins*) that regulate the activity of lymphocytes. The regulatory populations (helper, suppressor) of T lymphocytes also release a variety of interleukins that participate in intricate activation and suppression circuits. The study of the regulation of immune responses (immune regulation) is currently in an explosive phase, and it is obvious that only by improving our knowledge of the different steps involved in the control of a normal immune response can we hope to learn eventually how to manipulate them in disease states.

V. LYMPHOID TISSUES

Immune cells are present not only in the peripheral blood but also in specialized tissues (lymphoid tissues) that include the thymus, spleen, lymph nodes, Peyer's patches of the intestine, tonsils, and bone marrow. The role of the thymus in promoting the differentiation of T lymphocytes has been extensively studied, although a perfect understanding of thymic function has not yet been reached. The bone marrow is the source of precursors for all leukocytes and also the site where plasma cells tend to localize in humans. The spleen, lymph nodes, tonsils, and Peyer's patches appear to be structures where the initial stages of immune responses take place because they provide the ideal environment for the cell-to-cell interactions that are essential for the proper collaboration between and among different cell populations. It is also becoming clear that there is a constant *lymphocyte traffic* to and from different lymphoid organs, and it appears that such traffic is not a random event but rather closely controlled by specific receptors on immune cells and lymphoid tissues. This is an area that we are only beginning to understand and that may have significant correlations with pathological conditions affecting the lymphoid tissues (leukemias and lymphomas).

VI. A GENERAL OVERVIEW

One of the most difficult intellectual exercises in immunology is to try to understand the global function of the immune system. Its extreme complexity and the wide array of regulatory circuits involved in the control of its functions are formidable obstacles to our understanding. The diagram reproduced in Figure 1.1 attempts to synthesize some of the current general concepts concerning the different segments of the immune system, as activated by exposure to an antigen. In many cases, particularly if the antigen is of large size and complex nature (such as a bacterium), it will be eliminated by phagocytic cells such as the *granulocytes, monocytes*, and *macrophages*, whose main function seems to be to scavenge foreign particulate matter, cell debris, etc. But if this first barrier is not efficient in removing the antigen from the organism, the immune system will be mobilized. The first type of cell activated, in most cases, is the *helper T lymphocyte*, whose function is to assist the differentiation of effector cells. However, for the helper T cell to be activated, the antigen must first be processed by specialized phagocytic cells, the *macrophages*. The processed antigen is then presented to the T cell on the membrane of a macrophage or of some other cell

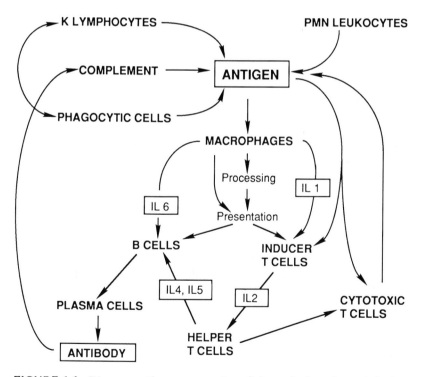

FIGURE 1.1 Diagrammatic representation of the main functions of the immune system, as triggered by exposure to a foreign antigen.

of the same lineage, collectively known as *antigen-presenting cells* (APC) or *accessory cells* (AC). Furthermore, the macrophage, once activated by the ingestion and processing of an antigen, releases soluble substances such as *interleukin 1*, which assist T cell differentiation. The activated helper T cell also secretes interleukins that act on a variety of cells, some on macrophages (further increasing their level of activation), others on effector cells. Two main types of effector cells will differentiate: *cytotoxic T cells*, which are very efficient in the elimination of virus-infected cells, and *B cells*, which upon activation by antigen and helper T cells evolve into *plasma cells*. The plasma cells are engaged in the synthesis of large amounts of antibody; this antibody will bind to the antigen, activate the complement system, and promote the lysis or phagocytosis of the antigen. Also, the antibody bound to a cellular antigen is the signal that appears to allow a second type of killing mediated in this case by cytotoxic cells that recognize the bound antibody (*K lymphocytes*). This last process is known as *antibody-dependent cell-mediated cytotoxicity* (*ADCC*). Finally, once the antigen is removed, negative feedback mechanisms become predominant, turning off the immune response. This is one of the functions of a third population of T cells, the *suppressor T cells*. This general view, complicated as it may appear to the beginner, is extremely oversimplified. The regulatory circuits are complex and poorly understood, and the effector mechanisms that we have discussed are but a few of those that are better characterized. For example, in the area of tumor immunology, a variety of effector cells, including natural killer cells (NK cells), lymphokine-activated killer cells (LAK cells) and tumor-infiltrating lymphocytes (TIL) have been proposed as playing essential roles. However, very little is known about their identity and mechanisms of activation and antitumor activity.

VII. CLINICAL IMMUNOLOGY

Immunological concepts have found ample application in medicine. The exquisite specificity of the antigen-antibody reaction has been extensively applied to the development of diagnostic assays; and the therapeutic use of interleukins, activated cytotoxic cells, monoclonal antibodies, anti-idiotypic antibodies, and immunotoxins are being extensively investigated. Immunotherapy, once derided as little less than wishful thinking, is coming of age rapidly. Human pathology, on the other hand, has provided a wide array of experiments of nature through which clinical immunologists have been able to examine the consequences of malfunction of the immune system. First and foremost, the study of children with deficient development of the immune system (immunodeficiency diseases) has provided solid evidence for the existence of several functional compartments in the immune system of humans and has allowed the definition of the relative importance of those different segments of the immune system in the defense against infectious agents. The emergence of the acquired immunodeficiency symdrome (AIDS) has underscored the delicate balance that is maintained in the healthy individual between the immune system and infectious agents. The AIDS virus, by destroying the helper T cell population, disturbs such balance and opens the door to the most unusual infections by the most uncommon agents.

The importance of the still poorly understood mechanisms that suppress the reactivity of the immune system against self is dramatically illustrated by the autoimmune diseases, in which the immune system reacts against cells and tissues that may initially have been recognized as modified self (for example, as a consequence of a viral infection). Even reactions against nonself antigens have been proven to have pathological consequences to the responding individual, if and when the delicate balance that keeps the immune system from overreacting is broken (hypersensitivity states).

Immunology and oncology have also been developing in close parallel. On the one hand, it is known that cells of the immune system can become malignant, and considerable basic knowledge has been derived from the study of malignant lymphocytes, plasma cells, and their products. On the other hand, the idea that the immune system may play an important role in the elimination of neoplastic cells is very attractive. This putative antitumor defense is believed to involve a variety of cell types, some better defined than others. In particular, LAK cells and NK cells have received considerable attention. Both are of uncertain lineage, recognize tumor cells through unclear mechanisms, and are able to destroy tumor cells in vitro, leading to their eventual elimination. The transfusion of LAK cells or of activated NK cells can improve the survival of animals and humans with malignant tumors. A considerable effort is under way to research new ways to manipulate the immune system in patients with cancer, usually with the goal of inducing the immune system to eliminate residual tumor cells that persist after surgery or chemotherapy.

In the remaining chapters of this book we shall abundantly illustrate the productive interaction that has always existed in immunology between basic concepts and clinical applications. In fact, no other biological discipline illustrates better the importance of interaction between basic and clinical scientists; in this probably lies the main reason for the prominence of immunology as a biomedical discipline.

2

Tissues and Cells in the Immune Response

GABRIEL VIRELLA, CHRISTIAN C. PATRICK, and JEAN-MICHEL GOUST

One of the most striking characteristics of the immune system is the diversity of cells and factors that play different roles in the several stages of the immune response. The lymphocytes play the key role in the recognition of nonself, undergoing as a consequence a series of complex events that leads to the various manifestations of the immune response. They are also the main cells involved in the control and regulation of immune responses. The monocytes, macrophages, and related cells participate in the inductive stages of the immune response, by processing and presenting antigens in a favorable way for their recognition by lymphocytes. In the late stages of the immune response, these same cells play an important role by killing or by ingesting and digesting nonself elements previously targeted for destruction. This chapter deals with the diverse cellular elements involved in immune reactions and their organization in specialized tissues.

I. LEUKOCYTIC CELLS

A. Lymphocytes

The lymphocytes (Fig. 2.1a) occupy a very special place among the leukocytes that participate in one way or another in immune reactions because of their ability to interact specifically with antigenic substances. In a normal individual, lymphocytes are able to react specifically against exogenous antigens which are recognized as nonself, but do not respond to the antigens of the body's own

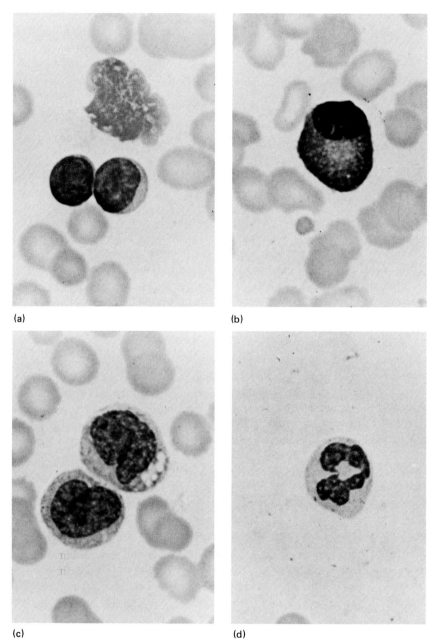

(a)   (b)

(c)   (d)

FIGURE 2.1   Morphology of the main types of human leukocytes. (a) lymphocyte, (b) plasma cell, (c) monocyte, (d) granulocyte. (*Source*: Reproduced with
permission from Reich P. R., *Manual of Hematology*. Upjohn, Kalamazoo,
Michigan, 1976.)

tissues (self). These properties (*specificity* and *discrimination of self vs. non-self*) are the main characteristics defining the normal immune response.

The lymphocyte differentiates from stem cells in the bone marrow and fetal liver into two main functional classes. One class is composed of lymphocytes that have the capacity to produce antibodies, designated as *B lymphocytes* or *B cells*. The designation derives from the bursa of Fabricius, a lymphoid organ, located close to the caudal end of the gut in birds, that plays a key role in their differentiation. A mammalian counterpart to the avian bursa has not yet been found. Some investigators believe that the bone marrow is the most likely organ for B cell differentiation, while others propose (by analogy with birds) that the gut-associted lymphoid tissues (GALT) play this role. The other major class of lymphocytes, termed *T lymphocytes* or *T cells* (for thymus-derived), is concerned with a variety of functions, such as the regulation of immune responses, and various effector functions, (cytotoxicity and lymphokine production being the main ones) that are the basis of *cell-mediated immunity* (*CMI*). A major characteristic of the cytotoxicity mediated by T cells is that the target cells must be genetically identical to the cytotoxic cells. In other words, T cell cytotoxicity is limited by histocompatibility antigens (see Chapter 3). The actual destruction of target cells seems to be largely a function of the release of *perforins*. These molecules are inserted in the target cell membrane, where they form transmembrane pores, causing the loss of the osmotic balance essential for cell life.

Lymphocytes are predominantly recirculating cells, easily accessible for collection and study given their abundance in the peripheral blood. Based on their membrane markers, lymphocytes can be classified into three groups: *B cells, T cells* and *non-B, non-T cells*. The B cells or B lymphocytes have membrane immunoglobulin, which functions as a receptor for antigen and, after antigenic stimulation, will differentiate into plasma cells that produce and export antibody. The B cells are localized in specialized lymphoid tissues (spleen, lymph nodes, bone marrow). T lymphocytes, originally identified in humans by their receptor for sheep red cells, are plurifunctional cells, and several subpopulations with separate functions have been recognized. *Helper* and *suppressor T lymphocytes* are involved in the induction and regulation of immune responses, while *cytotoxic T lymphocytes* are the effector cells in many cell-mediated immune responses. Recently, two new subpopulations of T cells have been defined on the basis of their membrane antigens: *helper-inducer* and *suppressor-inducer*. These subpopulations are believed to play important roles in the regulation of the immune response. However, this clear-cut functional differentiation between T and B cells can be questioned on the basis of data showing that, at least in vitro and in special circumstances, B cells can participate in immunoregulatory circuits, exhibiting helper and suppressor functions usually ascribed to T lymphocytes. B lymphocytes can also play the role of *antigen-presenting cells*, which is usually attributed to cells of monocytic/macrophage lineage.

Lymphocytes are morphologically distinct depending upon their stage of functional differentiation. Upon contacting a foreign substance, a resting small T lymphocyte with surface receptors specific for the substance rapidly undergoes *blastogenic transformation* into a large lymphocyte (13-15 μm). This large lymphocyte (lymphoblast) then subdivides to produce an expanded population of medium (9-12 μm) and small lymphocytes (5-8 μm) with the same antigenic specificity. A B lymphocyte, after antigenic stimulation, will also undergo blastic transformation but will eventually differentiate into a plasma cell.

B. Plasma Cells

Plasma cells are morphologically characterized by their eccentric nuclei with clumped chromatin, and a large cytoplasm with abundant rough endoplasmic reticulum (Fig. 2.1b). No membrane immunoglobulin can be detected, but plasma cells carry specific membrane antigens defined by serological means (such as the PC antigens). They are functionally specialized in antibody production and secretion, rarely found in peripheral blood, mostly "fixed" in lymphoid tissues (e.g., the lymph nodes, and in man they are particularly abundant in the bone marrow), and divide very poorly, if at all.

C. K, NK and LAK Cells

Among the population of cells that are classified as lymphocytes by classical morphological criteria, there are cells that do not express either T or B cell markers. *Killer, (K) natural killer (NK)*, and *lymphokine-activated (LAK) cells* are classifed as non-T, non-B lymphocytes; the true nature and lineage of these cells is controversial and it is not clear whether they constitute three different populations or one single population with different effector mechanisms.

K cells are able to lyse target cells previously coated with IgG antibody in vitro. They express immunoglobulin receptors on their cell membrane, through which they connect with the target cell-bound antibody. Their mechanism of killing has not been fully characterized, although it appears to involve the release of perforins. This *antibody-dependent cellular cytotoxicity (ADCC)* can also be mediated in vitro by nonlymphocytic cells such as eosinophils and neutrophils, but the precise physiological significance of ADCC is not clear.

The natural killer (NK) cells appear to be found mostly among cells described as large lymphocytes with granular cytoplasm, and very little is known about their recognition system and killing mechanisms. These cells are defined by their ability to kill cultured tumor cells in a non-MHC-restricted manner and have been best characterized in the mouse, where they appear to play an important role in antitumor defense. Their mechanisms of killing depend on the release of perforins and other unidentified factors.

A third non-T, non-B population has been recently defined, based on immunotherapeutic studies in which lymphocytes were incubated in vitro with large concentrations of interleukin 2, a major soluble mediator (or lymphokine) released by activated T lymphocytes. As a consequence of this treatment a population of lymphoid cells acquires the ability to lyse fresh tumor cells as well as some cell lines resistant to NK cells, this population of cytotoxic cells is designated as lymphokine-activated cells (LAK). These cells have been also shown to appear in the circulation of humans treated with interleukin 2. LAK cells appear to be a somewhat heterogenous population, some cells expressing T cell markers and the majority expressing the same markers as NK cells. Therefore, it is believed that the majority of LAK cells are equivalent to a functionally activated population of NK cells. LAK cells are also able to participate in ADCC; this feature argues in favor of the theory that K, NK and LAK cells are just different functional stages of a single cell type.

D. Monocytes and Macrophages

The *monocyte* (Fig. 2.1c) is considered a leukocyte in transit through the blood which when fixed in a tissue will become a *macrophage*. Monocytes and macrophages, as well as granulocytes (see below), are able to ingest particulate matter (microorganisms, cells, inert particles) and for this reason are said to have phagocytic functions. The phagocytic activity is greater in macrophages, which, together with monocytes, also play an important role in the immune response by processing complex antigens and concentrating the processed antigen on the cell membrane. In this form, the antigen is recognized by helper T lymphocytes. Bone-marrow-derived cells sharing certain functional properties with monocytes and macrophages are present in skin (Langerhans cells), kidney, brain (microglia), capillary walls, and lymphoid tissues. One type of monocyte-derived cell, the *dendritic cell* (Fig. 2.2), is present in the spleen and lymph nodes, particularly in follicles and germinal centers. This cell, apparently of monocytic lineage, is not phagocytic, but it appears particularly suited to carry out the antigen-presenting function by concentrating antigen on its membrane and keeping it there for relatively long periods of time, a factor that may be crucial for a sustained immune response. A similar role seems to be played by *interdigitating cells* located in the paracortical areas. These cells are believed to be lymph-node fixed Langerhans cells. All antigen-presenting cells express one special type of histocompatibility antigen, designated as Ia (I-region-associated) (see Chapter 3). The expression of Ia antigens is essential for interaction with helper T cells.

Also, all antigen-presenting cells produce a soluble factor, interleukin 1, which assists T cell proliferation.

E. Granulocytes

Granulocytes are a collection of white blood cells with lobulated nuclei and granules in their cytoplasm that are visible with special strains. *Neutrophils, eosinophils*, and *basophils* are included in this group of cells. Neutrophils are also referred to a *polymorphonuclear (PMN) leukocytes* (Fig. 2.1d). They comprise the largest subpopulation of white blood cells and have two types of cytoplasmic granules with bactericidal activity. These cells are attracted by chemotactic factors to areas of inflammation, where they engulf and destroy foreign substances such as bacteria; and represent an important primary line of defense. Great numbers of PMN may die in this process; dead PMN and their debris become the primary component of pus. Nonimmunological mechanisms have also been shown to lead to ingestion by phagocytic cells (phagocytosis), perhaps reflecting phylogenetically more primitive mechanisms of recognition.

The eosinophil's granules stain orange-red with the use of cytologic stains containing eosin. These cells are found in high concentrations in allergic reactions and during parasitic infections, and their roles in both areas will be discussed in later chapters.

The basophil stains metachromatically because of its granules, which contain histamine and heparin. The tissue-fixed mast cell is very similar to the basophil even though they appear to evolve from different precursor cells. Both the basophil and the mast cell are involved in antiparasitic immune mechanisms and with allergic reactions.

II. IMMUNE TISSUES

The immune system is organized on several special tissues, collectively designated as *lymphoid* or *immune tissues*. These tissues, as shown in Figure 2.3, are distributed throughout the entire body, and can be subdivived into primary and secondary lymphoid tissues based on the premise that the ability to produce lymphocytes is characteristic of primary lymphoid tissues.

Table 2.1 shows the relative percentages of T and B cells within human immune tissues. The percentage of T and B cells in peripheral blood totals approximately 90%, with the remaining 10% being non-T, non-B lymphocytes. The thymus, being the primary lymphoid organ where T lymphocytes differentiate, contains almost exclusively T cells. The thoracic duct contains 90% T cells and 10% B cells. B cells tend to remain fixed in tissues predominating over T cells in the bone marrow and in the gut-associated lymphoid tissues, while T cells, which have a longer life span than B cells, are the major recirculating cell in the

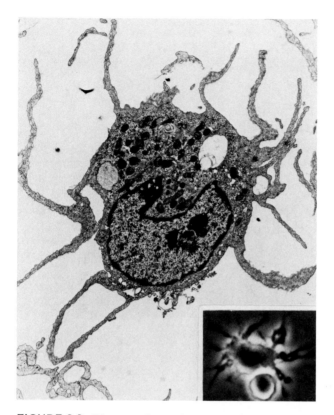

FIGURE 2.2   Electron photomicrograph of a dendritic cell isolated from a rat lymph node (×5000). The inset illustrates the in vitro interaction between a dendritic cell and a lymphocyte as seen in phase contrast microscopy (×300). (*Source*: Reproduced with permission from Klinkert, W. E. F., Labadie, J. H., O'Brien, J. P., Beyer, L. F., and Bowers, W. E. *Proc. Natl. Acad. Sci. USA 77*: 5414, 1980.)

lymphatic circulation and the predominant type of lymphocyte in the lymph nodes.

  Some lymphoid tissues achieve a remarkable degree of organization and can be designated as *lymphoid organs*. The most ubiquitous of the lymphoid organs are the lymph nodes, which are located in groups along major blood vessels and loose connective tissues. Figure 2.4 shows the intimate relations between the lymphatic and the circulatory system. Afferent lymphatics from interstitial

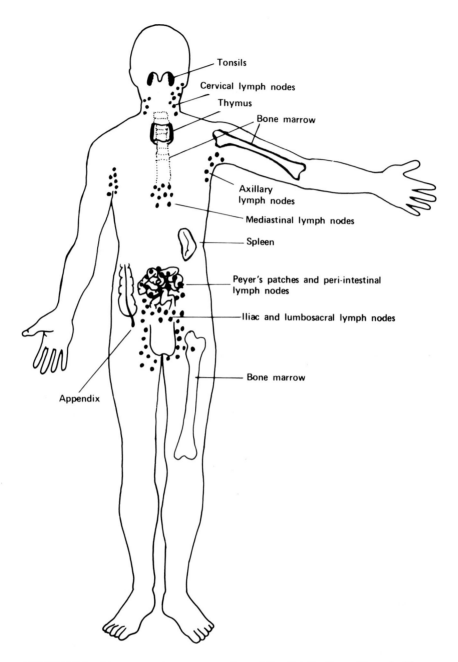

FIGURE 2.3 Diagrammatic representation of the distribution of lymphoid tissues in humans. (*Source*: Modifed from Mayerson, H. S. *Sci. Am. 208*:80, 1963.)

spaces drain into lymph nodes, which "filter" these fluids, removing foreign substances. "Cleared" lymph from below the diaphragm and the upper left half of the body drains via efferent lymphatics, emptying into the thoracic duct for subsequent drainage into the left innominate vein. Cleared lymph from the right side above the diaphragm drains into the right lymphatic duct with subsequent drainage into the origin of the right innominate vein. Peripheral blood, in turn, is filtered by the spleen and the liver, the spleen having organized lymphoid areas and the liver being rich in Kupfer cells, which are macrophage-derived phagocytes.

Other mammalian lymphoid organs and tissues include the thymus, the spleen, GALT (including the tonsils, Peyer's patches, and the appendix), and aggregates of lymphoid tissue in the respiratory and genitourinary tracts.

A. Lymph Nodes

The lymph nodes are extremely numerous and are disseminated all over the body. They measure 1 to 25 mm in diameter and play a very important role in the initial or inductive states of the immune response. In a sense, lymph nodes can be compared to a network of filtration and communication stations where antigens are trapped and messages interchanged between the different cells involved in the immune response. This interchange is favored by the dual circulation of the lymph nodes, which receive both lymph and arterial blood flow. Afferent lymphatics draining peripheral interstitial spaces enter the capsule of the node and open into the subcapsular sinus. The lymph, with its cellu-

TABLE 2.1 Distribution of T and B Lymphocytes in Humans

Immune tissue	Lymphocyte distribution (%)[a]	
	T cell	B cell
Peripheral blood	80	10[b]
Thoracic duct	90	10
Lymph node	75	25
Spleen	50	50
Thymus	100	< 5
Bone marrow	< 25	> 75
Peyer's patch	10-20	70

[a]Approximate values.
[b]The remaining 10% correspond to non-T, non-B lymphocytes.

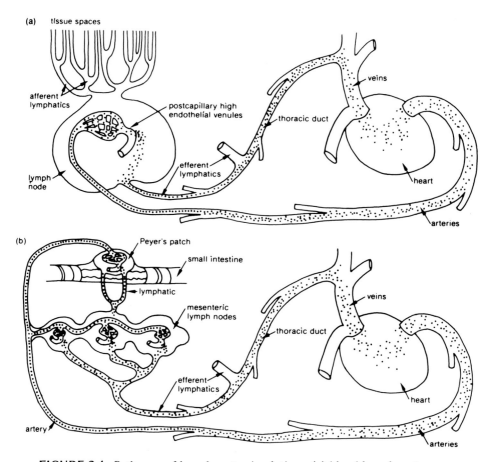

FIGURE 2.4 Pathways of lymphocyte circulation: (a) blood lymphocytes enter lymph nodes, adhere to the walls of specialized postcapillary venules, and migrate to the lymph node cortex. Lymphocytes then percolate through lymphoid fields to medullary lymphatic sinuses and then to efferent lymphatics, which in turn collect into major lymphatic ducts in the thorax, which then empty into the superior vena cava; (b) the gut-associated lymphoid tissues (Peyer's patches and mesenteric lymph nodes) drain into the thoracic duct, which also empties into the superior vena cava; (c) the spleen receives lymphocytes and disburses them mainly via the blood vascular system (inferior vena cava). (*Source*: Reproduced with permission from Hood, L. E., Weissman, I. L., Wood, W. B., and Wilson, J. H. *Immunology*, 2nd Ed. Benjamin/Cummings, Menlo Park, California, 1984.)

lar elements, percolates from this subcapular sinus to the efferent lymphatics via cortical and medullary sinuses, and the cellular elements of the lymph have ample opportunity to migrate into the lymphocyte-rich cortical structures during their transit through the nodes. The artery that penetrates through the hilus brings peripheral blood lymphocytes into the lymph node; these lymphocytes can also leave the vascular bed at the level of the *high endothelial venules* located in the *cortical* and *paracortical areas* (the latter area is also known as the *deep cortex*). The cortex and deep cortex are densely populated by lymphocytes, in constant traffic between the lymphatic and the systemic circulation. In the cortex, at low-power magnification, one can distinguish roughly spherical areas containing densely packed lymphocytes, areas termed *follicles* or *nodules* (Fig. 2.5). The predominant type of lymphocyte in the follicle is the B cell (hence the follicles are designated as *T-independent areas*), but macrophages, dendritic cells, and some T cells are also present. The follicles are very densely packed with small lymphocytes in lymph nodes not actively involved in an immune response, and in this state they are designated as *primary follicles*. In a lymph node draining an area in which an infection has taken place, one will find larger, less dense follicles, termed *secondary follicles*, containing clear *germinal centers* where B cells are actively dividing as a result of antigenic stimulation. Finally, in the paracortical area, which is not as densely populated as the follicles, T lymphocytes are the predominant cell population, and for this reason the paracortical area is designated as *T-dependent*. Interdigitating cells are also present in this area, where they present antigen to the constantly circulating T cells.

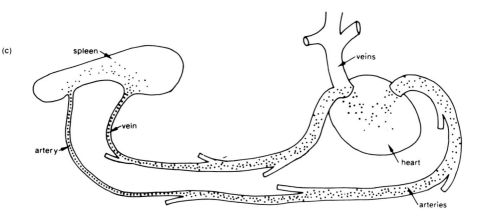

FIGURE 2.4 (Continued)

B. Spleen

The *spleen* is the lymphoid organ associated with filtering or clearing of particulate matter, infectious organisms, and aged or defective formed elements in the blood stream. The spleen has two components, namely the white and the red pulp. The *white pulp* is a secondary lymphoid organ and is composed of lymphoid tissue surrounding small arteries called central arteries (periarteriolar lymphatic sheath). In the white pulp, T cells are in close proximity to the arteriole, whereas the B cell germinal centers lie more peripherally (Fig. 2.6).

The *red pulp* performs the function of filtering the blood. It is composed of the cords of Bilroth and venous sinuses. The red pulp is located distally to the white pulp after the central arterioles narrow to become penicillar arteries. Blood leaving the white pulp enters the red pulp's splenic cords, where numerous macrophages serve a filtering function. Blood exits the penicillar arteries and enters the venous sinuses by an unknown mechanism. Regardless of the precise organization of the splenic circulation, blood is filtered to remove particulate matter and formed elements, i.e., microorganisms, and senescent or deformed erythrocytes (e.g., spherocytes, ovalocytes). Blood then exits the venous sinuses and enters the venous system. Given the anatomical proximity of the white and red pulp, it appears very likely that antigen-processing macrophages may migrate into the white pulp and initiate an immune response by interacting with lymphocytic cells.

C. Thymus

The thymus is the only clearly individualized primary lymphoid organ in mammals. It is believed to play a key role in determining the differentiation of T lymphocytes. The thymus, whose structure is diagrammatically illustrated in Figure 2.7, is located in the superior mediastinum, anterior to the great vessels. It has trabeculae composed of connective tissue and epithelial cells extending from its capsule, dividing the organ into lobules. Each lobule has a *cortex* and a *medulla*. Lymphocyte aggregates, composed mainly of immunologically immature T cells, are located in the cortex, an area of intense cell proliferation. A small number of macrophages and plasma cells are also present in the cortex. The medulla is not as densely populated as the cortex; it contains predominantly T lymphocytes and has a larger epithelial cell-to-lymphocyte ratio than the cortex. Unique to the medulla are concentric rings of squamous epithelial cells known as *Hassall's corpuscles*; their significance is unknown. The reticular epithelial cells in the thymus are derived from the same embryonic pouches that give rise to such endocrine glands as the thyroid and parathyroid and appear to be involved in the synthesis of a wide variety of thymic humoral factors. The precise location of mature thymocytes prior to their migration to the

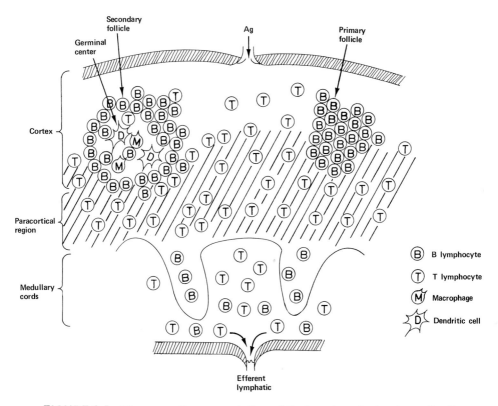

FIGURE 2.5 Diagrammatic representation of the lymph node structure. B cells are predominantly located on the lymphoid follicles and medullary cords (B-dependent areas), while T cells are mostly found in the paracortical area (T-dependent area).

peripheral blood and lymphoid tissues is controversial. Most authors believe that the cortex is an area of intense cell proliferation and death (only 1% of the cells generated in the thymus eventually mature and migrate to the peripheral tissues) and that the thymocytes reach full maturity in the medulla. However, recent experiments suggest that fully mature thymocytes tend to be found scattered throughout the cortex rather than in the medulla.

The precise mechanism whereby the thymus determines T cell differentiation is poorly understood and will be discussed in detail in later chapters. However, some of the soluble factors produced by the epithelial cells are believed to play an important role in the regulation and differentiation of T cells (e.g., *thymosin* and *thymopoietin*). Thus far, however, efforts to use these hormones or their

Periarteriolar
sheet

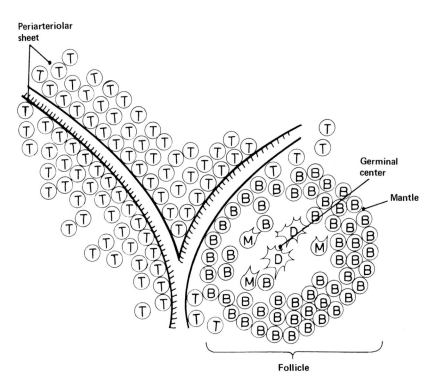

Germinal
center

Mantle

Follicle

FIGURE 2.6   Diagrammatic representation of the topography of the splenic lymphoid tissue. The lymphocytic periarteriolar sheet is a T-dependent area, while the B lymphocytes are localized on lymphoid follicles (B-dependent areas).

synthetic analogues in the treatment of primary or acquired cellular immunodeficiencies have met with limited success.

D. Gut-Associated Lymphoid Tissue (GALT)

Gut-associated lymphoid tissue is the designation proposed for all lymphatic tissues found along the digestive tract. Three major areas of GALT that can be identified are the tonsils (Fig. 2.8), the Peyer's patches, located on the submucosa of the small intestine (Fig. 2.9), and the appendix. In addition, scanty lymphoid tissue is present in the lamina propria of the gastrointestinal tract. The genitourinary tract, tracheobronchial tree, and mammary glands have lymphoid tissue similar to that found in the lamina propria. All of the mucosal-associated lymphoid tissues are unencapsulated and contain both T and B cells, the latter predominating. These tissues, together with the GALT, can be designated as *mucosal-associated lymphoid tissues* (*MALT*).

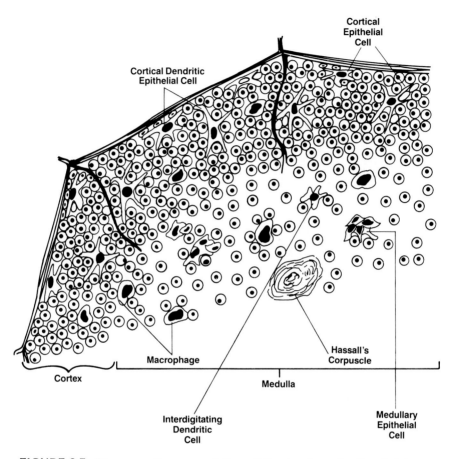

FIGURE 2.7 Diagrammatic representation of the structure of a thymic lobe. The densely packed cortex is mostly populated by T lymphocytes and by some cortical dendritic epithelial cells and cortical epithelial cells. The more sparsely populated medulla contains epithelial and dendritic cells, macrophages, T cells, and Hassall's corpuscles. (*Source*: Adapted from Butcher, E. C., and Weissman, I. L. Lymphoid tissues and organs. In *Fundamental Immunology*, W. E. Paul, Ed. Raven Press, New York, 1984.)

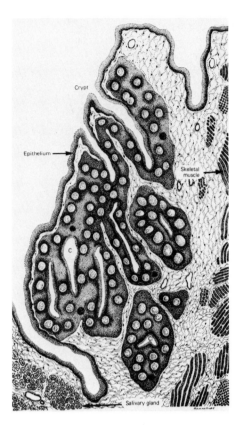

FIGURE 2.8   Diagrammatic representation of the histological structure of the tonsils. (*Source*: Reproduced with permission from Junqueira, L. C., Carneiro, J., and Contopoulas, J. *Basic Histology*, 2nd Ed. Lang, Los Altos, California, 1971.)

III.   LYMPHOCYTE RECIRCULATION AND HOMING

There is a constant traffic of lymphocytes throughout the body. Those cells circulating in the systemic circulation eventually enter a lymphoid organ, exit via the efferent lymphatic vessels, and reenter the systemic circulation (Fig. 2.4). There is also evidence that B lymphocytes circulate between different segments of the mucosal-associated lymphoid tissues, including the GALT, the mammary-gland-associated lymphoid tissue, and the lymphoid tissues associated with the respiratory tree and urinary tract. The recirculating ability seems better developed in mature lymphocytes, particularly in memory cells.

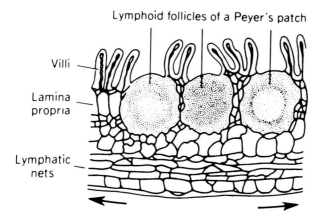

FIGURE 2.9 Diagrammatic representation of the topography of the lymphoid follicles of a Peyer's patch. (*Source*: Reproduced with permission from Kampmeier, O. F. *Evolution and Comparative Morphology of the Lymphatic System.* C. C. Thomas, Springfield, Illinois, 1969.)

The crucial step in the traffic of lymphocytes from the systemic circulation to a lymphoid tissue is the crossing of the endothelial barrier at specific locations. This seems to take place at the level of the *high endothelial venules* (*HEV*) of the lymphoid organs, which appear to be recognized by membrane receptors present on T and B lymphocytes. After adhering to an HEV, a lymphocyte will migrate through endothelial slits into the lymphoid organ parenchyma.

It is known that the lymphocyte constitution of lymphoid organs is variable (Table 2.1). T cells predominate in the lymph nodes, but B cells, mostly IgA-producing, predominate in the Peyer's patches and the GALT in general. This differential homing appears to be a consequence of specific interactions between lymphocytes and HEV. Most B lymphocytes recognize specifically the GALT-associated HEV and do not interact with the lymph-node-associated HEV, while most T lymphocytes recognize both the lymph-node-associated HEV and the GALT-associated HEV. Also, the ability to interact with HEV appears to be modulated by antigen stimulation. Immediately after antigen stimulation, the recirculating lymphocyte appears transiently to lose its capacity to recirculate. This loss of recirculating ability is associated with a tendency to self-aggregate (perhaps explaining why antigen-stimulated lymphocytes are trapped at the site of maximal antigen density) and to a temporary loss of the ability to interact with HEV. When activated lymphocytes recover the ability to interact with HEV they tend to do so in an area homologous to that where the antigenic stimulation took place. In other words, a lymphocyte that recognized an antigen in a peripheral lymph node will recirculate to another peripheral lymph node, while a lymphocyte that was stimulated at the GALT level will recirculate to the GALT.

The differentiation of T-dependent and B-dependent areas in lymphoid tissues is a poorly understood aspect of lymphocyte "homing." It appears likely that the distribution of T and B lymphocytes is determined by their interaction with nonlymphoid cells. For example, the interaction between interdigitating cells and T cells may determine the predominant location of T cells in the lymph node paracortical areas and periarteriolar sheets of the spleen, whereas the interaction of B cells with follicula dendritic cells may determine the organization of lymphoid follicles in the lymph node, spleen, and GALT.

SELF-EVALUATION

Questions

Choose the one *best* answer.

2.1   A patient born without the human bursa-equivalent would be expected to have all of the following conditions *except*

A. A lack of germinal centers in the lymph nodes.
B. An absence of circulating lymphocytes bearing surface immunoglobulins.
C. An absence of plasma cells in the spleen.
D. A depleted number of cells in the paracortical areas of the lymph nodes.
E. Atrophic tonsils.

2.2   Human T lymphocytes

A. Normally comprise about 90% of the small lymphocyte population in the thoracic duct.
B. In the lymph nodes are found mainly in the medullary cords.
C. Are found in well-organized primary follicles in the appendix.
D. Are responsible for antigen processing.
E. Have a large cytoplasm with abundant endoplasmic reticulum.

Match the listed properties and characteristics with the right type of lymphocytes. A, T lymphocytes; B, B lymphocytes, C, both; D, neither.

2.3   Are present in large numbers in the follicles and germinal centers of the lymph nodes.

2.4   Respond specifically to antigen stimulation.

2.5   Recirculate between different segments of the GALT.

2.6   Are the most abundant lymphoid cells in the thymus.

2.7   Are found in the white pulp of the spleen.

2.8   Concentrate antigen on their surfaces.

2.9   Predominate in the bone marrow.

2.10 Produce and secrete large amounts of immunoglobulins.

Answers

2.1   (D)   The lack of a bursal equivalent would result in virtually no differentiation of B cells and plasma cells, and this would be reflected in the peripheral blood and B-cell-rich lymphoid tissues. However, the paracortical areas of the lymph nodes are mostly populated by T cells and as such would not be affected.

2.2   (A)

2.3   (B)

2.4   (C)   *Both* B and T cells have specific recognition systems that allow them to respond to a single antigen or a small group of closely related antigens.

2.5   (B)

2.6   (A)

2.7   (C)   The white pulp of the spleen is organized in two different areas: the periarteriolar sheet (where T cells predominate) and the follicles (where B cells predominate).

2.8   (D)   This function is attributed to the dendritic cells found in the lymphoid follicles.

2.9   (B)

2.10 (D)   Immunoglobulin secretion is a property of the plasma cell that although derived from B cells has unique functions and membrane markers.

BIBLIOGRAPHY

Bier, O. G., da Silva, W. D., Gotze, D., and Motz, I. *Fundamentals of Immunology*. Springer-Verlag, New York, 1981. (Contains chapters called "Tissues and Cells of the Immune System" and "Activity of Immune Cells.")

Butcher, E. C. The regulation of lymphocyte traffic. In *Current Topics in Microbiology and Immunology 128*:85, 1986. (An updated and authoritative review of the topic.)

Golub, E. S. *Immunology: A Synthesis.* Sinauer, Sunderland, Massachusetts, 1987. (Contains extensive discussions on T and B lymphocyte characteristics and functions.)

Hood, L. E., Weissman, I. L., Wood, W. B., and Wilson, J. H. *Immunology,* 2nd Ed. Benjamin/Cummings, Menlo Park, California, 1984. (Contains an excellent section called "The Development of the Immune System.")

Paul, W. E. (Ed.). *Fundamental Immunology.* Raven Press, New York, 1984. (Includes an excellent section called "The Cells of the Immune System," in which lymphoid tissues and organs are also discussed.)

Phillips, J. H., and Lavier, L. L. Dissection of the lymphokine-activated killer phenomenon relative contribution to peripheral blood natural killer cells and T lymphocytes to cytolysis. *J. Experimental Medicine 164*:814, 1986.

Roitt, I., Brostoff, J., and Male D. *Immunology.* C. V. Mosby, St. Louis, Missouri, 1989. (Contains excellent sections called "Cells Involved in the Immune Response" and "The Lymphoid System" with profuse illustrations of excellent quality.)

Woodruff, J. J., Clarke, L. M., and Chin, Y. H. Specific cell-adhesion mechanisms determining migration pathways of recirculating lymphocytes. *Annual Review of Immunology 5*:201-222, 1987. (An updated revision of the lymphocyte "homing" mechanisms.)

3

Major Histocompatibility Complex

JEAN-MICHEL GOUST

I. INTRODUCTION

The major function of the immune system is to protect the organism from non-self material such as extracellular microorganisms. This function requires the recognition of nonself antigenic structures and the induction of an immune response through a set of cell-cell interactions involving macrophages, T lymphocytes, and B lymphocytes. Viruses and other intracellular parasites present a special problem to the immune system because of their being shielded from contact with immunocompetent cells. However, the immune system can recognize virally coded proteins expressed on the membrane of infected cells and destroy them, preventing viral multiplication. It had been suspected for a long time that viral antigens had to become an integral part of the host membrane, and alter what the immune system had learned to perceive as self, for such recognition to take place. This was very difficult to prove until the genes and molecules that the immune system identifies as self and modified-self were defined. It was eventually proven that the cellular antigens playing this role are the *histocompatibility antigens*, so designated because they also determine compatibility or rejection of transplanted tissues.

   Unless tissues or organs are transplanted between genetically identical individuals they are rapidly destroyed (rejected) by an immunological reaction. The definite proof that graft rejection is under *genetic control* was obtained in mice. A marked variation in graft survival was seen when skin was transplanted

31

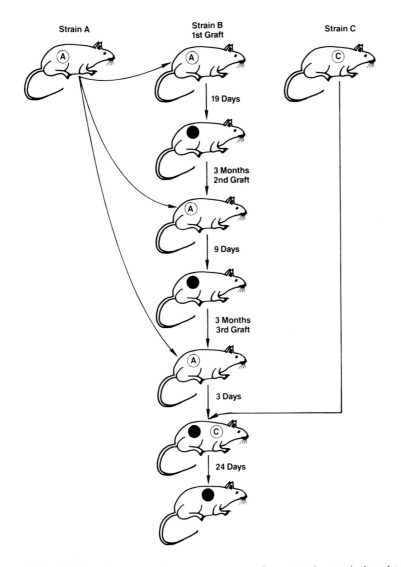

FIGURE 3.1 Diagrammatic representation of an experiment designed to demonstrate the memory and specificity of graft rejection. Memory is demonstrated by the progressive shortening of the time it takes for a mouse of strain B to reject consecutive skin grafts from a strain A donor. Specificity is demonstrated by the fact that although a mouse of strain B is able to reject a graft from strain A in accelerated fashion, if given a graft from a third, unrelated strain (C), rejection will take as long as the rejection the first graft from strain A. In other words, sensitization of mouse B to strain A was strain-specific and did not extend to unrelated strains.

among animals of different strains. The breeding of inbred stains of mice (after 20 or mor generations of brother/sister mating) made possible detailed studies of this genetic control. Members of a given inbred strain are virtually identical from the genetic point of view. No rejection is observed when skin is grafted among animals of the same inbred strain. However, the inbred animals are perfectly able to reject skin from animals of a different strain. On the other hand, the first generation hybrids (F1 hybrids), produced by mating animals of two genetically different strains, do not reject tissue from either parent, while the parents do reject skin from the F1 hybrids. These observations showed that the genetic differences explaining transplant rejection are due to codominant histocompatibility determinants. Further studies, diagrammatically summarized in Figure 3.1, showed that graft rejection shares two important characteristics with the classical humoral immune responses: *specificity* and *memory*.

Detailed studies of the animals used in skin graft experiments led to important discoveries. It was found that the animals receiving the graft developed antibodies that reacted specifically with skin and peripheral blood lymphocytes of the donor strain. These findings pointed to the sharing of antigens by different tissues of the donor animal. This possibility was confirmed through reverse immunizations, in which mice preinjected with lymphocytes obtained from a different strain would show accelerated rejection of a skin graft taken from the animals of the same strain from which the lymphocytes were obtained. It is now well established that most nucleated cells of the organism express histocompatibility antigens.

II. THE MAJOR HISTOCOMPATIBILITY COMPLEX

After many years of detailed genetic analysis it became clear that the system that determines the outcome of a transplant is complex and highly polymorphic. The study of inbred strains of mice also showed that the pattern of genetic segregation and inheritance of many traits (such as tail length, eye color, fur quality, several isoenzymes, and blood groups) was closely linked to the genetic transmission of histocompatibility antigens. For instance, there are eight blood groups in wild mice. The second (defined by the erythrocyte antigen 2 or Ea2) is strongly associated with the histocompatibility gene complex, which was thus named *H2 complex* (H for histocompatibility, 2 for the erythrocyte antigen #2). It was also observed that this system contained antigens of variable strength. The major antigens are responsible for most graft rejection responses and trigger a stronger immune response than others, which are designated as minor.

For many years, this field remained a branch of experimental immunology. Then investigators observed that the serum of multiparous women contained antibodies agglutinating their husband's lymphocytes. These *leukoagglutinins* were also found in the serum of multitransfused individuals, even when the donors were compatible with the transfused individual for all the known blood groups. The antigens responsible for the appearance of these antibodies were thus present on leukocytes and received the designation of *HLA* (*human leukocyte antigens*). The *H2 complex* in mice, the *HLA system* in humans, and equivalent systems in other species are generically designated as *major histocompatibility complex* (*MHC*).

III. CLASSIFICATION AND DETECTION OF HLA ANTIGENS

Six different loci of the HLA system have been identified and are designated as HLA-A, HLA-B, HLA-C, and HLA-DP, HLA-DQ, and HLA-DR (the last three corresponding to different loci of what is known as the D/DR region). Each locus has multiple cells, ranging from 6 in the case of HLA-C to more than 40 in the case of HLA-B. Each allele is designated by a number (e.g., HLA-B27). The D/DR region, which has three subloci, is the most polymorphic. The antigenic specificities associated with the different alleles of these loci are recognized by two types of techniques.

The *serological technique* uses lymphocytotoxic antibodies of known specificity (obtained from multiparous females or from recipients of multiple transfusions) in the presence of complement. Monoclonal antibodies have also been raised against HLA specificities and may be more widely used in the future. These antibodies identify several groups of HLA antigens, which are therefore designated as *serologically defined*. The antigens originally identified serologically were classified in three major groups, HLA-A, HLA-B, and HLA-C), and they are found on most nucleated cells. They are also designated as *class I MHC antigens*. Recently, two additional antigenic groups, the DQ and DR antigens, have been defined serologically.

The *mixed lymphocyte culture* (*MLC*) *assay* uses cell-cell interaction to determine differences not detectable with antisera. In the homozygous typing cell test, irradiated (non-dividing) cells from one individual, homozygous at the D/DR locus, will induce a very strong proliferation of T lymphocytes from another individual phenotypically identical at the HLA-A, B, and C loci level but carrying different D/DR antigens. This proliferation is detected by increased incorporation of [^{3}H] thymidine, which measures blastogenesis of the responding cells. The HLA antigens recognized in this assay are coded by the DP region and by associations of DQ and DR genes. For example, the MLC can distinguish several subgroups among individuals typed as DR4-DQw3. The DP, DQ, and DR subloci constitute the human *class II MHC*.

Mankind is highly outbred, and not all the alleles coded by the HLA genes have yet been found. This is exemplified by the fact that some individuals express unknown specificities at some loci (usually class II) that the typing laboratory reports as blank. Also, new HLA antigens are continuously discovered. To avoid unnecessary confusion HLA antigens are assigned a numerical designation by regularly held workshops of the World Health Organization. At first the designation is preceded by a *w*, indicating a provisional assignment. For example, DQw3 designates an antigenic specificity of the DQ locus that has been tentatively designated as w3 by a workshop. When worldwide agreement is reached that this is really a new specificity, the *w* is dropped. A method rapidly gaining widespread acceptance is to determine the presence of the gene coding for a given allele with its DNA probe. This approach is expected to alleviate the current ambiguities of the serological techniques and the technical difficulties of the MLR.

IV. CELLULAR DISTRIBUTION OF THE MHC ANTIGENS

A. Class I Antigens

Immunofluorescence and cytotoxicity assays demonstrate that in mice the *class I antigens* (Table 3.1), coded by the murine H2K, D and L genes, are expressed on all nucleated cells with only two exceptions: neurons and striated muscle cells. They are particularly abundant on the surface of lymphocytes (1,000 to 10,000 molecules/cell). The distribution of HLA-A, B, and C antigens in humans is identical to that of the murine class I antigens.

TABLE 3.1 The Main Characteristics of MHC Antigens Classes

Characteristics	Class I	Class II	Class III
Designation	H molecules	Ia molecules	C3 activators
Loci (mouse)	K, D, TL	I (A, E)	S (C4)
Loci (man)	A, B, C	DP, DQ, DR	C4, C2, factor B
No. of alleles	>100	>20	>2
No. of specificities	>100	>50	>2
Distribution of gene products	All nucleated cells	Lymphocytes, macrophages	Serum; red cell membrane (Chido and Rogers antigens)

B. Class II Antigens

It must be stressed that all cells expressing class II MHC antigens simultaneously express class I MHC antigens. The *Ia* and *Ie* antigens of the mouse H2 complex and the *DP, DQ,* and *DR* antigens of the human HLA system are exclusively expressed in two groups of leukocytes: B lymphocytes and cells of the monocyte-macrophage family, which includes all antigen-presenting cells (Langerhans cells in the skin, Kupfer cells in the liver, microglial cells in the central nervous system, and interdigitating cells in the spleen). With the exception of activated suppressor T cells, thymus-derived lymphocytes do not express class II antigens.

C. Class III Antigens

This group includes proteins of the complement system and other related proteins. They are coded by the S locus in mice and the *C2, C4* and *factor B* loci in humans. These loci are located between class I and class II MHC genes, and this proximity led to the creation of a third class of MHC gene products. However, their biological significance is quite unrelated to that of class I and class II MHC gene products. The class III antigens are mainly proteins found in serum, but the *Chido and Rogers erythrocyte antigens* are closely related to C4 from the structural point of view.

V. CHROMOSOMAL LOCALIZATION OF THE MHC; REGIONS AND SUBREGIONS

The mapping of the MHC region has been established based on the study of crossover gene products and on *in situ* hybridization studies with DNA probes. The MHC genes are located on *chromosome 17* of the mouse and on *chromosome 6* of humans. In both cases the MHC genes are located between the centromere and the telomere of the short arm of the respective chromosomes. The detailed maps of the H2 and the HLA systems are shown in Figure 3.2. In both species, the number of subregions is roughly the same, and occupy 0.5 (mice) and 1.8 centimorgans (humans) of their respective chromosomes. The larger size of the human HLA region suggests that it may include more genes and is probably more polymorphic than the murine H2. In mice, the H2 complex is subdivided into three loci. The H2-K locus and the H-2L/H-2D loci (class I genes) are separated by the I region, which includes two loci: I-A and I-E (class II genes). One additional locus, locus S, codes for the C4 molecule of the complement system (class III genes) and is located between the H-2K and H-2D loci. The organization of the HLA gene complex in humans is similar. However, in humans, the class II genes are closer to the GLO1 locus (coding for one isoenzyme of glioxylase) and are followed by several loci coding for proteins

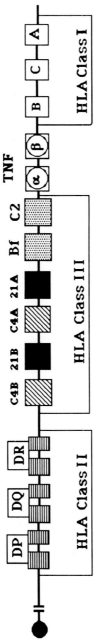

FIGURE 3.2 Simplified map of the region of human chromosome 6 where the HLA locus is located. The HLA class III loci include the genes for several complement components as well as the genes for 21 α and 21 β hydroxylase. The genes for tumor necrosis factors (TNF) α and β have also been located to chromosome 6 but are not considered as part of the HLA complex.

related to the complement cascade, such as Bf, C2 and C4 (class III genes), and
by the HLA, B, and C loci (class I genes). However, studies of the DNA found
in the entire H2 or HLA region revealed that it includes non-MHC genes such as
those coding for tumor necrosis factors α and β (TNF-α, TNF-β, see Chapter 11),
which are located near the C4 genes. In addition, the two C4 alleles are sepa-
rated from each other by the genes coding for the enzyme 21 α hydroxylase
(Fig. 3.2).

VI. BIOCHEMICAL AND STRUCTURAL STUDIES OF MHC ANTIGENS

A. Class I Antigens

The H2 or HLA molecules coded by MHC class I genes have molecular weights
that may vary from antigen to antigen from 43,000 to 48,000. They are formed
by a single peptide with a long extracellular region divided into three domains,
named $\alpha 1$, $\alpha 2$, and $\alpha 3$, followed by a short transmembrane, hydrophobic region
of 24 amino acids and an intracytoplasmic "tail" composed of about 30-35
amino acids, which includes the carboxyterminus and is attached to cytoskeletal
structures. *$\beta 2$ microglobulin*, a 12,000 dalton protein coded by a gene located
on *chromosome 15*, is postsynthetically and noncovalently associated with the
major polypeptide chain. Studies of the amino acid sequences of this polypeptide chain and of the nucleotide sequences of the exons of the various domains
of class I MHC antigens in mice and humans shows that most of the amino acid
and nucleotide changes responsible for the differences between alleles occur in
the $\alpha 1$ and $\alpha 2$ domains. The $\alpha 3$ domain shows much less genetic polymorphism
and, together with $\beta 2$ microglobulin, appears to support the deployment of the
more polymorphic $\alpha 1$ and $\alpha 2$ domains. The tridimensional structure of the
HLA class I antigens has been determined by x-ray crystallography (Fig. 3.3).
The most polymorphic areas of the molecule are located within and around a
groove formed at th junction of the $\alpha 1$ and $\alpha 2$ domains.

B. Class II Antigens

Although a remarkable degree of tertiary structure homology seems to exist
between class I and class II gene products (Fig. 3.4), there are important
differences in their primary structure. First, class II gene products are not
associated with $\beta 2$ microglobulin. Second, they consist of two distinct polypeptide chains, a light chain (β, MW 28,000), which is usually associated with
the greatest degree of genetic polymorphism, and a less polymorphic heavy
chain (α, MW 33,000). Each polypeptide chain has two extracellular domains
($\alpha 1$ and $\alpha 2$, $\beta 1$ and $\beta 2$), a short transmembrane domain, and a cytoplasmic tail.
The NH2 (or distal) terminals, $\alpha 1$ and $\beta 1$, contain hypervariable regions. Al-

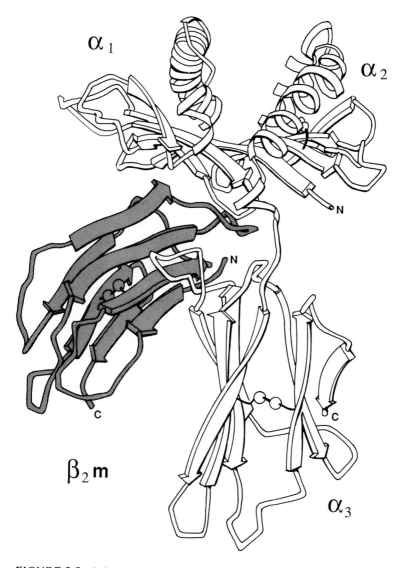

FIGURE 3.3   Schematic representation of the spatial configuration of the HLA-A2 molecule, based on x-ray crystallographic data. The diagram shows the immunoglobulinlike domains ($\alpha 3$, $\beta 2$m) at the bottom and the polymorphic domains ($\alpha 1$, $\alpha 2$) at the top. The indicated C terminus corresponds to the site of papain cleavage; the native molecule has additional intramembrane and intracellular segments. The $\alpha 1$ and $\alpha 2$ domains form a deep groove that is identified as the antigen recognition site. (Modified from Bjorkman et al., *Nature 329*:506, 1987.)

Class I   Class II

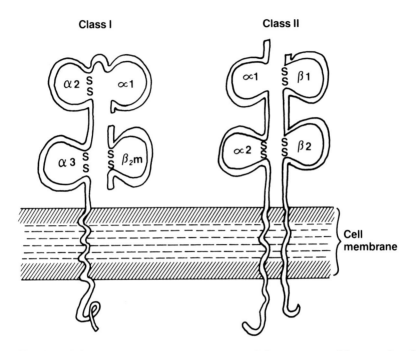

FIGURE 3.4   Diagrammatic representation of the structure of human class I and Class II histocompatibility antigens. (*Source*: Modified from Hood, L. E., et al. *Immunology*, 2nd Ed. Benjamin/Cummings, Menlo Park, California, 1984.)

though the three-dimensional structure of class II antigens has not yet been established, computer models using the primary sequence suggest that the $\alpha 1$ domains of class I and II should have similar α helical structures, and that the $\beta 1$ domains of class II HLA antigens should resemble the $\alpha 2$ domain of the class I HLA antigens. It also appears likely that the junction of $\beta 1$ and $\beta 2$ domains forms a groove similar to the one formed by the $\alpha 1$ and $\alpha 2$ domains of class I MHC antigens.

VII. GENETIC RULES OF INHERITANCE IN THE MHC

The MHC antigens are alloantigens (from the Greek αλλοσ, different); they distinguish individuals within a given species. Since there are so many alleles, there is only an extremely remote chance that two unrelated humans will be found who share an individual set of MHC antigens. Their expression is governed by two fundamental rules.

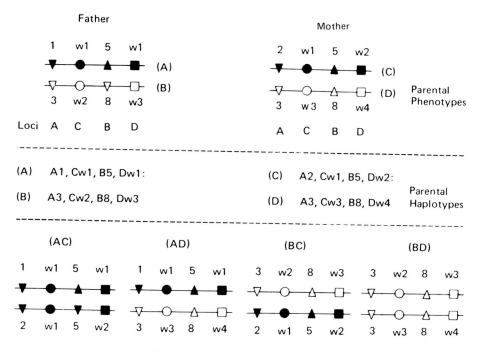

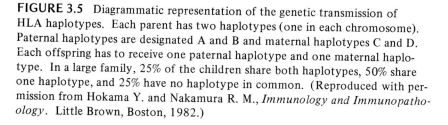

Four possible haplotypes of the offspring

FIGURE 3.5 Diagrammatic representation of the genetic transmission of HLA haplotypes. Each parent has two haplotypes (one in each chromosome). Paternal haplotypes are designated A and B and maternal haplotypes C and D. Each offspring has to receive one paternal haplotype and one maternal haplotype. In a large family, 25% of the children share both haplotypes, 50% share one haplotype, and 25% have no haplotype in common. (Reproduced with permission from Hokama Y. and Nakamura R. M., *Immunology and Immunopathology*. Little Brown, Boston, 1982.)

Rule 1. Each antigenic specificity of any given MHC locus is determined by one structural gene. For each locus, a given individual may be homozygous or heterozygous. In the first case, both DNA strands of the chromosome carry the same structural gene for that locus and the cells of the individual express one single antigenic specificity. In contrast, the cells of an individual heterozygous for a given locus will express the set of specificities inherited from each parent, which are coded by the two DNA strands of the same chromsome. In other words, both pecificities for each locus will be expressed by every individual cell of a heterozygous individual. Therefore, the MHC genes are *codominant* at the cell level, and there is no allelic exclusion, as observed in the case of immuno-globulin genes (see Chapter 7).

Rule 2. Individuals are able to respond to an MHC alloantigen that they do not express, but they cannot respond to an alloantigen that they do express.

The polymorphism of the HLA system revealed by serological means is very extensive. Multiple antigenic determinants are coded by different alleles within each gene complex or locus. The set of alleles that an individual carries at each locus on a single chromosome forms the haplotype, transmitted as a single unit except in very rare cases of recombination within the complex.

Figure 3.5 shows an example of haplotype inheritance within the HLA com-plex in humans. All the alleles of any individual being codominant (Rule 1), it follows that both haplotypes that form an individual genotype will be expressed. HLA or H2 *phenotype* is a term often used in tissue typing to indicate all the alleles detected in a given individual, e.g., Al,2; B8,27; Dw3,-; DR23,-. The hyphen indicates that only one antigen of a particular locus can be typed and that therefore the individual either is homozygous or possesses an antigen that cannot be typed because no appropriate reagents are available. Family studies are the only way to distinguish between these two possibilities.

VIII. LINKAGE DISEQUILIBRIUM

In an outbred population in which matings take place at random, the frequency of finding a given allele at one HLA locus associated with a given allele at a second HLA locus should simply be the product of the frequencies of each individual allele in the population. However, certain combinations of alleles (i.e., certain haplotypes) occur with a higher-than-expected frequency. Thus many HLA antigens occur together on the same chromosome more often than is expected by chance. This phenomenon is termed *linkage disequilibrium*. As an example, the HLA-A1 allele is found in the Caucasian population with a frequency of 0.158, and the HLA-B8 allele is found with a frequency of 0.092. The A1, B8 haplotype should therefore be found with a frequency of 0.158 × 0.092 = 0.015. In reality, it is found with a frequency of 0.072. The linkage disequilibrium is expressed as the difference (Δ) between the observed and the expected frequencies of the alleles, i.e., 0.072 - 0.015 = 0.057.

IX. EVOLUTIONARY CONSERVATION OF THE MHC

When it became possible to purify and determine the amino acid sequences of the MHC antigens, it became clear that they were highly conserved through-out all mammalian species. A very high degree of homology has been found be-tween mice and humans, HLA-A and B antigens sharing up to 70% of their amino acids with class I antigens of the murine H2 complex. This structural conservation in evolution is considered as evidence for their primordial role in the immune response: The individuals expressing the genes least efficient in the fight against infections will not survive. It is also striking that a strong homology also exists between HLA antigens and immunoglobulin molecules. It is believed that both immunoglobulin and HLA genes derive from a common ancestral gene that served as a source for evolutionarily advantageous genes.

X. MHC AND THE GENETIC CONTROL OF IMMUNE RESPONSES

The MHC complex has, therefore, a biological significance that transcends the determination of the fate of a transplant between nonidentical individuals. Using inbred strains of mice and guinea pigs as experimental models, it was shown that the amplitude of the response to a given antigen is genetically controlled: Some strains are high responders while others are low responders to specific antigens. These quantitative differences in the amplitude of the response are under the control of genes closely linked to MHC class II genes that constitute the *immune-response associated region* of the MHC. The specific mouse leukocyte antigens coded by those genes have received the generic designation of *Ia* (meaning *I*mmune response *a*ssociated). The D/DR region plays an equivalent role in humans, and the term *Ia antigens* is also frequently used as a designation for human MHC II gene products.

XI. FUNCTIONS OF THE MHC IN THE IMMUNE RESPONSE

The current views on the role of the MHC can be summarized by stating that cell-associated antigens are recognized by T cells only if complexed to MHC antigens. This essential role of MHC antigens was first established in the mid-1970s for the cell-mediated immune responses to viruses. *For effector (cytotoxic) cells to kill virally-infected cells efficiently, target and effector cells have to share identical class I MHC antigens.* In other words, the killing of a target cells is MHC restricted.

It is believed that the "groove" of the HLA MHC class I molecule is a most likely site for binding of endogenously produced antigens. For example, viral proteins being synthesized in the cytoplasm of infected cells would bind intracytoplasmically to newly synthesized HLA molecules. This HLA-viral antigen complex would then be transported to the infected cell's membrane where it would be recognized the precursors of cytotoxic T cells as *self plus X*. This specific interaction of a given T cell subset with a particular class of antigen-modified MHC molecule is central to the functions of the immune system and is responsible for the phenomenon of MHC restriction.

TABLE 3.2 Examples of Associations Between Particular Diseases and the MHC in Humans[a]

Disease	Linked HLA region determinant	Disease risk of persons who bear determinant (relative) to disease risk in the population at large = 1)	Description of disease
Inflammatory diseases			
Ankylosing spondylitis	B(27)	100–200	Inflammation of the spine, leading to stiffening of vertebral joints
Reiter's syndrome	B(27)	40	Inflammation of the spine, prostate, and parts of eye (the uvea)
Acute anterior uveitis	B(27)	30	Inflammation of the iris and ciliary body
Juvenile rheumatoid arthritis (type II)	B(27)	10–12	A multisystem inflammatory disease of children characterized by rapid onset of joint lesions and fever
Psoriasis	B(13)	4–5	An acute, recurrent, localized inflammatory disease of the skin (usually scalp, elbows, and knees), often associated with arthritis
Celiac disease	B(8) D(Dw3)	9–10	A chronic inflammatory disease of the small intestine; probably a food allergy to a protein in grains (gluten)

Disease	Locus	Relative risk	Description
Multiple sclerosis	D(DR2)	5	A progressive chronic inflammatory disease of brain and spinal cord that causes hardening (sclerosis) and loss of function in affected foci
Rheumatic fever	DR(antibody 833)	4–5	An autoimmune disease wherein antibodies raised during β-hemolytic streptococcal pharyngitis cross-react with heart tissue to give rise to damaging myocarditis and valculitis
Endocrine diseases			
Addison's disease	D(DR3)	4–5	A deficiency in production of adrenal gland cortical hormones
Diabetes mellitus	D(DR3,DR4)	2–5	A deficiency of insulin production; pancreatic islet cells usually absent or damaged
Miscellaneous diseases			
Narcolepsy	DR2	100	A condition characterized by the tendency to fall asleep unexpectedly.

Source: Modified from Hood, L. E., Weissman, I. L., Wood, W. B., and Wilson, J. H. *Immunology*, 2nd Ed. Benjamin/Cummings, Menlo Park, California, 1984.

It has been experimentally demonstrated that cytotoxic T cells recognize antigen-modified class I antigens on their targets while helper and inducer T cells interact with antigen-presenting cells carrying on their surface a complex formed by processed antigen and HLA class II antigens. It thus appears that the essential function of the MHC is to provide binding sites for endogenous and processed antigens, allowing their recognition by T cells. The polymorphism of MHC genes would be required to generate the large number of binding sites necessary to accommodate a large variety of antigenic molecules. Irrespective of whether these antigenic molecules are endogenously produced or the result of the processing of exogenous antigens, they will have two functionally distinct regions. One, designated as the *aggretope*, determines the binding to the MHC molecule. This probably corresponds to a few oligopeptides shared by many different proteins, but it still seems very likely that some aggretopes may have a much better fit with some MHC molecules than others. From this it follows that the repertoire of MHC molecules of a given individual may control the ability to respond well or not to a specific antigen. If an MHC molecule able to bind the aggretope of a particular antigen with high affinity is expressed in the individual's T lymphocytes, the individual will be a high responder to the antigen in question. If, on the contrary, the binding of the aggretope to MHC molecules is rather loose, the individual will be a low responder. Thus the magnitude of the immune response will be directly determined by the closeness of fit between aggretope and MHC molecules. The second important region in the antigenic molecule is the one that will interact with the antigen receptors and is designated as *epitope*. The aggretope, tightly bound to the MHC molecule, will not be seen by immunocytes. The epitope, although immobilized by the interaction with the MHC molecule, is accessible to the immune system.

Most of the research concerning MHC restriction and its molecular basis has been, of necessity, carried out with experimental animals (particularly mice), and there is some uncertainty about the degree to which the concepts emerging from experimental work can be fully applied to humans. However, a considerable amount of concordant data has been generated from in vitro studies using human cells, and it appears more and more likely that the rules established in mice may be general biological rules.

XII. MHC AND DISEASES

Considering the essential role played by MHC gene products in the control of the immune response, it seems logical that genetically determined susceptibility to many diseases should be associated with the expression of a given HLA antigen or cluster of antigens (Table 3.2). This could be due to five possible mechanisms.

First, the genetic control of the immune response depends on MHC genes. Because HLA antigens have binding sites for processed antigens from common pathogens, the ability to respond adequately to that pathogen is dependent on the conformation of the HLA molecule and genetically determined by MHC genes. In other words, the immune response genes in the D/DR region would determine a degree of fit between the aggretopes of the antigens and the MHC class II gene products. A very close fit between aggretope and MHC II molecules is probably essential for optimal antigen presentation to T cells, therefore determining an immune response of high magnitude. If a particular antigen could only bind weakly to the available MHC class II molecules, the immune response would be negatively affected and would be of low magnitude. In the case of infectious agents, a high responder individual is better protected than a low responder, and the low responder may be more susceptible to the disease caused by that agent.

Second, all the human diseases in which autoimmune phenomena have been identified are strongly linked to D/DR antigens. Carrying those D/DR antigens associated with autoimmune diseases implies only an increased susceptibility to the disease. The individual may remain asymptomatic for life, or an encounter with a given pathogen may trigger an immune response that ends by recognizing some autologous molecule structurally similar to an epitope carried by this pathogen. The genes of the DQ locus appear to be the most closely linked to autoimmune diseases. For example, the susceptibility to insulin-dependent diabetes and the autoimmune response against pancreatic islet cells are determined by allelic polymorphisms of the β chain of the DQ antigen. Since the DQ antigens seem to be preferentially involved in the interactions with helper/inducer T cells, this observation suggests that abnormalities in these interactions may predispose to autoimmunity.

Third, it has been suggested that HLA antigens may act as receptors for some intracellular pathogens. These pathogens would interact with specific HLA antigens in the cell membrane, would infect the cells carrying those antigens, and could determine long-lasting changes in cell functions. This could be the case in ankylosing spondylitis and related disorders (acute anterior uveitis, Reiter's syndrome) in which 80 to 100% of the affected individuals are HLA-B27. However, the pathogenic agents responsible for this group of diseases have not been identified to date.

Fourth, another proposed mechanism is the molecular mimicry between antigenic determinants in infectious agents and HLA antigens. For example, *Yersinia psuedotuberculosis* has been shown to contain epitopes cross-reactive with HLA-B27. Therefore an immune response directed against this bacterium could lead to an autoimmune reaction against self. Why this reaction would affect specific joints, however, is not clear.

Fifth, the very strong association of various forms of 21 hydroxylase deficiency responsible for congenital adrenal hyperplasia with various HLA haplotypes (HLA -Bw 47, DR7), and other data obtained in classical genetic studies, suggest that this disorder is determined by alleles of a single locus. Eventually it was demonstrated that the genes coding for 21-hydroxylase are located on chromosome 6, close to the genes coding for the alleles of the complement fragments C4-A and C4-B (Figure 3.2). Thus the 21-hydroxylase genes are physically linked to MHC genes, with which they show strong linkage disequilibrium. A similar explanation may account for the very strong associations between HLA-DR2 and narcolepsy, HLA-Bw35 and hemochromatosis, and HLA-B27 and ankylosing spondilitis. The chromosomal segment on which the HLA genes are located is large enough to include many other yet unidentified genes whose presence is only suspected by the strong associations with diseases that could be determined by genes transmitted in linkage disequilibrium with MHC genes. More extensive mapping and sequencing of the short arm of chromosome 6 may answer these questions.

SELF-EVALUATION

Questions

Choose the one best answer.

3.1   Immune response (Ir) genes
      A. Are linked to the X chromosome.
      B. Control V region amino acid sequence variability in immunoglobulins.
      C. Are believed to be part of the histocompatibility gene complex.
      D. Control common region allotypes of immunoglobulins.
      E. Are found in all animals, from sponges to humans.

3.2   Which of the following is not coded for by MHC genes?
      A. β2-microglobulin.
      B. Type I HLA antigens.
      C. Type II HLA antigens.
      D. C4.
      E. Chido and Rogers erythrocyte antigens.

3.3   The HLA phenotypes of a married couple are (man) A1,3;Cw1,w2;B5,8, Dw 1,w3 and (woman) A2,3,Cw1,w3,B5,8,Dw2,w4. Which of the following phenotypes would definitely not be possible in an offspring of this couple?
      A. A1,2,Cw1-,B5-,Dw1,w2.
      B. A2,3;Cw1,w2;B5,8;Dw2,w3.
      C. A1,3,Cw1,w3;B5,8;Dw1,w4.
      D. A1-;Cw1,w2;B5-;Dw1,w3.
      E. A3-,Cw3,w3,Bi,-;Dw3,w4.

3.4 Class I HL-A antigens
   A. Are defined by the MLC assay.
   B. Code for complement proteins.
   C. Are restricted to lymphocytes and monocytes.
   D. Include $\beta2$ microglobulin as one of their constitute chains.
   E. Are closely associated with the immune response genes.

3.5 Predisposition to develop diabetes mellitus is associated with _____ alleles.
   A. HLA-A.
   B. HLA-B.
   C. HLA-DP.
   D. HLA-DQ.
   E. HLA-DR.

3.6 The frequency of the HLA-A1 and HLA-B8 alleles in the general population is 0.158 and 0.092, respectively. Assuming that these alleles are transmitted independently (without linkage disequilibrium), the expected frequency of the A1,B8 haplotype would be
   A. 0.072.
   B. 0.057.
   C. 0.030.
   D. 0.015.
   E. 0.003.

3.7 A resting T cell will express on its surface antigens coded by HLA genes of class
   A. I, II and III.
   B. I and II.
   C. I and III.
   D. I only.
   E. II only.

3.8 Over 80% of the patients with ankylosing spondilitis are positive for
   A. HLA-DW3.
   B. HLA-B8.
   C. HLA-B27.
   D. HLA-B7.
   E. HLA-A5.

3.9 Cells not expressing class I HLA antigenic products include
   A. Monocytes.
   B. B lymphocytes.
   C. Skin cells.
   D. T lymphocytes.
   E. Striated muscle cells.

3.10   The association of congenital adrenal hyperplasia with HLA-Bw47/HLA-
DR1 is explained by
A. Immune stimulation of the adrenal gland by an autoimmune response.
B. The close association between MHC Class III genes and the gene coding
for 21 is hydroxylase.
C. Stimulation of the adrenal gland by cachectin.
D. Infection of adrenal cells by a pathogen that uses B247/DR1 as recep-
tors.
E. Statistical coincidence.

Answers

3.1   (C)   In man, the D/DR locus either corresponds to the immune response
genes or is closely linked to them.

3.2.   (A) $\beta2$ microglobulin is coded by a gene in chromosome 15 and becomes
associated with the heavy chain of HLA I antigens postsynthetically.
The Chido and Rogers antigens are related to C4 and synthesized
under control of type III HLA genes.

3.3   (D)   The phenotype should include specificities 2 or 3 for locus A and
W2 or W4 for locus D (one specificity being of paternal origin and
the other of maternal origin).

3.4   (D)   MLC defines some of the class II antigens (DP locus).

3.5   (D)

3.6   (D)   The frequency of the A,B haplotype equals the product of the frequencies of each antigen in the general population.

3.7   (D)

3.8   (C)

3.9   (E)   Class I antigens are expressed in most nucleated cells, except nervous tissue cells and striated muscle cells.

3.10   (B)   The 21 is hydroxylase genes are closely located to the MHC class III
genes in chromosome 6, showing strong linkage disequilibrium with
various HLA specificities.

BIBLIOGRAPHY

Bjorkman, P. J., Saper, M. A., Samroui, B., Bennett, W. S., Strominger, J. L.,
and Wiley, D C. Structure of the human class I histocompatibility antigen,
HLA-A2. *Nature 329*:506, 1987.

Hood, L. E., Weissman, I. L., Wood, W. B., and Wilson, J. H. *Immunology*, 2nd Ed. Benjamin/Cummings, Menlo Park, California, 1984. (The structure, genetics, and biological role of the MHC are discussed in detail in this text.)

Klein, J. The Histocompatibility-2 (H-2) Complex. In *The Mouse in Biomedical Research*, Vol. 1, H. L. Foster, J. D. Small, and J. G. Fox (Eds.). Academic Press, New York, 1981, p. 120.

Klein, J. *Immunology: The Science of Self-Nonself Discrimination*. John Wiley & Sons, New York, 1982.

Klein, J., Juretic, A., Baxevanis, C. N., and Nagy, Z. A. The traditional and new version of the mouse H-2 complex. *Nature 291*:455, 1981.

Litwin, S. D. (Ed.). *Human immunogenetics. Basic principles and clinical relevance*. Marcel Dekker, New York, 1989.

Marx, J. L. What T cells see and how they see it. *Science, 242*:863, 1988.

Sachs, D. H. The major histocompatibility complex. In *Fundamental Immunology*, W. E. Paul (Ed.). Raven Press, New York, 1984, p. 303.

Schwartz, R. H. The role of gene prodicts of the major histocompatibility complex in T cell activation and cellular interactions. In *Fundamental Immunology*, W. E. Paul (Ed.). Raven Press, New York, 1984, p. 379.

Todd, J. A., Bell, J. I., and McDevitt, H. O. $HLA-DQ\beta$ gene contributes to susceptibility and resistance to insulin-dependent diabetes mellitus. *Nature 329*: 599, 1987.

White, P. C., New, M. I., and Dupont, B. Congenital adrenal hyperplasia. *N. Eng. J. Med. 316*:1519, 1987.

4

Antigenicity and Immune Recognition

GABRIEL VIRELLA

One of the most important aspects of the fundamental knowledge of the immune response is the understanding of the mechanisms whereby a given substance is recognized as "foreign" and the sequence of subsequent events that lead from such recognition to the full stimulation of immunocompetent cells and induction of specific effector mechanisms that result in the elimination of the foreign substance. The concepts of antigenicity, immunogenicity, and immune recognition are the cornerstones of our understanding, which is still very superficial, of this important question.

I. ANTIGENICITY AND IMMUNOGENICITY

Antigenicity is the property of a substance (an *antigen*) that allows it to react with the products of a specific immune response (*antibodies*, specifically *sensitized T lymphocytes*).

Immunogenicity is the property of a substance (an *immunogen*) that endows it with the capacity to provoke a specific immune response. All immunogens are antigens, but the reverse is not true. For example, certain low-molecular-weight substances termed *haptens* can elicit a specific immune response only when coupled to a larger immunogenic *carrier* molecule. However, once an antihapten antibody is produced, it can combine with soluble hapten molecules, free of carrier protein.

II. ANTIGENIC DETERMINANTS

Most immunogenic substances are either macromolecules or cell components. In either case, only a restricted portion of the immunogen actually binds to the antibody. This part of an antigen that fits the antibody combining site is called an *antigenic determinant* or *epitope*.

The maximum size of an antigenic determinant is about 3000 cubic Å, about the size of four amino acids or four to five sugar molecules. The amino acids forming an antigenic determinant do not need to be contiguous in the polypeptide chain. The only requirements is that they be *spatially contiguous*; two distant regions in the polypeptide chain can be brought together by the tertiary folding of the protein to constitute a site. A polypeptide with 100 amino acids may have as many as 14 to 20 nonoverlapping determinants. However, a typical 100-amino-acid globular protein is folded over itself, and most of its structure is hidden from the outside. Only surface determinants will usually be accessible for recognition by immunocompetent cells and for interactions with antibodies (Fig. 4.1).

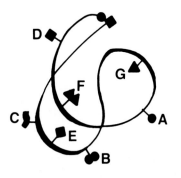

FIGURE 4.1 Diagrammatic representation of a globular protein that has several different antigenic determinants that are externally located and accessible to the immune system (A, B, C, D) and others that are buried and will not be easily recognized (E, F, G).

III. CHEMICAL NATURE OF IMMUNOGENS

Many different substances can induce immune responses. Proteins and polysaccharides are potent immunogens, relatively small polypeptidic chains and nucleic acids can, given the right circumstances, also be immunogenic.

A. Proteins

Large proteins (molecular weight greater than 10,000) containing a wide diversity of antigenic determinants are among the most potent immunogens. Bacterial toxins, enzymes, and heterologous serum proteins are examples of strongly immunogenic proteins. The protein moiety of lipoprotein molecules can also be immunogenic, while the lipid portion is usually not recognized by the immune system.

B. Polysaccharides

These are probably among the most important natural antigens, since either pure polysaccharides or the sugar moieties of glycoprotein, lipopolysaccharides, glycolipid-protein complexes, etc., are immunogenic. In nature, many microorganisms have polysaccharide-rich capsules or cell walls; and a variety of mammalian antigens, such as the erythrocyte antigens (A, B, O, Le, H), are polysaccharides.

C. Nucleic Acids

These usually are not immunogenic, but if they are coupled to a protein (forming a nucleoprotein) they can induce antibody formation. The spontaneous formation of nucleoproteins could be one of the initial steps involved in the autoimmune responses to DNA and RNA that characterize some of the so-called autoimmune diseases (e.g., systemic lupus erythematosus).

D. Polypeptides

Hormones such as insulin, although relatively small in size (MW 1500), are usually immunogenic when isolated from one species and administered over long periods of time to an individual of a different species.

IV. HAPTENS AND CARRIERS

Haptens are defined as small substances that, by themselves, are not immunogenic but that are recognized specifically by preformed antibody. To some extent, haptens are equivalent to antigenic determinants that can be added to carrier proteins. Landsteiner, Pauling, and others discovered in the 1930s and 1940s that small aromatic groups such as aminobenzene sulphonate, aminobenzene arsonate, and aminobenzene carboxylate could be chemically coupled to immunogenic proteins (*carriers*). When these conjugates were injected into animals, the resulting antibodies were able to react specifically with each hapten; however, if the haptens were injected without carriers, no antibodies were produced.

More recently, the chemical group dinitrophenyl (DNP) has been extensively used as a hapten; indeed, most of our knowledge about T-B cell cooperation has originated on immunization studies using DNP-protein conjugates. Also, drug-protein conjugates have been used to produce antibodies to a wide variety of drugs and are the basis for numerous drug assays (e.g., plasma digoxin levels). Furthermore, the hypersensitization to some drugs, chemicals, and metals is believed to result from spontaneous coupling of the active substance to an endogenous protein, creating a hapten-carrier situation. One example of this mechanism is the spontaneous coupling of the penicilloyl derivative of penicillin to a host protein, which is probably the first step toward developing a hypersensitivity reaction to penicillin.

V. CHARACTERISTICS ASSOCIATED WITH IMMUNOGENICITY

A. Foreignness

As a rule, only substances recognized as nonself will trigger the immune response. Microbial antigens and heterologous proteins are obviously nonself and strongly immunogenic. However, low levels of antibodies and of sensitized T lymphocytes reacting with self components have been deteced in most normal individuals, probably playing a beneficial role by promoting the elimination of aged or damaged cells. Much higher levels of autoantibodies are present in patients with autoimmune disorders, as we shall discuss in detail in later chapters.

B. Molecular Size

The most potent immunogens are macromolecular proteins (MW > 100,000). Molecules smaller than 10,000 daltons are usually weak immunogens. Also many small antigenic molecules tend to elicit cellular reactions (T-cell-mediated) rather than antibody production.

C. Chemical Structure and Complexity

Positively charged (basic) amino acids, such as lysine, arginine, and histidine are repeatedly present in the antigenic sites of lysozyme and myoglobin, while aromatic amino acids (such as tyrosine) are found in two of albumin's six antigenic sites. Therefore, it appears that basic and aromatic amino acids may contribute more strongly to immunogenicity than other amino acids; basic proteins with clusters of positively charged amino acids are strong immunogens. There is also a direct relationship between antigenicity and chemical complexity: aggregated or chemically polymerized proteins are much stronger immunogens than their soluble monomeric counterparts.

VI. FACTORS ASSOCIATED WITH THE INDUCTION OF AN IMMUNE RESPONSE

A. Genetic Constitution of the Animal

Different animal species or different strains of one species show different degrees of responsiveness to a given antigen. In humans, different individuals can behave as high responders or low responders to any given antigen. The genetic control of the immune response has been well documented in animals by studying the immune response to well-defined antigens in inbred strains of rats, mice, guinea pigs, etc. In guinea pigs, for example, the ability to respond to poly-L-lysine has been found to be inherited as an autosomal dominant trait. Both in guinea pigs and in mice it has been possible to characterize *immune response* *(IR) genes*, part of the *MHC* system, which control the immune response. In humans, the IR genes are believed to be class II genes of the MHC (Chapter 3).

B. Method of Antigen Administration

A given dose of antigen may elicit no detectable response when injected intravenously but may elicit a strong immune response if injected intradermally. This last route of administration results in slow removal and prolonged antigenic stimulation; these are important conditions for immunogenicity. The presence of Langerhans cells in the dermis, which are extremely effective as antigen-presenting cells, is believed to be a significant factor in determining the strong responses obtained when antigens are injected intradermally.

C. Use of Adjuvants

Adjuvants are agents that when administered along with an antigen can cause any of three effects. They can

1. Enhance the immune response of an immunogen.
2. Alter the nature of an immune response to a given immunogen.
3. Elicit an immune response by themselves.

In experimental work, the most commonly used adjuvant is complete Freund's adjuvant (CFA), a water-in-oil emulsion with killed mycobacteria in the oil phase. Water-in-oil emulsions by themselves (Freund's incomplete adjuvant), bacterial endotoxins, aluminum hydroxide, synthetic polynucleotides, and other microorganisms, such as killed *Bordetella pertussis*, bacillus Calmette-Guerin (BCG), and *Corynebacterium parvum*, have also been used, the last two in humans, to boost the activity of a patient's immune system.

The mechanism of action of adjuvants is not clearly understood, but a delayed release of antigen, nonspecific inflammatory effects, and the activation of monocytes and macrophages appear to be the most important factors. For example, muramyldipeptide (MDP), which is the active moiety of *Mycobacterium tuberculosis* and of BCG, has potent adjuvant activity and can be shown to stimulate a variety of macrophage functions.

VII. IMMUNOPOTENCY AND IMMUNODOMINANCE

The capacity of a region of an antigenic molecule to serve as an antigenic determinant and induce the production of specific antibodies is known as *immunopotency*. From our discussion on antigenic determinants it clearly results that immunopotent regions have to be accessible (i.e., externally exposed side chains or regions), hydrophilic, and rich in positively charged amino acids such as lysine and arginine. It is interesting to note that the recognition of a given region as immunopotent is also genetically controlled. For example, the insulin molecule is known to have two main epitopes, and it has been shown that different guinea pig strains may react preferentially to one and not to the other. Similar observations have been obtained in studies of the response of different strains of mice to synthetic polypeptides.

A given antigenic determinant or epitope may be composed of several peptides or sugar moieties. However, some of the peptide or sugar residues appear to have a stronger influence on the reactivity with a corresponding antibody than others, or, in other words, some peptides or sugars are *immunodominant*. For example, two antigenic determinants may differ only by a positively charged amino acid present in one and absent in the other. Such charged amino acids have a great influence in the conformation of the determinant, and the antibodies raised against these otherwise similar structures may not cross-react. The charged amino acid is, therefore, considered to be immunodominant. A corollary of this concept is that an immunodominant amino acid or sugar must be easily accessible to the immune system. The terminal amino acids of a polypeptide side chain, for example, are likely to be immunodominant.

VIII. A CLASSIFICATION OF ANTIGENS FROM
THE HOST PERSPECTIVE

Antigens can basically be subdivided into those of exogenous origin and those that are of endogenous origin. Most of the antigens to which we react are of exogenous origin; they include microbial antigens, pollens, pollutants, and medications. Our immune system has as its objective their elimination, because they are clearly nonself, but in some instances the immune response itself may have a deleterious effect (hypersensitivity states).

By definition, our response to our own self antigens normally is very limited. Our autoantigens (autologous antigens) are endogenous, and their recognition can be the cause of severe pathological stiuations (autoimmune diseases), although it may also have an important role in normal catabolic processes (i.e., anti-red-cell antibodies may help in eliminating senescent erythrocytes). A remarkable group of endogenous antigens are those incorrectly designated as xenoantigens or heteroantigens (literally, antigens from a different species). Normally any living being expresses only antigens of its own species. However, in patients suffering from viral diseases, particularly infectious mononucleosis, antibodies that react with herbivore red cells appear in the circulation. It is believed that the viral infection somehow induces or specifies the expression of a new antigen on the surface of infected cells, closely related to the blood group A oligosaccharide and also to blood group antigens present in herbivores. This antigen is recognized as nonself and elicits an immune response, and the resulting antibody appears to be directed against herbivore red cells, i.e., against a determinant from a different species (e.g., sheep).

IX. ALLOANTIGENS

A most significant group of antigens is that of the *alloantigens*, i.e., antigenic determinants that distinguish one individual from another. These are endogenous antigens, and they basically define the antigenic makeup of the cells and tissues of an individual. Classical examples are the A, B, and O blood group antigens: some individuals carry the A specificity, others are B, AB, or do not express either A or B (O). Other examples of alloantigens are the histocompatibility antigens of nucleated cells and tissues, the platelet (Pl) antigens, and the immunoglobulin allotypes.

Normally we do not produce antibodies against our own or any other alloantigens. Their production can result from unknown causes, as in autoimmunity, or from sensitization. Women may become sensitized to red cell or immunoglobulin alloantigens during pregnancy. Transfusion of whole blood can induce sensitization against cellular or immunoglobulin alloantigens. Organ transplantation usually results in sensitization against histcompatibility alloantigens expressed in the transplanted organ.

X. IMMUNE RECOGNITION

For an immune response to be initiated, the antigen must be recognized as nonself by the immunocompetent cells. This phenomenon is called *immune*

recognition. It is calculated that as many as 10^6-10^8 different antigenic specificities can be recognized by the immune system of a normal human, and it is
believed that a normal individual has an equal number of different small families
(clones) of immunocytes bearing receptors for those different antigens. Each
immunocompetent cell expresses on its membrane multiple copies of a receptor
for one single antigen; when stimulated, each cell will proliferate and differentiate into a population (clone) of daughter cells carrying the same receptor. The
recognition of antigens by immunocompetent cells depends on the stimulation
of several distinct cell populations (clones), each one carrying *clonally restricted*
receptors for one specific determinant, by the several different antigenic determinants or epitopes expressed on the antigen. In B cells, these specific receptors
are surface-bound immunoglobulins, particularly IgD and monomeric IgM molecules. The T cell receptor is constituted by two polypeptide chains, termed
α and β, with similar molecular weight (40-45,000). The two chains have a
short transmembrane segment that extends into the cytoplasm; they are joined
by a disulfide bridge outside the transmembrane segment and have an extracellular segment with a variable and a constant domain (Fig. 4.2). Considerably more
diversity exists among β chains than among α chains. The β chains appear to be
coded by a multigene family that includes genes for regions homologous to the
V, C. D, and J regions of human immunoglobulins, these will be discussed in
Chapter 5 ("Immunoglobulin Structure"). At this point, we should recall that
the stimulation of a T cell requires the presentation of processed antigen by an
accessory cell sharing MHC antigens with the responding T cell. The helper T
cells, for example, are apparently able to respond to the antigen only when it is
associated to a class II MHC antigen (I-region-associated antigen or Ia in mice).
Specific regions of the α and β chains of the T-cell receptor have a significant
homology with the immunoglobulin variable regions that are involved in antigen binding. It has been hypothesized that the recognition of the complex
formed by antigen and HLA takes place mainly through only one of the variable domains of either the α or the β chain. In the example shown in Figure 4.2,
the β chain variable domain interacts both with the antigen and with a complementary surface on the Ia β_1 domain, while in other T-cell clones the Vα domain
may be used for antigen binding. According to this model, the same T-cell receptor interacts both with antigen and with the nonpolymorphic region of the
α_1 and β_1 domain of the Ia antigen (Fig. 4.2). This dual interaction would
allow the cross-linking of T-cell receptors, which is essential for the onset of
T-cell stimulation. Taking as basis x-ray crystallography studies of MHC antigens (see Chapter 3) it has been proposed that the processed antigen is bound
to a grove determined by the variable regions of the α_1 and β_1 domains of a
class II MHC antigen (Ia). The binding site of the TcR would recognize the antigen while other regions of the TcR Vα and Vβ domains would interact with the

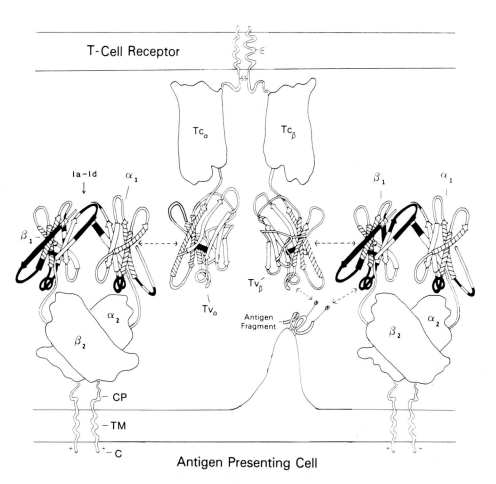

FIGURE 4.2 A hypothetical model for the T cell receptor (TcR) recognition of antigen in association with MHC class II Ia glycoproteins. Two Ia molecules are shown on the antigen-presenting cell, each composed of a β chain (β_1 and β_2 domains) and an α chain (α_1 and α_2 domains). CP, connecting peptide; TM, transmembrane region; C, cytoplasmic region. The antigen represents a membrane-associated cytochrome fragment with a C-terminal lysine residue at 103 interacting with the β_1 domain and another lysine residue at 99 proposed to interact with TcR. The TcR has disulfide-linked β and α chains with corresponding variable (TVβ, TVα) and constant (TCβ, TCα) domains. The TcR V-domains are shown interacting with two Ia molecules; alternative models of binding to a single Ia molecule (TCα-α_1, for example) have not been ruled out. (Reproduced, with permission, from Norcross, M. A. and Kanehisa, M. The predicted structure of the Ia domain: A hypothesis for the structural basis of MHC-restricted T cell recognition of antigens. *Scand. J. Immunol. 21*:511, 1985.)

α_1 and β_1 domains of the Ia antigens. Both types of interactions (TcR-Ag and TcR-Ia) have to occur if an effective stimulating signal is to be delivered to the T cells.

The antigen receptors in B and T cells are present in unstimulated cells, because it is through the interaction between the antigen and its corresponding receptor that cell stimulation will result. At the end of an immune response the total number of antigen-specific clones will remain the same, but the number of cells in those clones that participated in the response will have increased several fold. This increased residual population of antigen-specific cells is long-lived, and it is believed to be the origin of the phenomenon known as immunological memory, which will be discussed in later chapters.

XI. T-DEPENDENT AND T-INDEPENDENT ANTIGENS

Antigens can be divided into two groups according to the involvement of T cells in their recognition: *T-dependent* and *T-independent*. This functional definition is mostly based on experimental work carried out with inbred mice, and it cannot be considered as an absolute fact in all species (there may be a continuous gradation from T dependency to T independence, rather than two discrete groups of antigens), but enough evidence has been obtained, even in man, to accept and use this as a working classification of antigens.

T-dependent antigens (such as proteins and viruses) are made up of a large number of different antigenic determinants; little repetition occurs among them. In contrast, most T-independent antigens appear to be polysaccharides composed of repeating units of a small number of oligosaccharides (Fig. 4.3).

Two theories concerning the signaling by T-independent antigens have been proposed. One theory is that a T-independent antigen can stimulate B cells by means of two receptors, the antigen-specific receptor (membrane immunoglobulin) and a mitogen receptor (most T-independent antigens being often mitogens are able to stimulate B cells nonspecifically). The association of these two signals would then trigger antibody production. The second theory is that the direct stimulation of B cells is possible when the antigen presents multiple repeats of the same epitope, allowing the cross-linking of membrane immunoglobulins. The antibody produced, in most cases, is IgM. The switch to IgG production that is seen in most immune responses does not occur with T-independent antigens, and immunological memory is not generated.

XII. THE HAPTEN-CARRIER PHENOMENON

Most of our understanding of immune recognition derives from experiments carried out with hapten-carrier complexes, allowing the study of the hapten-carrier phenomenon. Most often, the hapten used has been the 2-dinitrophenyl

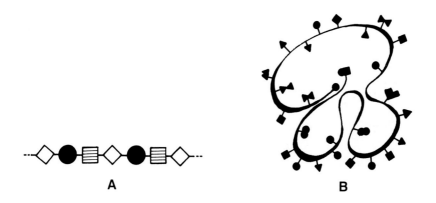

FIGURE 4.3   Diagrammatic representation of the structural differences between T-dependent and T-independent antigens. T-independent antigens (A) are polysaccharides and lipopolysaccharides in which the immunogenic structures are repeating sequences of a limited number of sugars (represented by the blocks of different shapes in the diagram). T-dependent antigens, such as macromolecular proteins (B) comprise a large number of different, rarely repeating, antigenic structures.

(2-DNP) radical; the most popular carriers have been complex proteins, such as human and bovine serum albumin (HSA, BSA), ovalbumin (OVA), and bovine gammaglobulin (BGG).

If an animal is primed with DNP-OVA, a primary immune response to the immunizing complex is obtained. The immunized animal will produce antibodies both to the hapten and to the carrier. A recall challenge with DNP-OVA will trigger a secondary response against both hapten and carrier, of higher magnitude. But if the primed animal is challenged with the same hapten coupled to a different carrier (DNP-BGG), a secondary response to DNP is not observed (Fig. 4.4). On the other hand, if the animal is primed with ovalbumin alone and a secondary challenge with DNP-OVA is given, a secondary response to DNP is obtained (Fig. 4.5). In this context, the term *secondary* is applied to the anti-DNP response because of its magnitude, but it does not imply that the animal had been previously exposed to the hapten.

These observations suggest that (a) carrier and hapten are recognized independently, (b) immunologic memory is largely determined by the carrier moiety; (c) once a memory response is elicited by the carrier, the antihapten response will be of the high magnitude characteristic of secondary responses. Experiments with thymectomized animals or in animals that had been sublethally irradiated and later reconstituted with either B cells or T cells proved that T

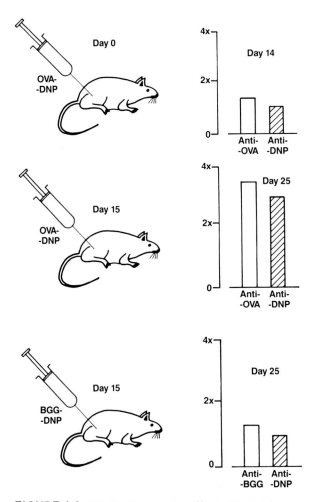

FIGURE 4.4 The hapten–carrier effect. To obtain a secondary immune response to DNP, the animal needs to be immunized and challenged with the same DNP–carrier combination; a change in the carrier will result in an anti-DNP response of identical magnitude to that obtained after the initial immunization. The memory response, therefore, appears to be carrier-determined.

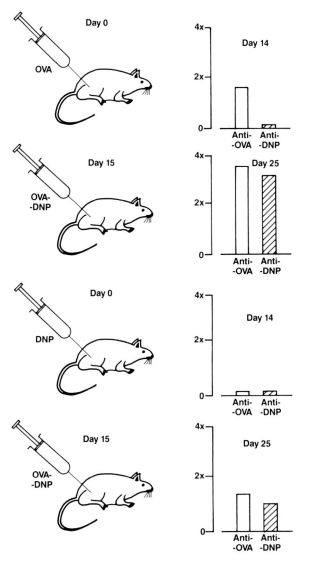

FIGURE 4.5 Further proof of the carrier dependency of the secondary antibody response to a hapten-carrier conjugate was obtained by studying the effects of primary immunization with carrier or hapten alone on a booster response with the hapten-carrier conjugate. A primary immunization with OVA was followed by a secondary response to both hapten and carrier when the animals were challenged with OVA-DNP. A primary immunization with DNP did not induce anti-DNP antibodies and the animal reacted to the challenge with OVA-DNP as if it were a primary immunization to either carrier or hapten.

cells are responsible for the recognition of the carrier and B cells for the recognition of the hapten. In other words, T helper cells have the ability to recognize the carrier molecule and to assist the antihapten response of the B cells. The magnitude of the antihapten response appears to reflect the mass of helper T cells activated by the carrier, whose help is obviously not antigen-specific.

Most immune responses involve complex antigens that are simultaneously recognized by T helper and by B cells, perhaps after some degree of processing or binding by macrophages. The complex interactions between antigens and these three types of cells that result in the triggering of the immune response have been the objects of a large number of theories and inerpretations.

XIII. THE TRIGGERING OF AN IMMUNE RESPONSE BY A T-DEPENDENT ANTIGEN

In spite of the enormous progress of immunology in the last decades, our understanding of some of the most essential steps in the immune response is still largely incomplete.

Most immune responses to complex T-dependent antigens require the participation of several cell types. The first cells that appear to play an important role are the *macrophages* and other antigen-presenting cells. Macrophages are probably able to recognize antigens through non-antibody-dependent as well as through antibody-dependent mechanisms. Non-antibody-dependent recognition mechanisms are likely to play a major role in primary responses and include phagocytosis through sugar receptors or complement receptors (complement being activated by the alternative pathway by many microorganisms and soluble substances). In the case of microorganism, macrophage processing involves the breakdown of the infectious agent and release of immunogenic subunits. In the case of complex proteins, processing involves unfolding and breakdown into small fragments.

The stimulation of resting T helper cells appears to be possible only when the antigen has been processed and is presented by an adequate *accessory cell*. The need for accessory cells derives from the fact that the T helper cells recognize the processed antigen when associated to class II MHC molecules. The processed antigen, bound or associated to a class II MHC antigen, will be recognized by the T cell antigen-receptor, which interacts both with the antigen and with the MHC determinant. In the case of macrophage processing, the antigen is internalized into an endosome, where it is broken into immunogenic fragments by acidic proteases. Those fragments are believed to interact with Ia (class II MHC) molecules lining the endosomic vesicle and are subsequently transported (bound to Ia) and inserted into the cell membrane (Fig. 4.6). The specificity of the Ia molecule is believed to be rather loose, but it is essential if the immune response is to develop. Specific Ia alleles are known to have the ability to associate with some immunogenic peptides and not with others. An animal genetically lacking a given Ia allele will not respond against the peptides that are usually associated with it. The mechanism of antigen presentation by cells not known to process antigen (such as the Langerhans cells of the epidermis and the dendritic cells of the lymphoid tissues) is unknown. Either those cells present antigen that may not require processing to interact with Ia, or they bind processed antigen that has been shed by macrophages. It is believed that antigen presenting cells may be able to retain the adsorbed antigens on their surfaces for long periods of time, continually interacting with other cells participating in the immune responses. The macrophage and other antigen-presenting cells also produce interleukin 1 (IL1), which promotes growth and differentiation of many cell types, including T and B lymphocytes. Both membrane-bound and soluble IL1 have been shown to be important in activating T cells in vitro, but it is difficult to ascertain which IL1 form is physiologically more important. Other nonspecific signaling mechanisms may also be significant in this early stage of T cell activation, including the interaction between glycoproteins expressed on the membranes of T cells and accessory cells (see Chapter 11).

Therefore, the resting T helper cell (or a T helper/inducer subpopulation) is stimulated specifically by the processed antigen associated to the class II MHC and nonspecifically by other cell-cell interactions and by interleukin 1 (Fig. 4.7). During T helper cell differentiation, T cells will acquire new functional properties, namely the capacity to express new membrane receptors and to synthesize and release lymphokines. The activated T cells start synthesizing a second interleukin (IL2, T cell growth factor) and express an interleukin 2 receptor. This interleukin 2 promotes further division and differentiation of the cell releasing it and of other antigen-stimulated T cells. The result is a tremendous expansion of the helper T cell population, which, as it further differentiates, may then produce other lymphokines that stimulate the growth and differentiation of other types of T and B cells.

The stimulation of B cells is equally complex (Fig. 4.8). It seems likely that the initial steps require close contact between all the relevant cells, i.e., the antigen-presenting cell, the helper T cell, and the B cell. The B cell recognizes a given epitope of the presented antigen by its membrane immunoglobulin. A major difference relative to the helper T cells is that the B cell recognizes the determinants expressed by the antigens in their native configuration rather than the determinants generated during antigen processing. Therefore, the B cells do not require the same degree of antigen processing as T cells; for effective B cell stimulation it may be sufficient to recognize epitopes in the unprocessed or partially processed antigen while adsorbed to a macrophage membrane. This duality in the specificity of T and B cells raises the question of how T-B cell cooperation is ensured. First, the simultaneous recognition of unprocessed and denatured antigen could take place in an antigen-loaded lymph node,

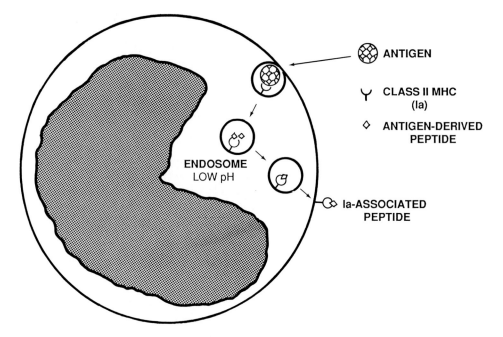

FIGURE 4.6   Diagrammatic representation of the main steps involved in antigen processing and presentation. A complex antigen (i.e., a foreign protein) is endocytosed and broken down by acid proteases released into the endosome. Denatured oligopeptide fragments of the protein are thus generated and bind to Ia molecules lining up the internal side of the endosomic vesicle. The peptide-Ia antigen complex is then transported and inserted into the cell membrane, where it may be easily recognized by helper T cells. Other antigenic fragments may be totally denatured by lysosomal proteases and lose their immunogenicity.

and because T cell help is mediated by soluble, nonspecific mediators, it is not essential that T and B cells react with identical epitopes. An alternative possibility is that the B cell, after receiving the first signal from binding nondenatured antigen, will internalize and process the antigen. Once the B cell has processed the antigen, it will express it in the membrane in association with an MHC class II product and allow direct interaction with a helper T cell, which in turn will help further differentiation of the B cell (Fig. 4.9). The current experimental evidence suggests that these two models are not mutually exclusive.

Helper T cells provide additional signals for B cell proliferation, such as interleukin 2 and other lymphokines. Functionally, these lymphokines can be divided into those that act in the early stages of B cell proliferation (B cell growth

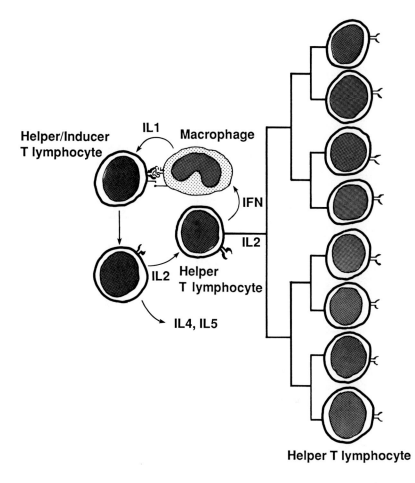

FIGURE 4.7 In the initial stages of an immune response, CD4(T4)$^{+}$ helper lymphocytes are stimulated by a complex set of interactions involving the T-cell antigen receptor and the Ia-processed antigen complex, the Ia antigen and the C4 molecule, the CD2 molecules expressed by the lymphocyte and the LFA-3 molecule expressed by the APC, and membrane-bound or soluble IL1 with its corresponding receptor on the T cell. As a consequence of activation, the CD4^{+} lymphocytes will express interleukin 2 receptors and release several soluble factors, including interleukin 2. IL2 will play a role in promoting further proliferation and differentiation of antigen-stimulated helper T cells.

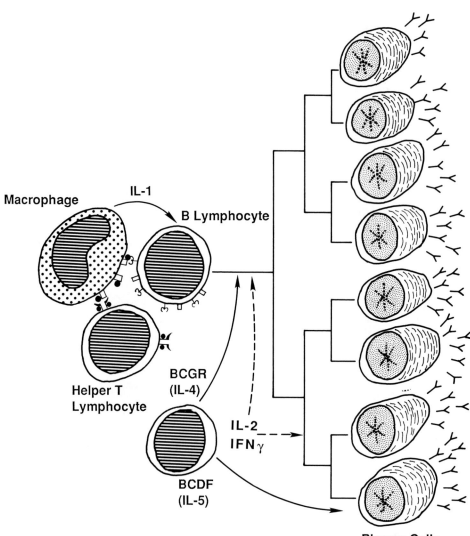

Macrophage

IL-1

B Lymphocyte

Helper T Lymphocyte

BCGR (IL-4)

IL-2 IFN γ

BCDF (IL-5)

Plasma Cells

FIGURE 4.8 The proliferation and differentiation of antibody-producing B cells results from a combination of several stimuli. The antigen (or a fragment conserving its native configuration), possibly adsorbed to the membrane of an antigen-presenting cell, provides a specific stimulus, while the activated helper T cells will provide a second stimulus. The interaction between helper T cells and B cells appears to be more efficient when all the involved cells (macrophages, helper T cells, and B cells) are clustered together, probably by allowing direct cell-to-cell transfer of interleukins. T cells do not recognize epitopes identical to those recognized by B cells; however, once activated, they can assist the proliferation of B cells by releasing growth and differentiation factors such as IL2, IL4, and IL5. IL6, which seems to play a role in the differentiation of B cells into antibody-producing plasma cells, is probably released by more than one cell type, including monocytes, macrophages, and T lymphocytes.

Helper T Lymphocyte

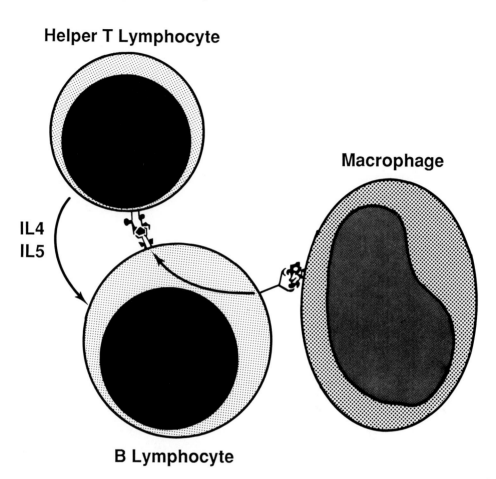

B Lymphocyte

FIGURE 4.9   A minimal model for B cell activation, as illustrated in this diagram, proposes that the B cell is stimulated by unprocessed antigen, which is subsequently processed and expressed in association with class II MHC (Ia) antigens. Helper T cells recognize the antigen processed and presented by the B cell and become activated, providing the B cell with the additional signals necessary for its proliferation and differentiation.

TABLE 4.1   Interleukins and Other Soluble Factors Assisting B Cell Differentiation

Early acting (proliferation factors)
    Interferon α
    Interferon β
    Interferon γ (?)
    Interleukin 2
    B cell growth factor I (BSF1, interleukin 4)
    B cell growth factor II (T cell replacing factor, interleukin 5)
Late acting (differentiation factors)
    Interferon γ (?)
    Interleukin 2
    B cell differentiation factor I
    B cell differentiation factor II (BSF2, interferon $\beta2$, interleukin 6)

factors) and those that act in the late stages of B cell differentiation (B cell differentiation factors). As summarized in Table 4.1, various mediators have been suggested to promote B cell proliferation and differentiation. In experimental animals, the most important appear to be interleukins 4 and 5, but activated B cells also express IL2 receptors, and a role for IL2 as a promoter of human B cell differentiation is possible. With the availability of pure interleukins produced by recombinant DNA technology, it has been possible to prove that several of the soluble factors listed in Table 4.1 can enhance human B cell responses to mitogens such as *Staphylococcus aureus* (Cowan I strain). In addition, IL4 has the unique property of inducing in vitro differentiation of IgE-producing cells. However, the in vivo role of these interleukins during an immune response has not yet been properly investigated.

The stimulation of a cytotoxic T cell response probably follows a similar sequence of events, but the resting cytotoxic T cell can only interact with a cell that has identical class I histocompatibility antigens. This is because the cytotoxic T cell receptor appears to recognize a complex formed by antigen shed by the infected or neoplastic cell and a class MHC I molecule. Interleukin 2 also plays a very important role in cytotoxic T cell activation and proliferation, at least in vitro. Whether IL2 or a specific differentiation factor plays the major role in promoting the functional differentiation of cytotoxic T cells in vivo is not yet totally clear. These question will be examined in detail in one discussion of cell-mediated immunity (see Chapter 11).

SELF-EVALUATION

Questions

Choose the one best answer.

4.1 Which of the following is not a requirement or characteristic of the inter-
actions between monocytes/macrophages and T lymphocytes;
A. Identity at the histocompatibility antigen level between the interact-
ing cells.
B. Processing of the antigen by the macrophage.
C. Presentation of processed antigen to the T lymphocyte.
D. Release of interleukins by both types of interacting cells.
E. Synthesis and secretion of antibody.

4.2 The induction of a "secondary" anti-DNP response after boosting an OVA-
primed animal with OVA-DNP proves that
A. Memory is hapten-specific.
B. OVA-stimulated memory cells assist the proliferation and differentia-
tion of B cell clones producing anti-DNP antibodies.
C. Memory is T-cell specific.
D. Memory is B-cell specific.
E. Memory B cells for DNP are induced by immunization with OVA.

4.3 All of the following are true statements concerning interleukin 2, except
A. It is released by macrophages.
B. It promotes the multiplication and differentiation of cytotoxic T cells.
C. It promotes the multiplication and differentiation of helper T cells.
D. It can be recognized by receptors present in activated B cells.
E. It is equivalent to T cell growth factor.

4.4 Which of the following are least likely to induce an immune response?
A. Polysaccharides.
B. Proteins.
C. Lipids.
D. Nucleic acids.
E. Proteins to which carbohydrate side chains are attached.

4.5 A rabbit has been immunized with DNP-BSA. Three weeks later you want
to induce an anamnestic response to DNP-BGG. This can be accomplished
by:
A. Passively administering anti-DNP antibodies prior to challenge with
DNP-BGG.
B. Boosting with DNP one week before immunization with DNP-BGG.
C. Transfusing purified lymphocytes from a rabbit primed with DNP at

least two days before challenge with DNP-BGG.
  D. Immunizing with BGG one week after the initial immunization with DNP-BSA.
  E. Passively administering anti-BGG antibodies before immunization with BGG.

4.6   What do you expect when you immunize a nude mouse (congenitally athymic) with type III pneumococcal polysaccharide?
  A. No immune response, either cellular or humoral.
  B. Production of significant amounts of IgG antibodies.
  C. Production of significant amounts of IgM antibodies.
  D. No evidence of specific antibody synthesis.
  E. Development of overwhelming pneumococcal sepsis.

4.7   Alloantigens
  A. Are genetic markers that differ in distribution in individuals of the same species.
  B. Are identically distributed in all individuals of the same species.
  C. Are antigens that define protein isotypes.
  D. Do not induce an immune response in animals of the same species.
  E. Are restricted, among immunoglobulins, to IgG.

4.8   Haptens
  A. Cannot bind to an antibody molecule unless coupled to a carrier.
  B. Are macromolecules.
  C. Are usually of polypeptidic nature.
  D. Are not immunogenic by themselves.
  E. Can only trigger humoral immune reactions.

4.9   Intrinsic antigen receptors are not found in the
  A. T cells of a nonimmune animal.
  B. B cells of a nonimmune animal.
  C. T cells of an immunized animal.
  D. B cells of an immunized animal.
  E. Macrophages during an immune response.

4.10 Which of the following will not enhance antigenicity?
  A. Intradermal injection.
  B. High speed centrifugation to eliminate aggregates.
  C. Injection of an antigen-adjuvant emulsion.
  D. Immunization on antigen obtained from a phylogenetically distant species to that of the animal immunized.
  E. Chemical polymerization of the antigen.

Answers

4.1 (E) The production of immunoglobulins is exclusive of B cells.

4.2 (B) If an OVA-primed animal produces large amounts of antibody to DNP after OVA-DNP boosting, it follows that OVA-stimulated memory cells helped not only B cells producing anti-OVA antibodies to differentiate but also the differentiation of anti-DNP-producing B cells.

4.3 (A) IL2 is released by stimulated T cells; IL2 receptors exist on the membrane of activated T cells and activated B cells.

4.4 (C)

4.5 (D) The development of a memory response (quantitatively amplified relative to the primary response) requires preimmunization with the carrier. Hence the animal needs to be previously immunized either with the same hapten-carrier conjugate used to induce the secondary immune response or to the carrier alone.

4.6 (C) Polysaccharides are T-independent antigens and induce responses of the IgM type in mice.

4.7 (A) As the A, B, O antigens or the immunoglobulin allotypes.

4.8 (D)

4.9 (E) The monocyte/macrophage cells may bind antigens through immunoglobulins bound to Fc receptors, C3b receptors, or sugar receptors, but they do not possess clonally restricted antigen-specific receptors as an intrinsic part of their membranes.

4.10 (B) Soluble proteins are less immunogenic than aggregated or polymerized proteins.

BIBLIOGRAPHY

Atassi, M. Z., Van Oss, C. J., Abrolom, D. R. (Eds.). *Molecular Immunology*. Marcel Dekker, New York, 1984. (Contains authoritative chapters discussing antigenicity and immune recognition from the structural point of view.)

Dinarello, C. A., and Mier, J. W. Lymphokines. *New England J. Med. 317*:940, 1987.

Germain, R. N. The ins and outs of antigen presentation. *Nature, 322*:687, 1986.

Hood, L. E., Weissman, I. L., Wood, W. B., and Wilson, J. H. *Immunology*, (2nd Ed. Benjamin/Cummings, Menlo Park, California, 1984. (Contains detailed discussions of cellular interactions and the role of the MHC.)

Kabat, E. A. *Structural Concepts in Immunology and Immunochemistry*. Holt, Rinehart & Winston, New York, 1968.

Klein, J. *Immunology: The Science of Self-Nonself Discrimination*. John Wiley & Sons, New York, 1982.

Moller, G. (Ed.). T cell-dependent and independent B cell activation. *Immunol. Rev. 99*. Minksgaard, Copenhagen, 1987.

Paul, W. E. *Fundamental Immunology, Second Edition*. Raven Press, New York, 1989. (Includes chapters discussing T and B cell receptors, lymphocyte activation, and cellular interactions.)

Unanue, E. R., and Allen, P. M. The basis for the immunoregulatory roles of macrophages and other accessory cells. *Science 236*:557, 1987.

5

Immunoglobulin Structure

GABRIEL VIRELLA

I. ANTIBODIES AS PROTEINS

As mentioned in previous chapters, one of the most obvious consequences of the injection of a foreign, nonself, substance into a vertebrate is the production of antibodies specifically able to combine with the antigen. As early as the turn of the century, German scientists led by Paul Ehrlich had characterized the antigen-antibody reaction as a chemical reaction, defined its unique specificity, and identified antibodies as proteins. Information concerning the precise structure of the antibody molecule started to accumulate in the 1930s, as new technological developments were applied to the study of the general characteristics of antibodies. By the early 1940s antibodies had been characterized electrophoretically as *gammaglobulins* (Fig. 5.1) and also classified into large families by their sedimentation coefficient determined by analytical ultracentrifugation (7S and 19S antibodies).

The next significant advance in the study of immunoglobulin structure resulted from a combination of factors: (1) plasma cells were identifed as the cells responsible for antibody production; (2) multiple myeloma was characterized as a malignant proliferation of plasma cells synthesizing large amounts of homogeneous gammaglobulins, which are relatively easy to purify from patient's serum and urine; (3) new techniques for protein separation were developed (e.g., chromatography, gel filtration), allowing the isolation of large

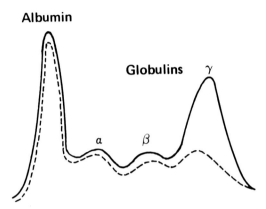

FIGURE 5.1 Electrophoretic separation of serum from a rabbit hyperimmunized with ovalbumin before (———) and after (- - - -) removal of antibody molecules by specific precipitation with ovalbumin. (Modifed from Tiselius, A. and Kabat, E. A., *J. Exp. Med. 69*:119, 1939.)

amounts of purified immunoglobulins (or of fragments thereof) from patients with multiple myeloma; (4) purified immunoglobulins and their fragments were injected into rabbits and other animals, and it was soon possible to identify antigenic differences between myeloma proteins from different patients; this was the basis for the initial identification of the different classes and subclasses of immunoglobulins and the different types of light chains.

II.   IMMUNOGLOBULIN G (IgG):
THE PROTOTYPE IMMUNOGLOBULIN MOLECULE

IgG, a 7S immunoglobulin, is the most abundant immunoglobulin in human serum and in the serum of most mammalian species. It is also the immunoglobulin most frequently detected in large concentrations in multiple myeloma patients. For this reason it was the first immunoglobulin to be purified in large quantities and to be extensively studied from the structural point of view. The basic knowledge about the structure of the IgG molecule was obtained from two types of experiments.

A.   Proteolytic Digestion

The incubation of purified IgG with papain, a proteolytic enzyme extracted from the latex of *Carica papaya*, results in the splitting of the molecule into two fragments that differ both in charge and in antigenicity. These fragments

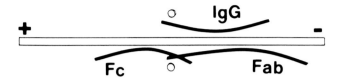

FIGURE 5.2 Immunoelectrophoretic separation of the fragments resulting from papain digestion of IgG. A papain digest of IgG was first separated by electrophoresis, and the two fragments were revealed with an antiserum containing antibodies that react with different portions of the IgG molecule.

can be easily demonstrated by immunoelectrophoresis (Fig. 5.2), a technique that separates proteins by charge in a first step, allowing their antigenic characterization in a second step (as explained in greater detail in Chapter 14).

B. Reduction of Disulfide Bonds

If the IgG molecule is incubated with a reducing agent containing free SH groups and fractionated by gel filtration in conditions able to dissociate noncovalent interactions, two fractions are obtained. The first fraction corresponds to polypeptide chains of MW 55,000 (heavy chains); the second corresponds to polypeptide chains of MW 23,000 (light chains) (Fig. 5.3).

The sum of the data obtained by proteolysis and reduction experiments resulted in the conception of a diagrammatic two-dimensional model for the IgG molecule (Fig. 5.4).

Papain digestion, splitting the heavy chains in the hinge region (so designated because this region of the molecule appears to be stereoflexible), results in the separation of two Fab fragments and one Fc fragment per IgG molecule (Fig. 5.5). The Fab fragments are so designated because they contain the antigen binding site, while the Fc fragment received this designation because it can be easily crystallized. If the disulfide bond joining heavy and light chains in the Fab fragments is split, one can separate a complete light chain from a fragment that comprises about half of one of the heavy chains, the NH2 terminal half. This portion of the heavy chain contained in each Fab fragment has been designated as the Fd fragment. A second proteolytic enzyme, pepsin, splits the heavy chains beyond the disulfide bonds that join them at the hinge region, producing a double Fab fragment or $F(ab')_2$ (Fig. 5.6), while the Fc portion of the molecule is digested into peptides.

The comparison of Fc, Fab, $F(ab')_2$ and whole IgG molecules shows both important similarities and important differences between the whole molecule and its fragments. Both Fab and $F(ab')_2$ contain antibody binding sites, but

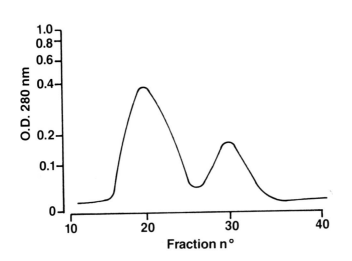

FIGURE 5.3   Gel filtration of reduced and alkylated IgG (MW 150,000) on a dissociating medium. Two protein peaks are eluted, the first corresponding to MW 55,000 and the second corresponding to MW 23,000. The 2:1 ratio of protein content between the high MW and low MW peaks is compatible with the presence of identical numbers of two polypeptide chains, one of which being about twice as large as the other.

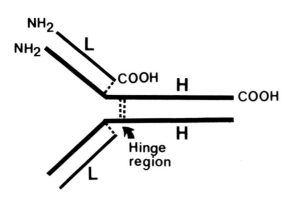

FIGURE 5.4   Diagrammatic representation of the IgG molecule.

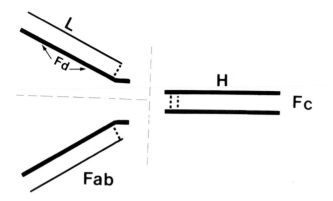

FIGURE 5.5   The fragments obtained by papain digestion of the IgG molecule.

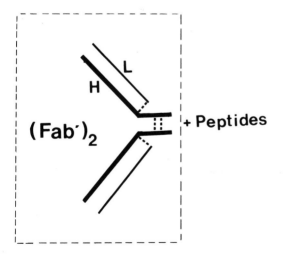

FIGURE 5.6   The fragments obtained by pepsin digestion of the IgG molecule.

while the intact IgG molecule of the F(ab')$_2$ are bivalent, the Fab fragment is monovalent. Therefore, a Fab fragment can bind to an antigen, but it cannot cross-link two antigen molecules. An antiserum raised against the Fab fragment reacts mostly against light chain determinants; the immunodominant antigenic markers for the heavy chain are located in the Fc fragment. The F(ab')$_2$ fragment is identical to the intact molecule in its antigen-binding properties, but it lacks the ability to fix complement, bind to cell membranes, etc., which are determined by the Fc region of the molecule.

III. THE STRUCTURAL AND ANTIGENIC HETEROGENITY OF HEAVY AND LIGHT CHAINS

The combination of structural and serological studies carried out mostly with monoclonal proteins isolated from patients with plasma cell malignancies and their fragments resulted in the definition of several antigenic groups of immunoglobulins and their polypeptide chains.

Five classes or isotypes of immunoglobulins were identified from antigenic differences of the heavy chains and designated as *IgG* (the classical 7S immunoglobulin), *IgA*, *IgM* (the classical 19S immunoglobulin), *IgD*, and *IgE*. IgG, IgA and IgM together constitute over 95% of the whole immunoglobulin pool in a normal human being and are designated as major immunoglobulin classes. The light chains also proved to be antigenically heterogeneous, and two main types were defined, *kappa* and *lambda*. Each immunoglobulin molecule is constituted by a pair of identical heavy chains and a pair of identical light chains; hence, a given immunoglobulin molecule can have either kappa or lambda chains but not both. A normal individual will have a mixture of immunoglobulin molecules in his serum, some with kappa chains (e.g., IgGκ), others with lambda chains (e.g., IgGλ). Normal serum IgG has a 2:1 ratio of kappa chain over lambda chain-bearing IgG molecules. The major characteristics of the five immunoglobulin classes are summarized in Table 5.1.

As shown in the table, antigenic differences between the heavy chains of IgG and IgA exist and define subclasses of those immunoglobulins. The most important structural and biological characteristics of IgG and IgA subclasses are listed in Tables 5.2 and 5.3.

In the case of IgG subclasses, it is noteworthy that IgG1 and IgG3 are more efficient in terms of complement fixation and have greater affinity for monocyte receptors. Those properties can be correlated with a greater degree of biological activity, both in normal antimicrobial responses, in which these properties have direct consequences in opsonization and bacterial killing, and in pathological conditions, in which the formation of immune complexes containing IgG1 and IgG3 antibodies is more likely to have pathogenic consequences.

TABLE 5.1 Major Characteristics of Human Immunoglobulins

	IgG	IgA	IgM	IgD	IgE
Heavy chain class	+	+	–	–	–
H-chain subclass	$\gamma_1,\gamma_2,\gamma_3,\gamma_4$	α_1,α_2	–	–	–
L-chain type	κ and λ	κ and λ	κ and λ	κ and λ	κ and λ
Sedimentation coefficient	7S	7S,9S,011	19S	7-8S	8S
Polymeric forms	No	Dimers, trimers	Pentamers	No	No
Molecular weight	150,000	(160,000)n	900,000	180,000	190,000
Carbohydrate	3%	12%	7.5%	12%	12%
Serum concentration (mg/dl)	600-1300	60-300	30-150	3	0.03
Intravascular distribution	45%	42%	80%	75%	51%

TABLE 5.2 IgG Subclasses

	IgG1	IgG2	IgG3	IgG4
% of total IgG in normal serum	60%	30%	7%	3%
Half-life (days)	21	21	7	21
Complement fixation*	++	+	+++	–
Placental transfer	++	++	++	++
Affinity for monocyte and PMN receptors	+++	+	++++	+
MW Heavy chain	52,000	52,000	58,000	52,000

*By the classical pathway.

TABLE 5.3   IgA Subclasses

	IgA1	IgA2
Distribution	Predominates in serum	Predominates in secretions
Proportions in serum	85%	15%
Allotypes	?	Asm(1) and A2m(2)
-S-S-H:L	+	−in A2m(1); + in A2m(2)
MW heavy chain	56,000	52,000

The IgG3 subclass has the greatest number of structural and biological differences relative to the remaining IgG subclasses. Basically most differences appear to result from the existence of an extended hinge region (which accounts for the greater MW) and with a large number of disulfide bonds (estimates of their number vary between 5 and 15). This extended and probably rigid hinge region seems to be easily accessible to protelytic enzymes, and this lability of the molecule is likely to account for its considerably shorter half-life.

As for IgA subclasses, it is interesting to note that a subpopulation of IgA2 molecules carrying the A2m(1) allotype is the only example of a human immunoglobulin molecule lacking the disulfide bond between heavy and light chains. The IgG2 A2m(1) molecule is held together through noncovalent interactions between heavy and light chain.

IV. PRIMARY STRUCTURE OF THE HEAVY AND LIGHT CHAINS OF IgG: THE DOMAIN CONCEPT

The light chains of human immunoglobulins are composed of 211 to 217 amino acids and are usually devoid of carbohydrates. As mentioned above, there are two major antigenic types of light chains (κ and λ); when the amino acid sequences of light chains of known types were compared, it became evident that two regions could be distinguished in the light chains molecule: a *variable region* comprising the portion between the amino terminal end of the chain and residue 108, and a *constant region*, extending from residue 109 to the carboxy terminus (Figure 5.7). The constant regions were found to be almost identical in light chains of the same type, but they differ markedly in κ and λ chains. It is assumed that the difference in antigenicity between the two types of light chains is directly correlated with the structural differences in constant regions. The amino acid sequence of the variable regions is different even in proteins of the same antigenic type, and early workers thought that this sequence would be totally individual to any single protein. With increasing data, it became evident that some proteins shared similarities in their variable regions, and it has been

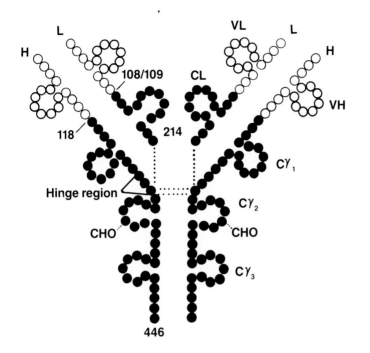

FIGURE 5.7   Schematic representation of the primary and secondary structure
of human IgG. The light chains are constituted by about 214 amino acids and
two regions, variable (first 108/109 amino acids, white beads in the diagram)
and constant (remaining amino acids, black beads in the diagram). Each of these
regions contains a loop formed by intrachain disulfide bonds and containing
about 60 amino acids, which are designated as variable domain and constant
domain (VL and CL in the diagram). The heavy chains have slightly longer variable regions (first 118 amino acids, white beads in the diagram), with one variable region domain (VH) and a constant region that contains three loops or
domains ($C\gamma_1$, $C\gamma_2$ and $C\gamma_3$), numbered from the NH2 terminus to the COOH
terminus.

possible to define variable region subgroups for the light chains. It also has been
found that any given variable region subgroup can be found in association with
both major constant regions (κ and λ).

The heavy chain of IgG is about twice as large as a light chain; it is constituted by 450 amino acids, and here too a variable and a constant region can be
identified. The variable region is constituted by the first 115 amino acids

(counted as usual from the amino terminal), and subgroups of these regions can also be identified. The constant region is almost three times larger; it starts at residue 116 and ends at the carboxy terminus (Figure 5.7). The maximal degree of homology is found between constant regions of IgG proteins of the same subclass.

The immunoglobulin molecule contains several disulfide bonds formed between contiguous residues. Some of them join two different polypeptide chains (interchain disulfide bonds), keeping the molecule together. Others (intrachain bonds) join different areas of the same polypeptide chain, leading to the formation of "loops." These loops and adjacent amino acids constitute the immunoglobulin domains (Figure 5.7). Variable regions have a single domain which is involved in antigen binding. The variable regions are designated VH in the case of heavy chains and VL in the case of the light chains. Light chains have one single constant region domain (CL), but heavy chains have several constant region domains (three in the case of IgG; four in the case of IgM and IgE). The constant regions are generically designated as CH1, CH2, and CH3, or if one wishes to be more specific, they can be identified by the class of immunoglobulins to which they belong, by adding the symbol for each heavy chain class $(\gamma,\alpha,\mu,\delta,\epsilon)$. For example, the constant region domains of the IgG molecule can be designated as $C\gamma_1$, $C\gamma_2$, and $C\gamma_3$.

Different functions and properties have been assigned to the different domains and regions of the heavy chains. For instance, $C\gamma_2$ is the domain involved in complement fixation, while $C\gamma_3$ is believed to be the domain responsible for binding to cell membranes. The hinge region is located between CH1 and CH2; this is the most frequent point of attack by proteolytic enzymes, although the precise splitting point varies from enzyme to enzyme.

V. THE ANTIBODY-COMBINING SITE

The binding of antigens by antibody molecules takes place in the Fab region, and it is basically a noncovalent interaction that requires a good fit between the antigenic determinant and the antigen-binding site on the immunoglobulin molecule. The antigen-binding site appears to be formed by the variable region of both heavy and light chains, folded in close proximity forming a cleft where an antigenic determinant or epitope will fit (Fig. 5.8). Structural studies of the variable regions have shown that certain sequence stretches vary widely from protein to protein, even among proteins sharing the same type of variable regions. For this reason, these highly variable stretches have been designated as *hypervariable regions*. It seems likely that these regions play a critical role in determining antibody specificity.

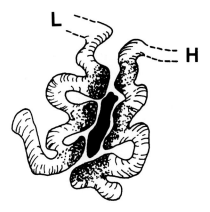

FIGURE 5.8 Diagrammatic representation of the hypothetical structure of an antigen binding site. The variable regions of the light and heavy chains would be folded in such a way that the hypervariable regions (darker areas in the diagram) would come into close apposition and define a pouch with a shape that would accommodate an antigenic determinant with a sterically complementary configuration.

VI.   IMMUNOGLOBULIN M: A POLYMERIC MOLECULE.
THE J CHAIN

IgM is basically constituted by five subunits (monomeric subunits, IgMs) similar to IgG, i.e., constituted by two light chains (κ or λ) and two heavy chains (μ). The heavy chains are larger than those of IgG by about 20,000 daltons, corresponding to an extra domain on the constant region (Cμ4).

A third polypeptide chain can be revealed by adequate methodology in most IgM molecules—the J chain. This is a small polypeptide chain of 15,000 daltons, also found in polymeric IgA molecules. One single J chain is found in any polymeric IgM or IgA molecule, irrespective of how many monomeric subunits are involved in the polymerization. It has been suggested that this chain plays some role in the polymerization process, but this is disputed because some polymeric IgM molecules lack the J chain.

VII.   IMMUNOGLOBULIN A: A MOLECULARLY HETEROGENEOUS
IMMUNOGLOBULIN. SECRETORY COMPONENT

Circulating IgA is molecularly heterogeneous, constituted by a mixture of monomeric, dimeric and larger polymeric molecules. In a normal individual over 70-90% of serum IgA is monomeric.

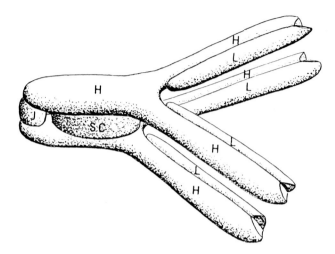

FIGURE 5.9 Structural model of the secretory IgA molecule.

Monomeric IgA is similar to IgG, constituted by two heavy chains (α) and two light chains (κ or λ). The heavy chains are slightly larger than those of IgG by about 5,000 daltons, but they do not contain an extra domain. The dimeric and polymeric forms of IgA found in circulation are covalently bonded synthetic products containing J chains.

IgA is the predominating immunoglobulin in secretions. Its presence there is not merely accidental; it reflects a selective transport across the mucosa. The mechanism of transport has not been fully characterized, but it is known that only polymeric IgA molecules are transported. Secretory IgA molecules contain a unique polypeptide chain, designated as *secretory component* (SC) (Fig. 5.9). This chain is synthesized by epithelial cells in the mucosa and attached to dimetic IgA postsynthetically. The molecular weight of secretory component has been estimated at 75,000. In the human species, it is always covalently bonded to IgA, but in other species it may be covalently bound or noncovalently associated to IgA.

VIII. THE MINOR CLASSES OF IMMUNOGLOBULINS: IgD AND IgE

IgD and IgE were the last immunoglobulins to be identified, because of their low concentrations in serum. Both are monomeric immunoglobulins, similar to IgG, but their heavy chains are larger than γ chains. IgE has five domains in the heavy chains (one variable and four constant); the precise number for IgD has not been firmly determined.

IgD is usually the predominant immunoglobulin class in the B lymphocyte membrane, where it probably plays the role of antigen-receptor. The role of circulating IgD, in contrast, is not clear.

IgE is an extremely important immunoglobulin because of its biological properties. Its biological role appears to be predominantly related to antiparasitic responses, but its main clinical relevance is related to allergic reactions. IgE has the unique property of binding to Fc receptors on the membranes of mast cells and basophils. The binding of IgE to those receptors has an extremely high affinity ($7.7 \times 10^9 \cdot mol^{-1}$), about 100-fold greater than the affinity of IgG binding to monocyte receptors. This high affinity binding of IgE to cell membranes is the basis for its designation as homocytotropic antibody and is responsible for its role in allergic reactions. In allergic individuals, if those IgE molecules have a given antibody specificity and react with the antigen while attached to the basophil or mast cell membranes, they will trigger the release of histamine and other substances that cause the symptoms of allergic reactions.

The biological activity of IgE (i.e., ability to bind to basophil or mast cell receptors) is lost after heating at $56°C$ for 30 minutes. Circular dichroism studies demonstrated that heating changes the configuration of Cϵ3 and Cϵ4 domains, a finding that suggests that those domains are predominantly involved in the binding to the basophil and mast cell receptors. IgE is the most thermolabile immunoglobulin, and it is the only one that loses biological activity after heating at $56°C$ for 30 minutes.

SELF-EVALUATION

Questions

Choose the one best answer.

5.1 Which of the following is a specific property of secretory IgA in relation to human serum IgA?
A. Presence of J chain.
B. Existence of dimeric forms.
C. Activation of the alternative pathway after aggregation.
D. Increased resistance to proteolytic enzymes.
E. Reaction with anti-IgA2 antiserum.

5.2 Each of the following statements concerning papain cleavage of IgG is correct except
A. The Fab fragment is divalent.
B. The Fc fragment contains part of the heavy chain.

C. The Fab fragment contains both heavy chain and light chain determinants.

D. The Fc fragment interacts specifically with certain lymphoid cell receptors.

E. Antisera prepared against the Fc fragment are specific for the IgG class of immunoglobulins.

5.3   The antigen-binding sites of an antibody molecule are located at
A. The constant region of heavy chains.
B. The constant region of light chains.
C. The variable region of heavy chains.
D. The variable region of light chains.
E. The variable regions of both heavy and light chains.

5.4   The immunoglobulin class that binds with very high affinity to membrane receptors on basophils and mast cells is
A. IgG.
B. IgA.
C. IgM.
D. IgD.
E. IgE.

5.5   A preparation of pooled human IgG injected into rabbits will not induce the production of antibodies against
A. Kappa light chains.
B. Lambda light chains.
C. Gamma heavy chains.
D. Gamma 3 heavy chains.
E. J chain.

5.6   The higher molecular weight of IgG3 molecules relative to all other IgG molecules is due to
A. An extra constant region domain.
B. The attachment of J chain to its COOH terminus.
C. Extracellular aggregation
D. An extended hinge region.
E. A high carbohydrate content.

For question 5.7-5.10, match in the following figure (Fig. 5.10) the regions indicated by letters with the corresponding descriptions listed below.

5.7   The region involved in binding to macrophage Fc receptors.

5.8   The region most susceptible to attack by proteolytic enzymes.

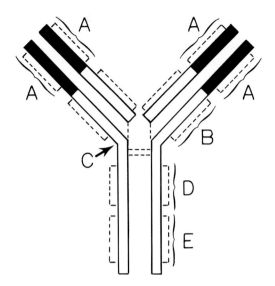

FIGURE 5.10

5.9   The region containing the binding sites for complement.

5.10 The region that determines the specificity of a given antibody molecule.

Answers

5.1   (D)   The coupling of secretory component to secretory IgA dimers increases its in vitro resistance to proteolytic enzymes.

5.2   (A)   The Fab fragments obtained with papain contain one single antigen binding site, while the $F(ab')_2$ fragments obtained with pepsin are divalent.

5.3   (E)

5.4   (E)

5.5   (E)   J chain is only found in polymeric immunoglobulins (IgM and IgA).

5.6   (D)   The hinge region of IgG3 is 8,000-10,000 daltons larger than the hinge regions of all other IgG molecules.

5.7   (E)   The $C\gamma_3$ domain.

5.8   (C)   The hinge region.

5.9   (D)   The $C\gamma_2$ domain.

5.10   (A)   The variable domains of the hand L chains.

BIBLIOGRAPHY

Atassi, M. A., Van Oss, J., and Absolom, D. R. (Eds.). *Molecular Immunology*.
   Marcel Dekker, New York, 1984. (A comprehensive textbook with excellent
   chapters on immunoglobulin isolation and characterization and on immunoglobulin structure and function.)
Capra, J. D. and Kehoe, J. M. Hypervariable regions, idiotypy, and the antibody
   combining site. *Adv. Immunology 20*:1, 1975.
Clark, W. R. The *Experimental Foundations of Modern Immunology*. John
   Wiley & Sons, New York, 1980. (A good discussion on how knowledge about
   immunoglobulin structure evolved.)
Edelman, G. M. and Gall, W. E. The antibody problem. *Ann. Rev. Biochem.*
   38:699, 1969. (A classical review with emphasis on the primary structure of
   IgG and its functional domains.)
Glynn, L. E. and Steward, M. W. (Eds.). *Immunochemistry: An Advanced
   Textbook*. John Wiley & Sons, New York, 1977. (Contains chapters on
   structure and function of immunoglobulins, antigen-combining region of
   immunoglobulins, and origin of antibody diversity.)
Nisonoff, A. *Introduction of Molecular Immunology*. Sinauer, Sunderland,
   Massachusetts, 1982. (Has excellent discussions of immunoglobulin struc-
   ture and antibody diversity.)
Tomasi, T. B. *The Immune System of Secretions*. Prentice-Hall, Englewood
   Cliffs, New Jersey, 1976.

6

Biosynthesis, Metabolism, and Biological Properties of Immunoglobulins

GABRIEL VIRELLA

After having discussed the structure of immunoglobulins, we shall approach three major questions in this chapter: how immunoglobulin molecules are synthized and assembled; what the fate is of the immunoglobulins once secreted; and what other important properties, other than binding to antigen, are specific to immunoglobulins. We already know that the production of immunoglobulin molecues is the most distinctive feature of B cells. Resting B lymphocytes synthesize only small amounts of immunoglobulins that mainly become inserted into the cell membrane. Plasma cells, the most differentiated B cells, are considered as end-stage cells arrested at the late G1 phase. Plasma cells consequently show very limited mitotic activity but are specialized to produce and secrete large amounts of immunoglobulins.

I. SYNTHESIS AND ASSEMBLY OF IMMUNOGLOBULIN MOLECULES

The synthetic capacity of the plasma cell is reflected by its abundant cytoplasm, extremely rich in endoplasmic reticulum (Fig. 6.1). Normally, heavy and light chains are synthesized in separate polyribosomes of the plasma cell. The amounts of H and L chains synthesized on the polyribosomes are usually balanced so that both types of chains will be combined into complete IgG molecules, without surpluses of any given chain. The assembly of a complete IgG molecule can be achieved by two different pathways:

93

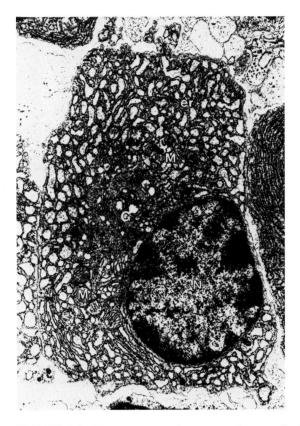

FIGURE 6.1 Ultrastructure of a mature plasma cell. Note the eccentric nucleus with clumped chromatin, the large cytoplasm containing a well-developed perinuclear Golgi apparatus (G), mitochondria (M), and abundant, distended, endoplasmic reticulum (er). The plasma cell partially shown at the right has abundant flattened endoplasmic reticulum. (Reproduced with permission from Tanaka, Y. and Goodman, J. R. *Electron microscopy of human blood cells*, Harper & Row, New York, 1972.)

$$H + H \rightarrow H_2, \quad L + L \rightarrow L_2, \quad H_2 + L_2 \rightarrow H_2 L_2$$

or

$$H + L \rightarrow HL, \quad HL + HL \rightarrow H_2 L_2$$

When plasma cells undergo malignant transformation, this balanced synthesis of heavy and light chains persists in most cases, but in about one third of the cases synthesis may be grossly aberrant. The most common aberration is the synthesis of an excess of light chains. In human plasmocytomas this is reflected by the elimination of the excessively produced light chains of a single isotype in the urine (Bence Jones proteinuria). However, traces of κ and λ light chains are eliminated by most normal individuals, suggesting that even normally there is a very small synthetic surplus of light chains.

The described synthetic pathway applies to single-unit immunoglobulins (IgG, IgD, IgE, monomeric IgA1 proteins) with the exclusion of IgA2 A2m(1) proteins. These, lacking the disulfide bridge joining H and L, have to be assembled by one single pathway:

$$H + H \rightarrow H_2, \quad L + L \rightarrow L_2, \quad H_2 + L_2 \rightarrow H_2 L_2$$

II. SYNTHESIS OF POLYMERIC IMMUNOGLOBULINS. THE J CHAIN

Polymeric immunoglobulins (IgM, IgA) have one additional polypeptide chain, the J chain. This is synthesized by *all* plasma cells, including those that produce IgG. However, it is only incorporated to polymeric forms of IgM and IgA. It is thought that the J chain has some role in initiating polymerization, as shown in Figure 6.2

IgM proteins are basically assembled, as are IgG proteins, to their monomeric subunits. Five of these will be combined in the final pentameric molecule. This

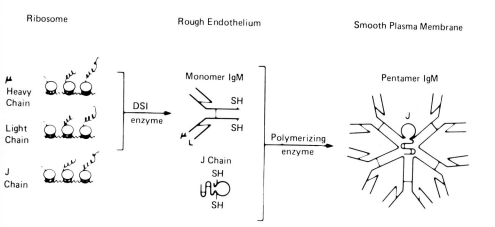

FIGURE 6.2   Schematic representation of IgM synthesis in a pentamer IgM-secreting cell. DSI, disulfide interchanging enzyme. (Reproduced with permission from Koshland, M. E. Molecular aspects of B cell differentiation. *J. Immunol. 131*:i, 1983.)

assembly seems to coincide with secretion in some cells, in which only monomeric subunits are found intracellularly, while in other cells the pentameric
forms can be found intracellularly.

III. SYNTHESIS AND ASSEMBLY OF SECRETORY IgA

Secretory IgA is an unusual protein, as it appears to be assembled in two stages,
each one taking place in a different cell. Dimeric IgA, containing two monomeric subunits and a J chain joined together by disulfide bridges, is predominantly synthesized by submucosal plasma cells, although a minor portion may
also be synthesized in the bone marrow. The secretory component on the
other hand, is synthesized in the epithelial cells, where the final assembly of
secretory IgA takes place. Secretory IgA must also flow back to the bloodstream, for small amounts are found in the blood of normal individuals. Higher
levels of secretory IgA in blood are found in certain conditions, such as liver
disease. This may be related to a clearing role of the liver with regard to dimeric IgA that backflows from the gut through the mesenteric lymph vessels.
Such IgA molecules appear to be taken up by hepatocytes, secreted into the
bile, and then channeled back into the gut. If the excretion mechanism is compromised, secretory IgA assembled in the hepatocyte backflows into the systemic circulation.

IV. BIOLOGICAL FUNCTIONS OF THE SECRETORY COMPONENT

Two different biological functions have been postulated for the secretory component (SC). Firstly, it has been shown that SC is present on the surface of
mucosal cells, it has been postulated that at that location it acts as a receptor
for the J chain of dimeric IgA. The binding of dimeric IgA seems to be the first
step in the final assembly and transport process of secretory IgA. Surface-bound
IgA is internalized, and SC is covalently bound to the molecule, probably by
means of a disulfide-interchanging enzyme that will break intrachain disulfide
bonds in both IgA and SC and promote their rearrangement to form interchain
disulfide bonds joining SC to an α chain. After this takes place, the complete
IgA molecule is secreted (Fig. 6.3). Basically, the same transport mechanisms
are believed to operate at the hepatocyte level. The hepatocyte produce SC,
bind and internalize dimeric IgA reaching the liver through the portal circulation, assemble complete secretory IgA, and secrete it to the bile.

In IgA-deficient individuals, IgM with coupled SC can be present in external
secretions. It is believed that the same basic transport mechanisms, involving
binding of IgM to the mucosal cell through its J chain as initial step, is responsible for assembly and transport of secretory IgM. IgM is not found in the secretions of individuals with normal IgA-associated J chain. Perhaps this is a conse-

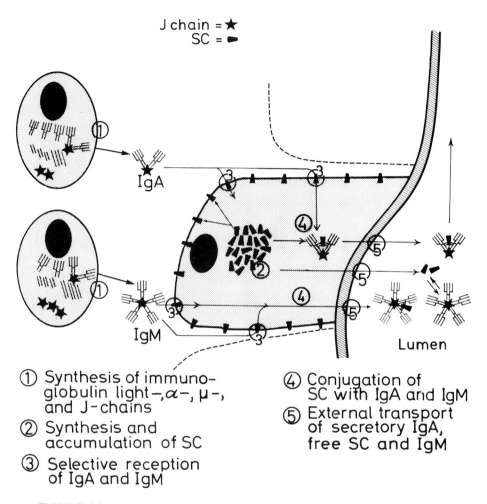

J chain = ★
SC = ▬

IgA

IgM

Lumen

① Synthesis of immuno-
globulin light –,α–, μ –,
and J-chains

② Synthesis and
accumulation of SC

③ Selective reception
of IgA and IgM

④ Conjugation of
SC with IgA and IgM

⑤ External transport
of secretory IgA,
free SC and IgM

FIGURE 6.3 Schematic representation of the mechanisms involved in the synthesis and external transfer of dimeric IgA. According to this model, SC acts as a specific receptor for J-chain-containing immunoglobulin molecules; SC-Ig complexes are internalized, and in the presence of a disulfide interchanging enzyme, covalent bonds are established between SC and the immunoglobulin. The complex is then secreted to the gland lumen. If the individual is IgA deficient, IgM may become involved in a similar process. (Reproduced with permission from Brandtzaeg, P. and Baklien, K. Intestinal secretion of IgA and IgM: A hypothetical model. In *Immunology of the Gut*, Ciba Found. Symp. 46 (new series), Elsevier/Excerpta Medica/North-Holland, New York, 1977).

quence of steric hindrance of the IgM-associated J chain, which would only be able to interact effectively with membrane-associated SC in the absence of competition from dimeric IgA molecules.

The second function proposed for SC is that of a stabilizer of the IgA molecule. This concept is based on experimental observations showing that secretory IgA or dimeric IgA to which SC has been noncovalently associated in vitro are more resistant to the effects of proteolytic enzymes than monomeric or dimeric IgA molecules devoid of SC. One way to explain these observations would be to suggest that the association of SC with dimeric IgA molecules renders the hinge region of the IgA monomeric subunits less accessible to proteolytic enzymes. From a biological point of view it would be advantageous for antibodies secreted into fluids rich in proteolytic enzymes (both of bacterial and of host origin) to be resistant to proteolysis.

V. IMMUNOGLUBULIN METABOLISM

Several techniques have been used for metabolic studies of immunoglobulins. The most common and accurate consists in injecting an immunoglobulin labelled with a radioisotope (^{131}I is preferred for the labeling of proteins to be used for metabolic studies because of its fast decay rate) and following the plasma activity curve. Potassium iodide has to be administered during turnover studies to block the thyroidal uptake of iodine that would interfere with the normal catabolism of the labeled immunoglobulin. Figure 6.4 reproduces an example of a metabolic turnover study. After an initial phase of equilibration, the decay of circulating radioactivity follows a straight line in a semilogarithmic scale. From this graph several parameters can be calculated. The most commonly used is the *half-life*, which corresponds to the time elapsed for a reduction to half of the IgG concentration after equilibrium has been reached. Other parameters frequently determined are the *synthetic rate* and the *fractional turnover rate* (which is the fraction of the plasma pool catabolized and cleared into urine in a day).

The metabolic properties of immunoglobulins can be summarized as follows:

1. IgG is the immunoglobulin class with the longest half-life (21 days) and lowest fractional turnover rate (4-10%/12 hr) with the exception of IgG3, which has a considerably shorter half-life (7 days), close to that of IgA (5-6 days) and IgM (5 days).

2. While most immunoglobulin classes are evenly distributed among the intra- and extra-vascular compartments, IgM, IgD, and to a lesser extent IgG3 are predominantly concentrated in the intravascular space.

3. The synthetic rate of IgA1 (24 mg/kg/day) is not very different from that of IgG1 (25 mg/kg/day), but the serum concentration of IgA1 is about

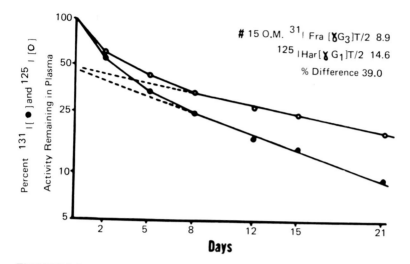

FIGURE 6.4   Plasma elimination curves of two IgG proteins, one typed as IgG1 (Har) and the other as IgG3 (Fra). The half-life can be determined from the stable part of the curve and its extrapolation (dotted line) as the time necessary for a 50% reduction of the circulating concentration of labeled protein. (Reproduced with permission from Spiegelberg, H. L., Fishkin, B. G., and Grey, H. M. Catabolism of human G immunoglobulins of different heavy chain subclass. *J. Clin. Invest. 47*:2323, 1968.)

1/3 of the IgG1 concentration. This is explained by a fractional turnover rate three times greater for IgA1 (24%/day).

4. The highest fractional turnover rate and shorter half-life are those of IgE (74%/day and 2.4 days, respectively).

5. The lowest synthetic rate is that of IgE (0.002 mg/kg/day compared to 20-60 mg/kg/day for IgG).

VI.   THE VARIATION OF THE CATABOLIC RATE OF IgG IN RELATION TO ITS SERUM CONCENTRATION

It has to be noted that IgG catabolism is very much influenced by the circulating concentration of this immunoglobulin. At high protein concentrations the catabolism will be faster, and at low IgG concentrations it will be slowed down. The most popular theory to explain these observations was proposed by Brambell. According to this author, when IgG is phagocytized by cells able to degrade it, some receptors will appear in the internal aspect of the endopinocytotic vesicles. Binding to such receptors will protect the molecule from degradation. At low

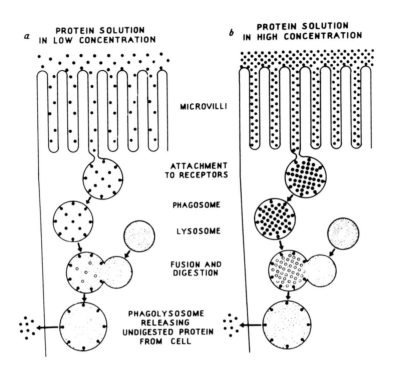

FIGURE 6.5   Schematic representation of Brambell's theory concerning the placental transfer of IgG and the relationship between concentration and catabolism of IgG. The diagram at the left shows that pinocytotic IgG will be partially bound to phagosome wall receptors and protected from proteolysis, being later released undigested. This mechanism would account for transplacental transfer. The diagram on the right side of the figure shows that if the concentration of IgG is very high, the number of IgG molecules bound to phagosome receptors will remain the same as when the concentration is low, while the number of unbound molecules will be much greater, and those will be eventually digested, resulting in a higher catabolic rate. (Reproduced with permission from Brambell, F. W. R. The transmission of immunity from mother to young and the catabolism of immunoglobulins. *Lancet* 2:1089, 1966.)

IgG concentrations most molecules will bind and the fraction of total IgG degraded will be small. The undegraded molecules will be released back into the extracellular fluids. At high IgG concentration the majority of IgG molecules will be unbound and degraded, resulting in a high catabolic rate (Figure 6.5).

VII. BIOLOGICAL PROPERTIES OF IMMUNOGLOBULINS

As stated in the previous chapter, two main functional regions can be distinguished in the immunoglobulin molecule: the Fab region, involved in antigenbinding, and the Fc region, which determines a variety of other functions that are listed in Table 6.1. Of particular physiological interest are the placental transfer, exclusive of IgG (all subclasses), complement fixation, and binding to Fc receptors.

A. Placental Transfer

In humans, the only major immunoglobulin transferred from mother to fetus across the placenta is IgG. The placental transfer of IgG is an active process; the concentration of IgG in the fetal circulation is often higher than the concentration in matched maternal blood. It is also known that a normal fetus synthesizes only trace amounts of IgG, depending on placental transfer for acquisition of passive immunity against common pathogens. Models explaining the selectivity of IgG transport have been proposed based on Brambell's receptor theory for IgG catabolism. The trophoblastic cells on the maternal side of the placenta would endocytose plasma containing all types of proteins but would have receptors in the endopinocytotic vesicles for the Fc region of IgG and not for any other immunoglobulin. Those proteins (e.g., IgG) bound to receptors would be protected from catabolism and through active reverse pinocytosis they would finally find their way to the fetal circulation.

B. Complement Fixation

Complement fixation can be achieved by two pathways, and different structural areas of the immunoglobulin molecule are probably involved in complement fixation by either pathway. At present all immunoglobulins have been found able to fix complement by one or the other pathway. However, there are some quantitative differences, and generally IgG1, IgG3, and IgM molecules are the most efficient in fixing complement, all of them through the classical pathway. Complement fixation has been already mentioned as being one of the main mechanisms through which antibodies trigger the destruction of target microorganisms or nonself cells.

C. Binding to Fc Receptors

Macrophages, neutrophils, and K lymphocytes can engulf or destroy target cells or microorganisms after recognizing the Fc fragment of specific antibodies bound to the surfaces of these cells or microorganisms. The recognition of the Fc region will direct the cytolytic and phagocytic functions of these cells, rendering them specific for the offending antigen that triggered antibody production.

TABLE 6.1 Biologic Properties of Immunoglobulins

	IgG1	IgG2	IgG3	IgG4	IgA1	IgA2	IgM	IgD	IgE
Serum concentration (mg/dl)	500–1200	80–400	30–200	3–20	50–200	0–20	50–200	0–40	0–0.2
Presence in normal secretions	−	+	−	−	+	+++	+	−	+
Placental transfer	+	+	+	+	−	−	−	−	−
Complement fixation									
Classical pathway	+++	+	+++	−	−	−	+++	−	−
Alternative pathway[a]	+	+	+	+	+	+	?	+	+
Reaction with Fc receptors on									
Macrophages	+	−	++	−	−	−	−	−	−
Neutrophils	+	−	++	−	−	−	−	−	−
Basophils/mast cells	−	−	−	−	−	−	−	−	+++
Platelets	+	+	+	+	−	−	−	−	−
Lymphocytes	++	?	++	?	−	−	+	−	−

[a]After aggregation.

Not all antibody molecules are able to react with the Fc receptors of these cells. The highest binding affinities for the Fcγ receptor is observed with IgG1 and IgG3 molecules. The binding of IgE to basophils and mast cells also involves an Fc receptor specific for IgE molecules; this binding has the highest affinity known for any Fc-receptor interaction. The basophil-bound IgE functions as a true cell receptor. When a membrane-bound IgE molecule binds the specific antigen against which it is directed, it triggers the release of histamine and other mediators from the cell it is attached to via the Fcγ receptor. The release of histamine and a variety of other biologically active compounds is the basis of the immediate hypersensitivity reaction, which is discussed in detail in Chapter 19.

SELF-EVALUATION

Questions

Choose the one best answer to the following questions.

6.1 The antibody not likely to be transmitted from mother to fetus across the placenta is
   A. IgG2 anti-tetanus toxoid.
   B. IgG4 anti-factor VIII.
   C. IgG1 anti-Rh.
   D. IgM anti-toxoplasma.
   E. Secretory IgA anti-poliovirus.

6.2 The Fab fragment of the IgG immunoglobulin
   A. Has the reaction site responsible for placental transfer.
   B. Has the reactive site responsible for complement fixation.
   C. Has the reactive site responsible for fixation to heterologous skin.
   D. Contains the antigen-binding site.
   E. Contains one single heavy chain domain.

6.3 The synthesis of J chain
   A. Occurs only in IgM-synthesizing plasma cells.
   B. Is a characteristic of plasma cells synthesizing polymeric immunoglobulins.
   C. Is common to all plasma cells.
   D. Takes place in cells other than plasma cells.
   E. Results from the malignant transformation of a plasma cell.

6.4 According to Brambell's theory, the key to the placental transfer of IgG is the
   A. High diffusibility of 7S antibodies.

B. Protection against proteolysis of proteins bound to receptors in the walls of pinocytotic vesicles.

C. Local production by subendothelial plasma cells on the maternal side of the placenta.

D. Existence of an uptake mechanism in trophoblast similar to that responsible for the transfer of IgA across mucosae.

E. Long half-life of maternal IgG.

6.5 The relatively greater resistance of secretory IgA to proteolytic enzymes is assumed to be a consequence of the

A. Binding of secretory component around the hinge region.

B. Predominantly dimeric nature of secretory IgA.

C. Increased resistance to protelysis of IgA2 molecules.

D. Anti-protease activity of secretory component.

E. Presence of J chain.

6.6 Which immunglobulin has a catabolic rate dependent on its circulating concentration?

A. IgG.

B. IgA.

C. IgM.

D. IgD.

E. IgE.

For questions 6.7-6.10, match the characteristic indicated with the immunoglobulin to which it is most specifically associated: (A) half-life of 7 days; (B) greatest fractional catabolic rate; (C) highest concentration in serum; (D) contains J chain; (E) two-step synthesis.

6.7 IgG1.

6.8 IgG3.

6.9 Dimeric IgA.

6.10 IgE.

Answers

6.1 (D) IgM antibodies are not transmitted across the placenta, while all IgG subclasses are.

6.2 (D) All biological properties of antibodies other than antigen binding are Fc-mediated.

6.3 (C)

6.4   (B)   Endocytosed and receptor-bound IgG will be protected from proteo-
            lysis.

6.5   (A)

6.6   (A)   Brambell's theory postulates that there is an inverse correlation
            between the circulating concentration of IgG and the proportion
            of IgG that is bound on the phagolysosome membranes and spared
            from degradation, hence, the catabolic rate will be directly propor-
            tional to circulating IgG concentrations.

6.7   (C)   IgG1 is the most abundant immunoglobulin in normal human serum.

6.8   (A)   IgG3 is more susceptible to proteolytic enzymes than other IgG pro-
            tein of subclasses 1, 2, and 4. This could explain its higher catabolic
            rate and shorter half-life.

6.9   (D)

6.10 (B)

BIBLIOGRAPHY

Brandtzaeg, P. Transport models for secretory IgA and secretory IgM. *Clin.
   Exp. Immunol. 44*:221, 1981.
Parkhouse, R. M. E. Biosynthesis of immunoglobulins. In *Immunochemistry:
   An Advanced Textbook*, L. E. Glynn and M. W. Steward (Eds.). John Wiley
   & Sons, New York, 1977.
Turner, M. W. Structure and function of immunoglobulins. In *Immunochem-
   istry: An Advanced Textbook*, L. E. Glynn and M. W. Steward (Eds.).
   John Wiley & Sons, New York, 1977.
Waldmann, T. A. and Strober, W. Metabolism of immunoglobulins. *Prog.
   Allergy 13*:1, 1969.

7

Genetics of Immunoglobulins

JANARDAN P. PANDEY

Immunoglobulin (Ig) molecules are encoded by three unlinked gene families—two for light (L) chains and one for heavy (H) chains—located on human chromosomes 2, 22, and 14, respectively. The "one gene (cistron), one polypeptide chain" concept, coined by Beadle and Tatum in the 1940s, still holds true for most proteins, for Ig molecules, however, this dogma of genetics does not fit with the known facts. As mentioned in the preceding chapters, each individual is able to produce one to several million different antibody molecules with different antigenic specificities, and this diversity corresponds to the extreme heterogeneity of the variable (V) regions in those antibody molecules, implying that each individual possesses a large number of structural genes for Ig chains. The allotypic determinants on the constant (C) region (see following discussion), on the other hand, segregate as a single mendelian trait, suggesting that there may be only one gene for each of the several Ig chain constant regions. To reconcile these seemingly contradictory observations, Dreyer and Bennet in 1965 proposed that the V and C regions are encoded by two separate genes that are brought together by a translocation event during lymphocyte development. Employing recombinant DNA technology, Hozumi and Tonegawa in 1976 obtained conclusive proof of this hypothesis (for his pioneering studies, Tonegawa was awarded the 1987 Nobel Prize in Medicine and Physiology).

I. IMMUNOGLOBULIN GENE REARRANGEMENT

It is well established that an Ig polypeptide chain is coded by multiple genes scattered along a chromosome of the germ-line genome. These widely separated gene segments are brought together (recombined) during B-lymphocyte differentiation to form a complet Ig gene.

The V region of an Ig molecule is coded by two gene segments for the κ and λ chains, designated as V and J (J for joining, because it joins V and C region genes); three segments are required for the V region of the H chains, V, J, and D (D for diversity, because it corresponds to the most diverse region of the H chain). To form a functional L- or H-chain gene, one or two gene rearrangements are needed: in the L chain, the V gene moves next to a J gene (on chromosome 2 or 22 in man); in the H chain gene, first the D and J regions are joined and next the V gene is joined to the D gene (on chromosome 14 in man). The VJ or VDJ segments and one of the C-gene complexes—Cκ or Cλ on chromosome 2 or 22, and Cμ, Cδ, Cγ3, Cγ1, Cα1, Cγ2, Cγ4, Cε, or Cα2 on chromosome 14—are then transcribed into mRNA containing VJ- or VDJ-coding sequences, the interconnecting noncoding sequences, and the coding sequence of one of the C genes. The intervening noncoding sequences are then excised, making a contiguous VJC or VDJC mRNA of the L and H chain genes, respectively (Figs. 7.1, 7.2). Gene rearrangements occur in a sequential order: H genes rearrange first, followed by κ and then λ genes.

It is believed that each germ line V gene carries a transcription promoter, but its expression seems to depend on a C region enhancer. For this reason, immunoglobulin synthesis (H or L chains) is detected only after the VDJ or VJ rearrangements, which bring the V region promoter into close proximity to the C region enhancer. During ontogeny and functional differentiation, the H chain genes may undergo further gene rearrangements that result in immunoglobulin class switching. As the B lymphocytes differentiate into plasma cells, one H-chain C-gene segment can be substituted for another without alteration of the VDJ combination (Fig. 7.3) In other words, a given V gene can be expressed in association with more than one H-chain class or subclass so that at the cellular level the same antibody specificity can be associated with the synthesis of an IgM immunoglobulin (characteristic of the early stage of ontogeny and of the primary response) or with an IgG immunoglobulin (characteristic of the mature individual and of the secondary response).

II. GENETIC BASIS OF ANTIBODY DIVERSITY

It has been calculated that an individual is able to produce at least 10^6 to 10^8 antibodies of different specificities. How this vast diversity is generated has long been one of the most intriguing problems in immunology. There are two

Kappa Light Chain

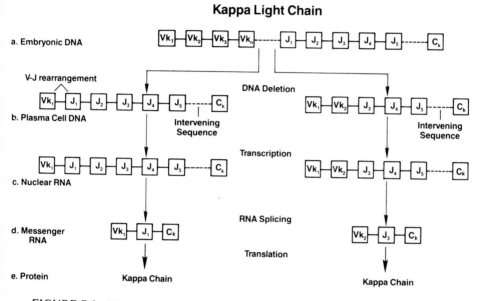

FIGURE 7.1 The embryonic DNA of chromosome 2 contains over 300 V genes, five J (joining) genes, and a C (constant) gene (a). The V and J genes code for the kappa chain's variable region, C for its constant region. In the left pathway, differentiation of the embryonic cell to a plasma cell results in deletion of the intervening V genes, so that Vκ1 is joined with the J_1 gene (b). The linked V$\kappa_1 J_1$ segment codes for one of over 1500 possible kappa light chain variable regions. The plasma cell DNA is transcribed into nuclear RNA (c). Splicing of the nuclear RNA produces messenger RNAs with the Vκ_1, J_1, and C genes linked together (d), ready for translation of a kappa light chain protein (e). The alternate pathway at right (c-d) shows another of the many possible pathways leading to a different kappa light chain with a different variable region specificity. (Modifed from David, J. R. Antibodies: Structure and function. In *Scientific American Medicine*. Scientific American, Inc., New York, 1980.)

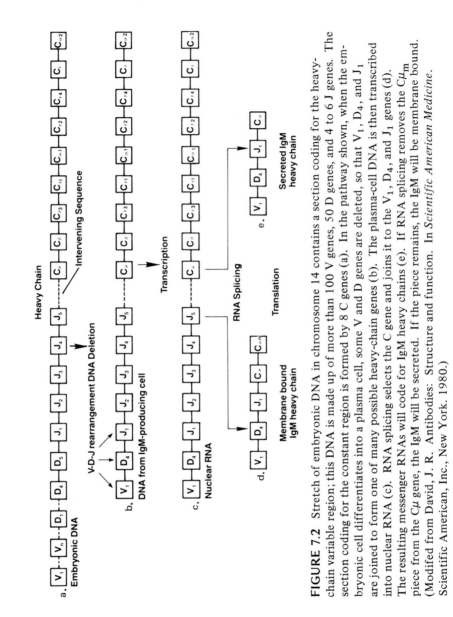

FIGURE 7.2 Stretch of embryonic DNA in chromosome 14 contains a section coding for the heavy-chain variable region; this DNA is made up of more than 100 V genes, 50 D genes, and 4 to 6 J genes. The section coding for the constant region is formed by 8 C genes (a). In the pathway shown, when the embryonic cell differentiates into a plasma cell, some V and D genes are deleted, so that V_1, D_4, and J_1 are joined to form one of many possible heavy-chain genes (b). The plasma-cell DNA is then transcribed into nuclear RNA (c). RNA splicing selects the C gene and joins it to the V_1, D_4, and J_1 genes (d). The resulting messenger RNAs will code for IgM heavy chains (e). If RNA splicing removes the $C\mu_m$ piece from the $C\mu$ gene, the IgM will be secreted. If the piece remains, the IgM will be membrane bound. (Modified from David, J. R. Antibodies: Structure and function. In *Scientific American Medicine.* Scientific American, Inc., New York. 1980.)

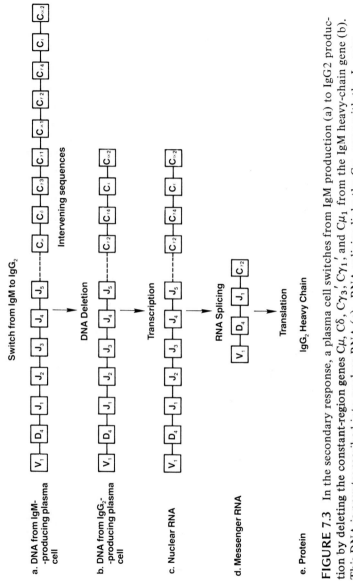

FIGURE 7.3 In the secondary response, a plasma cell switches from IgM production (a) to IgG2 production by deleting the constant-region genes $C\mu$, $C\delta$, $C\gamma_3$, $C\gamma_1$, and $C\mu_1$ from the IgM heavy-chain gene (b). This DNA is now transcribed into nuclear RNA (c). RNA splicing links the $C\gamma_2$ gene with the J_1 gene (d), and then the mRNA is translated into an IgG2 heavy chain (e). (Modified from David, J. R. Antibodies: Structure and function. In *Scientific American Medicine*. Scientific American, Inc., New York, 1980.)

possible mechanisms for this variability: either the information is transmitted from generation to generation in the germ line, or it is generated somatically during B-lymphocyte differentiation. Currently, after the dramatic progress that recombinant DNA technology has brought to this area, it is known that the following processes contribute to the generation of antibody diversity.

1. The *existence of a large number of V genes* and of a smaller set of D and J segments in the germ line DNA, which has probably been generated during evolution as a consequence of environmental pressure. In the mouse, sequence and cross-hybridization studies have shown that at least 100 VH genes exist in the germ line, which can be grouped into several families, each of these associated with different antibody specificities. A similar situation is likely to exist in man.

2. *Combinatorial association.* There are at least 100 V region genes for the heavy chain, and probably this is a conservative estimate. The total number of possible V genes is increased by the fact that any V segment can combine, in principle, with any of a number (4-6) of J segments, and with one of 50 different D segments. Imprecise joining of various V segments, creating sequence variation at the points of recombination, augments diversity significantly. In the case of the light chain, the number of V-region genes is estimated at 300, and they can also recombine with different J region genes. Last, random association of L and H chains plays an important role in increasing diversity. For example, random association of 1000 H chains and 1000 L chains would produce 10^6 unique antibodies. However, there is increasing evidence suggesting that gene rearrangements are not totally random, a fact that could drastically reduce our estimates of diversity directly resulting from germ-line associations and that reinforces the argument for the role of somatic mutations in generating antibody diversity.

3. *Somatic mutations.* Mutations as a source of antibody diversity were proposed in the 1950s. Experimental support for this hypothesis, however, was obtained only three decades later. Comparison of nucleotide sequences from murine embryonic DNA and DNA obtained from plasmacytomas revealed several base changes, suggesting occurrence of mutations during lymphocyte differentiation. Recent calculations of the mutation rate on B-cell precursors maintained in long-term culture are as high as 1 to 3×10^{-5} per base pair for each cell generation. There appear to be some special mutational mechanisms involved in Ig genes, because mutations accumulate only around the V genes and not around the C genes. In addition to these point mutations, certain enzymes can randomly insert and/or delete DNA bases. Such changes can shift the reading frame for translation (frameshift mutations) so that all codons distal to

the mutation are read out of phase and may result in different amino acids, thus adding to antibody diversity.

After years of controversy over which mechanism, germ line or somatic, is responsible for antibody diversity, immunologists have become convinced that both mechanisms contribute to the amplification of V region diversity. Their relative contribution, however, is not yet completely understood.

III. ANTIGENIC DETERMINANTS OF IG MOLECULES

Three main categories of antigenic determinants are found on the Ig molecules.

1. *Isotypes*. These determinants are present on all molecules of each class and subclass of immunoglobulin H chains and on each type of L chain; they are defined serologically by antisera directed against the constant regions of H and L chains. The antisera are produced in animals, which, upon injection of purified human immunoglobulins, recognize the structural differences between constant regions of H and L chains. Isotypic determinants are common to all members of a given species, hence they cannot be used as genetic markers. Their practical importance results from the fact that they allow the identification of classes and subclasses of immunoglobulins through the heavy chain isotypes and types of light chains (κ,λ). The L chain isotypes are shared by all classes and subclasses of normal immunoglobulins.

2. *Idiotypes*. The antigen-combining site in the V region of Ig molecules, in addition to determining specificity for antigen binding, can also act as an antigen and induce production of antibodies against it. Such antigenic determinants, usually associated with hypervariable regions, are called idiotypes.

3. *Allotypes*. These are hereditary antigenic determinants of Ig polypeptide chains that may differ between individuals of the same species. The loci controlling allotypic determinants are codominant (i.e., both are expressed phenotypically in a heterozygote) autosomal genes that follow mendelian laws. All allotypic markers that have so far been identified on human immunoglobulin molecules, with one exception (see later), are present in the C regions of H chains of IgG, IgA, IgE and on κ-type L chains. Because different individuals of the same species may have different allotypes, these determinants can be used as genetic markers.

A. Allotypes of H Chains of IgG: Gm Allotypes

Allotypes have been found on $\gamma 1$, $\gamma 2$, and $\gamma 3$ chains, but not as yet on $\gamma 4$. They are denoted as G1m, G2m, and G3m, respectively (*G* for IgG; the numer-

Pandey

TABLE 7.1 Currently Testable Gm Allotypes

Heavy chain subclass	Numeric	Alphanumeric
γ1	G1m(1)	(a)
	(2)	(x)
	(3)	(f)
	(17)	(z)
γ2	G2m(23)	(n)
γ3	G3m (5)	(b1)
	(6)	(c3)
	(10)	(b5)
	(11)	(b0)
	(13)	(b3)
	(14)	(b4)
	(15)	(s)
	(16)	(t)
	(21)	(g1)
	(24)	(c5)
	(26)	(u)
	(27)	(v)
	(28)	(g5)

als 1, 2 and 3 identify the subclass, the letter *m* stands for "marker"). At present, 18 Gm specificities can be defined—4 G1m, 1 G2m, and 13 G3m (Table 7.1). G1m(3) and G1m (17) are localized in the Fd portion of the IgG molecule, while the rest are in the Fc portion. In some cases it has been shown that the antigenic differences recognized as allotypic are a consequence of single amino acid substitutions on the heavy chains. For instance, G1m(3) chains have arginine at position 214 and G1m(17) chains have lysine at this position. A single H chain may possess more than one Gm determinant; G1m(17) and G1m(1) are frequently present on the Fd and Fc postions of the same chain in Caucasians.

The four C-region genes on human chromosome 14 that encode the four IgG subclasses are very closely linked. Because of this close linkage, Gm allotypes of various subclasses are transmitted as a group called *haplotypes*. Also, because of absolute linkage disequilibrium between the alleles of various IgG C-region genes, certain allotypes of one subclass are always associated with certain others of another subclass. For example, G1m(3) is controlled by the IgG1 gene, whereas G3m(5) and G3m(21) are controlled by the IgG3 gene. We should expect to find G1m(3) associated with G3m(5) as often as with G3m(21); in fact, in Caucasians a haplotype carrying G1m(3) is almost always associated with

G3m(5) and not with G3m(21). Every major ethnic group has a distinct array of Gm haplotypes. $Gm^{3,23,5,10,11,13,14,26}$ and $Gm^{1,7;..;5,10,11,13,14,26}$ are examples of common Caucasian and Black haplotypes, respectively. In accordance with a recommendation from the World Health Organization, haplotypes and phenotypes are written by grouping together the markers that belong to each subclass, by the numerical order of the marker and of the subclass; markers belonging to different subclasses are separated by semicolons, while allotypes within a subclass are separted by commas. Since G2m(23) is the only marker known on IgG2, its absence is denoted by two dots.

B. Allotypes of H Chains of IgA: Am Allotypes

Two allotypes have been discovered on human IgA2 molecules: A2m(1) and A2m(2). They behave as alleles of one another. No allotypes have been found on IgA1 molecules as yet. Individuals lacking IgA (or a particular IgA allotype) have in some instances been found to possess anti-IgA antibodies directed either against one of the allotypic markers or against the isotypic determinant. In some patients, these antibodies can cause severe anaphylactic reactions following blood transfusion containing incompatible IgA.

C. Allotype of H Chains of IgE: Em Allotypes

Only one allotype, designated as Em(1), has been described for the IgE molecule. Because of a very low concentration of IgE in the serum, Em(1) cannot be measured by hemagglutination-inhibition, the method most commonly used for typing all other allotypes. This marker is measured by radioimmunoassay using a monoclonal anti-Em(1) antibody.

D. Allotypes of K-Type L Chains: Km Allotypes

Three Km allotypes have been described so far: Km(1), Km(2), and Km(3). They are inherited via three alleles, Km^1, $Km^{1,2}$, and Km^3, on human chromosome 2. No allotypes have as yet been found on the λ-type L chains.

E. V-Region Allotype of H Chains: Hv(1)

The first allotypic determinant identified in the V region of human Igs is called Hv(1). It is located in the V region of H chains of IgG, IgM, IgA, and possibly also on IgD and IgE.

IV. DNA POLYMORPHISMS: RFLPs

Recently, several new genetic polymorphisms, detected directly at the DNA level, have been described in the Ig region. These are called *restriction fragment length polymorphisms (RFLPs)* because they result from variation in DNA base sequences that modify cleavage sites for restriction enzymes. RFLPs have been described in both V and C regions. Their significance is under active investigation.

V. ALLELIC EXCLUSION

One of the most fascinating observations in immunology is that Ig genes from only one of the two homologous chromosomes are expressed in a given B lymphocyte. Assuming that IgH chains are encoded by nine loci on chromosome 14, all nine alleles are turned off on one homologue and eight on the other; only one allele of each class or subclass is expressed in an individual B lymphocyte.

Two models have been proposed to explain allelic exclusion: *stochastic* and *regulated*. The main impetus for proposing the stochastic model was the finding that a high proportion of VDJ or VJ rearrangements are nonproductive, i.e., they do not result in a polypeptide chain. Therefore, according to this model, allelic exclusion is achieved because of a very low likelihood of a productive rearrangement on both chromosomes. According to the regulated model, a productive H or L chain gene arrangement signals the cessation of further gene rearrangements. This is also called feedback inhibition.

Results from recent experiments with transgenic mice (mice in which foreign genes have been introduced into the germline) favor the regulated model. It appears that a correctly rearranged H chain gene not only inhibits further H chain gene rearrangements but also gives a positive signal for the κ chain gene rearrangement. The rearrangement of the λ gene takes place only if both alleles of the κ gene are aberrantly rearranged. This mutually exclusive nature of a productive L gene rearrangement results in *isotypic exclusion*, i.e., a given plasma cell contains either κ or λ chains but not both.

Allelic exclusion is evident at the level of the Gm system. A given plasma cell from an individual heterozygous for Glm^{17}/Glm^3 will secrete IgG carrying either G1m(17) or G1m(3) but not both. Since this exclusion process is random, serum samples from such an individual will, of course, have both G1m(17) and G1m(3) secreted by different immunoglobulin-producing cells.

VI. IMMUNOGLOBULIN ALLOTYPES, IMMUNE RESPONSE, AND DISEASES

Several investigators have shown that immune responsiveness (both humoral and cellular) to certain antigens is influenced by particular Gm and Km allotypes or by genes in linkage disequilibrium with them. In addition, allotypes have been implicated in susceptibility to several diseases. Occasionally, two unlinked genetic systems—human leukocyte antigen (HLA) on chromosome 6 and Gm on chromosome 14—somehow interact to influence immune responsiveness and disease susceptibility. Associations reported thus far, however, are not strong enough to be of practical importance in medicine. This situation is likely to change when more RFLPs are used in association studies. For example, if the cleavage site for the restriction enzyme responsible for an RFLP is identical to the mutational site giving rise to the gene for disease susceptibility, we may have an absolute relationship between the presence of an RFLP allele and the disease. This information will be valuable in diagnosis, prognosis, and prophylaxis of the disease in question.

SELF-EVALUATION

Questions

Choose the one best answer:

7.1 Based on our current knowledge of the number of V, J, and D segments that constitute the V genes of H and L chains, the number of possible different specificities that can be generated by random association of genes and polypeptide chains is
A. 4×10^3.
B. 10^6.
C. 3.75×10^6.
D. 4×10^6.
E. 45×10^6.

7.2 The antibody specificity of a particular B cell
A. Is determined by the V region genes of the light chains.
B. Is not affected by the switch from one idiotype to another during B cell differentiation.
C. Is not affected by the switch from one isotype to another during B cell differentiation.
D. Is induced by interaction with antigen.
E. Is constantly changing because of somatic mutations.

7.3. The class-specific antigenic determinants of immunoglobulins are associated with the
A. J chain.
B. T chain.
C. H chain.
D. L chain.
E. Secretory component.

7.4 A human myeloma protein (IgM κ) is used to immunize a rabbit. The resulting antiserum is then absorbed with a large pool of IgM purified from

normal human serum. Following this absorption, the antiserum is found to react only with the particular IgM myeloma protein used for immunization, it is now defind as an anti-idiotypic antiserum. The specific portion(s) of the IgM myeloma protein with which this antiserum would react is/are
A. The constant region of the μ chain.
B. The constant region of the κ chain.
C. Variable regions of μ and κ chains.
D. The J chain.
E. None of the above.

In Question 7.5, the following data is presented at a paternity suit.

	G1m	Km
Mother	f	1,3
	(f,f)	(1,3)
Mr. X	z,f	1
	(z,f)	(1,1)
Child (3 years old)	f	1

7.5   Which of the following conclusions is correct?
A. Mr. X is the child's father.
B. Mr. X is not the child's father.
C. No conclusion about paternity is possible.
D. There was a mix-up in the samples.
E. The child is genetically unable to produce G1m(2) and Km(3) chains.

7.6   Somatic mutations can account for some degree of antibody diversity. These mutations
A. Occur at random in the different loci that control Ig synthesis.
B. Predominantly affect the κ genes.
C. Tend to involve the V genes only.
D. Scramble the order of genes and gene fragments.
E. Account for the C-gene switch during differentiation.

7.7   A haplotype is defined as
A. The sum of different allospecificities detected in a given individual.
B. Half of the allospecificities particular to a given individual.
C. A cluster of allospecificities transmitted with one of the parental chromosomes.
D. The order of genes coding for allotypic specificities in chromosome 6.
E. The sum of different genes involved in coding for an immunoglobulin polypeptide chain.

7.8   The Gm phenotype of a given individual is Gm 1,3,17;5. A single IgG1
      molecule of this individual may express the specificity
      A. Gm 1,3,17;5.
      B. Gm 5.
      C. Gm 1,3,17.
      D. Gm 1,17.
      E. Gm 3,17.

7.9   The generation of antibody diversity is best explained by
      A. Somatic mutation.
      B. Germ line diversity.
      C. Combinatorial association.
      D. A combination of germ line diversity, recombination events, and so-
         matic mutations.
      E. Adaptation to the environment.

7.10 The immunoglobulin G of an individual heterozygous for Gm markers will
      A. Express only half of the specificities that the genome can code for.
      B. Carry all allotypic specificities for the corresponding isotype in all
         molecules, because the allotypic loci are codominant.
      C. Carry half of the Gm specificities in some molecules and the other
         half in the remaining molecules.
      D. Carry a random distribution of isotype-associated allotypes, with vari-
         able expression from molecule to molecule, because of recombination
         events during differentiation.
      E. Carry light chains with different allotypic specificities and identical
         isotypes.

Answers

7.1   (E)   Assuming that there are 300 V segments and 5 J segments coding for
            the VL region, and 100 V segments, 50 D segments, and 6 J seg-
            ments coding for the VH region, and considering that both VH and
            VL play a role in determining antibody specificity and that the
            association of VH and VL regions is random, the total number of
            antibody specificities generated from this random association of
            different regions and segments can be calculated as 45×10^6. How-
            ever, there is evidence suggesting that the association is not entirely
            a random process, so that the diversity generated by this mechanism
            may be considerably less than the theoretical prediction.

7.2   (C)   One particular B cell may switch from one CH to another keeping
            the VH region constant.

7.3   (C)   The heavy chain isotypes define immunoglobulin classes and subclasses.

7.4   (C)   The idiotypic determinants are closely associated to the antigen
binding site, which is defined by the VH and VL regions.

7.5   (C)   The child is apparently homozygous for G1m(f) and Km(1). Since
both the mother and Mr. X carried the G1m(f) and Km(1) markers,
the child could belong to Mr. X, but it could also belong to any
other male carrying the same markers. (In general, paternity can be
excluded with certainty, but proved only to a probability of about
99%, by examining the traditional genetic markers—immunoglobulin
allotypes, blood groups, and HLA antigens. By employing the modern DNA "fingerprinting" methods, however, paternity can be
proven with almost 100% probability using one single test.)

7.6   (C)   Rather than being randomly distributed on the genome, somatic
mutations concentrate in the V-region genes.

7.7   (C)   Each child receives two haplotypes, one maternal and one paternal.
His genotype will be the sum of the two haplotypes.

7.8   (D)   Gm 5 is a G3m allotype (present on IgG3 molecules rather than in
IgG1 molecules); Gm 3 and 17 are alleles of a single locus and
normally are not present on the same molecule (allelic exclusion).
Gm 1 and 17 correspond to amino acid substitutions at two different sites for IgG1 and can be expressed simultaneously at different regions of one single γ1 chain.

7.9   (D)

7.10 (C)   As a consequence of allelic exclusion, each plasma cell only expresses one set of the alleles in the genome, but both sets of alleles
will be expressed by different cells.

BIBLIOGRAPHY

Alt, F. W., Blackwell, T. K., and Yancopoulos, G. D. Development of the primary antibody repertoire. *Science 238*:1079, 1987.
Caskey, C. T. Disease diagnosis by recombinant DNA methods. *Science 236*:
1223, 1987.
Grubb, R. and de Lange, G. G. (Ed.). Human Ig genetic markers. *Experimental
and Clinical Immunogenetics 6*:7, 1989. (The most up-to-date review of almost all aspects of human Ig allotypes.)
Kindt, T. J. and Capra, J. D. *The Antibody Enigma*. Plenum, New York, 1984.

(The most exhaustive discussion of the genetic determination of antibody diversity.)

Litwin, S. D. (Ed.). *Human Immunogenetics. Basic Principles and Clinical Relevance.* Marcel Dekker, New York, 1989.

Nisonoff, A. *Introduction to Molecular Immunology*, 2nd Ed. Sinauer, Sunderland, Massachusetts, 1984, p. 1.

Whittingham, S. and Propert, D. N. Gm and Km allotypes, immune response, and disease susceptibility. *Monographs in Allergy 19*:52, 1986.

Williamson, A. R. and Turner, M. W. *Essential Immunogenetics.* Blackwell, London, 1987.

8

Antigen-Antibody Reactions

GABRIEL VIRELLA

I. GENERAL CHARACTERISTICS OF THE ANTIGEN–ANTIBODY REACTION

In earlier chapters we have defined the nature of antigens and discussed in detail the structure of antibodies. This chapter will focus our discussion in the reactions involving antigens (Ag) and antibodies (Ab).

Antigens and antibodies bind through noncovalent bonds, in a manner not too different from that in which proteins bind to their cellular receptors or enzymes bind to their substrates. The binding is reversible and can be prevented by high ionic strength or extreme pH. The following intermolecular forces are involved in antigen-antibody binding:

A. Electrostatic Bonds

Electrostatic bonds result from the attraction between oppositely charged ionic groups of two protein side chains, for example, an ionized amino group (NH^{4+}) on a lysine in the antibody, and an ionized carboxyl group (COO^-) on an aspartate residue in the antigen.

B. Hydrogen Bonding

When the antigen and antibody are in very close proximity, relatively weak hydrogen bonds can be formed between hydrophylic groups (e.g., OH and C=O, NH and C=O, and NH and OH groups).

C. Hydrophobic Interactions

Hydrophobic groups, such as the side chains of valine, leucine, and phenyl-alanine, tend to associate because of van der Waals bonding and coalesce in an aqueous environment, excluding water molecules from their surroundings. As a consequence, the distance between them decreases, enhancing the energies of attraction involved. This type of interaction is estimated to contribute up to 50% of the total strength of the antigen-antibody bond.

D. Van der Waals Forces

Van der Waals forces depend on interactions between the electron clouds that surround the antigen and antibody molecules. The interaction has been compared to that which might exist between alternating dipoles in each molecule, alternating in such a way that at any given moment oppositely oriented dipoles will be present in closely apposed areas of the antigen and antibody molecules.

A general characteristic of all these types of interactions and bonds is their dependence on the close poximity of the Ag and Ab molecules. For that reason, the good fit between an antigenic determinant and an antibody combining-site determines the stability of the antigen-antibody reaction.

TABLE 8.1   Antigens Tested with Immune Serum for *Meta*-Aminobenzene Sulfonic Acid (Metanilic Acid)

	Antigens		
	ortho-	*meta-*	*para-*
Aminobenzene sulfonic acid	++	+++	+
Aminobenzene arsenic acid	0	+	0
Aminobenzoic acid	0	±	0

Reproduced with permission from Landsteiner, K. *The Specificity of Serological Reactions.* Dover, New York, 1962.

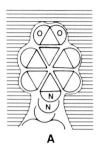

A

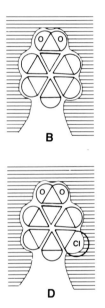

B

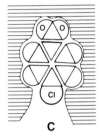

C

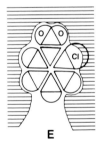

D

E

FIGURE 8.1 Diagrammatic representation of the "closeness of fit" between antigenic determinants and antibody binding sites. Antibodies were raised against the p-azobenzoate group of a protein-p-benzoate conjugate. The resulting anti-p-benzoate group reacts well with the original protein-p-benzoate conjugate (A) and with p-benzoate itself (B). If a chlorine atom (Cl) is substituted for a hydrogen atom at the p position, the substituted hapten will react strongly with the original antibody (C). However, if chlorine atoms are substituted for hydrogen atoms at the o or m positions (D,E), the reaction with the antibody is disturbed, because the chlorine atoms at those positions cause a significant change in the configuration of the benzoate group. (Modified from van Oss, C. J., in Rose, N., Milgrom, F., and van Oss, C. (Eds.). *Principles of Immunology*, 2nd Ed. Macmillan, New York, 1979.)

II. THE SPECIFICITY OF ANTIGEN-ANTIBODY REACTIONS

Most of the data concerning this topic was generated in studies of the immune response to closely related haptens. For example, if m-aminobenzene sulphonate is coupled to a carrier protein and injected into an experimental animal of a different species, and if the resulting antibodies are tested for their ability to bind to the ortho, meta and para isomers of the hapten and to related molecules in which the sulphonate groups is substituted by arsonate or carboxylate, it can be seen as shown in Table 8.1, that (1) best reactivity occurs with the injected hapten; (2) the hapten with the sulphonate group in the ortho position still reacts reasonably, but the para isomer reacts very poorly; and (3) the haptens produced by substitution of sulphonate by arsonate or carboxylate have a marked decrease of reactivity.

The results obtained in this type of experiment illustrate the exquisite specificity of the humoral immune response. It appears from these observations that the specificity is mainly determined by the overall degree of complementarity between antigenic determinant and antibody binding site; this complementarity also determines the affinity of the antigen-antibody reaction (Fig. 8.1).

III. ANTIBODY AFFINITY

In simple terms, antibody affinity can be defined as the attractive force between the complementary conformations of the antigenic determinant and the antibody combining site.

Experimentally, the reaction is best studied with antibodies directed against monovalent haptens. The reaction, as we know, is reversible, and it can be defined by

$$Ab + Hp \underset{k_2}{\overset{k_1}{\rightleftarrows}} AbHp \tag{1}$$

Here k_1 is the constant for association and k_2 the constant for dissociation. The k_1/k_2 ratio is the *intrinsic association constant* or *equilibrium constant* (K). This equilibrium constant represents the intrinsic affinity of the antibody binding sites for the hapten. High values for K will reflect a predominance of k_1 over k_2, or, in other words, a tendency for the antigen-antibody complex to be stable and not to dissociate.

The equilibrium constant can be defined by

$$k_1 [Ab] [Hp] = k_2 [AbHp] \tag{2}$$

$$K = \frac{k_1}{k_2} = \frac{[AbHp]}{[Ab] [Hp]} \tag{3}$$

where [Ab] corresponds to the concentration of free antibody-binding sites, [Hp] to the concentration of free hapten, and [AbHp] to the concentration of saturated antibody-binding sites.

The values for K, which can also be designated as the *affinity constant*, are usually determined by equilibrium dialysis experiments in which antibody is enclosed in a semipermeable membrane and dialysed against a solution containing known amounts of free hapten. Only the hapten diffuses across the membrane into the dialysis bag, where it will bind to antibody. Part of the hapten inside the bag will be free and part will be bound; the ratio of free to bound hapten depends on the antibody affinity. Upon equilibration, the amounts of free hapten are identical inside and outside the bag. The total amount of hapten inside the bag minus the concentration of free hapten outside the bag will be equal to the amount of bound hapten. If the molar concentration of antibody in the system is known, it becomes possible to determine the values of r (number of hapten molecules bound per antibody molecule) and c (concentration of free hapten).

Taking Eq. (3) as a starting point, if [AbHp] is divided by the total concentration of antibody, the quotient equals the number of hapten molecules bound per antibody molecule r, and the quotient of the number of vacant antibody sites [Ab] divided by the total concentration of antibody equals the difference between the maximum number of hapten molecules that can be bound by antibody molecules (n or valency) and the number of hapten molecules bound per Ab molecule r at a given hapten concentration c. Equation (3) can be rewritten as

$$K = \frac{r}{(n-r)c} \tag{4}$$

Equation (4) in turn can be rewritten as the Scatchard equation

$$\frac{r}{c} = Kn - Kr \tag{5}$$

By determining r and c concentrations in a series of experiments with dialysis membranes carried out at different total hapten concentrations, it becomes possible using Eq. 5 to construct what is known as a Scatchard plot, in which r/c is plotted against r (Fig. 8.2). From this plot it is obvious that at extremely high concentrations of unbound hapten (c), r/c becomes close to 0 and the plot of r/c against r will intercept r (number of hapten molecules bound per antibody molecule). For an IgG antibody the intercept value, which corresponds to the valency, is 2. It is also possible to determine the slope of the plot of r/c against r values, which corresponds to $-K$. Since the reactants (antibodies and haptens) are expressed in mole-liter^{-1}, the affinity constant is expressed as liter-mole^{-1} ($l \cdot mol^{-1}$).

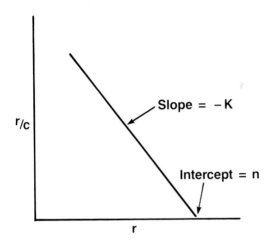

FIGURE 8.2 Diagrammatic representation of an ideal Scatchard plot between the quotient r/c (moles of hapten bound per mole of antibody r and the concentration of free hapten c and the concentration r of hapten bound per mole of antibody. The slope of the plot corresponds to the affinity constant, and the intercept corresponds to the number of hapten molecules bound per mole of antibody at a theroetically infinite hapten concentration (n or valency of the antibody molecule). (Modified from Steward, M. W., in Glynn, L. E. and Steward, M. W. (Eds.). *Immunochemistry: An Advanced Textbook*. John Wiley & Sons, New York, 1977.)

In most experimental conditions, an antiserum raised against one given hapten is composed of a restricted number of antibody populations with slightly different affinity constants. Under these conditions, it may be of practical value to calculate an average intrinsic association constant or average affinity (K_0) defined as the free hapten concentration required to occupy half of the available antibody binding sites (r = n/2. Substitution of n/2 for r in Eq. (4) leads to the formula $K_0 = 1/c$. In other words, the average affinity constant equals the reciprocal of the free antigen concentration when half the antibody sites are occupied by antigens. To give an idea of the magnitude of antibody affinity constants, high affinity antibodies have K_0 values as high as 10^{10} liter/mole. High affinity binding is believed to result from a very close fit between the antigen binding sites and the corresponding antigenic determinants which favor the establishment of strong noncovalent interactions between antigen and antibody.

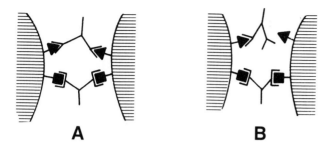

FIGURE 8.3 Diagrammatic representation of the avidity concept. The binding of antigen molecules by several antibodies of different specificities (A) stabilizes the immune complex, because it is highly unlikely that all Ag-Ab reactions dissociate simultaneously at any given point of time (B). (Modified from Roitt, I. *Essential Immunology*, 4th Ed. Blackwell, Scientific Publications, Oxford, 1980.)

IV. ANTIBODY AVIDITY

While the reaction of antibody and univalent haptens is defined in terms of affinity, *antibody avidity* can be defined as the strength of the binding of antibody to a complex antigen. Here we do not consider "antibody" as one single molecule but rather as a collection of antibody molecules that are produced in response to immunization with a complex immunogen. As mentioned in earlier chapters, all immunogenic molecules are multivalent, and in the corresponding immune response a variety of different antibodies will be formed. The avidity of the Ag-Ab reaction will be enhanced when several different antibodies bind simultaneously to different epitopes on the antigen molecule, cross-linking antigen molecules very tightly. Thus the closer antigen and antibody are to the optimal proportions for their interaction, the more stable their bonding will be, because of the bonus effect of multiple antigen-antibody bonds (Fig. 8.3); the increased stability of the antigen-antibody bonds corresponds to an increased avidity of the reaction.

V. SPECIFICITY AND CROSS-REACTIONS

When an animal is immunized with any antigen the resulting antisera may cross-react with another antigen partially related to that used for immunization, because of the sharing of epitopes with similar configurations between the two antigens. The avidity of a cross-reaction depends on the degree of structural

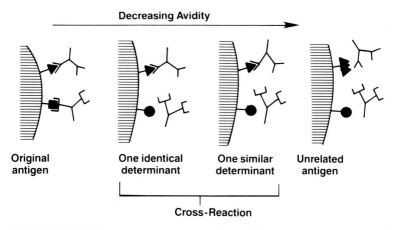

FIGURE 8.4 Diagrammatic representation of the concept of cross-reaction between complex antigens. An antiserum containing several antibody populations to the determinants of a given antigen will react with other antigens sharing common or closely related determinants. The avidity of the reaction will decrease with decreasing structural closeness, until it will no longer be detectable. The reactivity of the same antiserum with several related antigens is designated as cross-reaction. (Modifed from Roitt, I. *Essential Immunology*, 4th Ed. Blackwell, Scientific Publications, Oxford, 1980.)

similarity between the shared epitopes, when the avidity reaches a very low point, the cross-reaction will no longer be detectable (Fig. 8.4). This differential avidity between the original immunogen and other immunogens sharing epitopes of similar structure is responsible for the *specificity* of an antiserum, i.e., the property of an antiserum to recognize only one single antigen, or a few very closely related antigens.

VI. PRECIPITATION REACTIONS

A. Precipitation in Liquid Phase

When antigen and antibody are mixed in a test tube, one of two things may happen: both components will remain soluble, or variable amounts of Ag-Ab precipitate will be formed. If progressively increasing amounts of antigen are mixed with a fixed amount of antibody, a precipitin curve can be constructed. There are three areas to consider in a precipitin curve (Fig. 8.5):

1. *Antibody excess*. Free antibody remains in solution after centrifugation of Ag-Ab complexes.
2. *Equivalence*. No free antigen or antibody remain in solution. The amount of precipitated Ag-Ab complexes reaches its peak at this point.

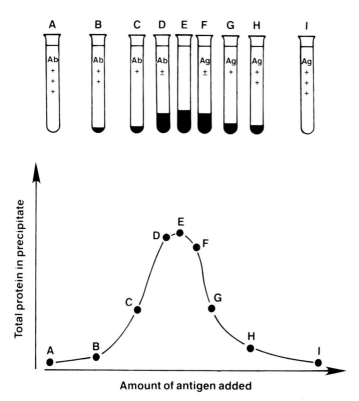

FIGURE 8.5 The precipitin curve. When increasing amounts of antigen are added to a fixed concentration of antibody, increasing amounts of precipitate appear as a consequence of the antigen-antibody interaction. After a maximum precipitation is reached, the amounts of precipitate begin to decrease. Analysis of the supernatants reveals that at low antigen concentrations there is free antibody left in solution (antibody excess); at the point of maximal precipitation, neither antigen or antibody is detected in the supernatant (equivalence zone); with greater antigen concentrations, antigen becomes detectable in the supernatant (antigen excess).

    3. *Antigen excess.* Free antigen is detected in the supernatant after centrifugation of Ag-Ab complexes.

These different expressions of the antigen-antibody reaction are explained by the *lattice theory*, according to which at equivalence the maximum cross-linking exists between Ag and Ab (Fig. 8.6).

    At great antibody excess, each antigen will tend to have antibody molecules bound to all its exposed determinants, and the number of antibody molecules

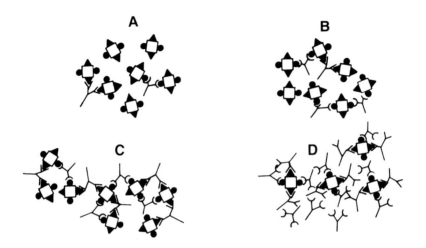

FIGURE 8.6   The lattice theory explaining precipitation reactions in fluid
media: at great antigen excess (A) each antibody molecule has all its binding
sites occupied, there is free antigen in solution, and the antigen-antibody complexes are very small ($Ag_2 Ab_1, Ag_1 Ab_1$). The number of epitopes bound per
antibody molecule at great antigen excess corresponds to the antibody valency.
With increasing amounts of antibody (B) larger AgAb complexes are formed
($Ag_3 Ab_2$, etc.), but there is still incomplete precipitation and free antigen in
solution. At equivalence, large AgAb complexes are formed, in which virtually
all Ab and Ag molecules in the system are cross-linked (C). Precipitation is
maximal and no free antigen or antibody is left in the supernatant. With increasing amounts of antibody (D) all antigen binding sites are saturated, but there is
free antibody left without binding sites available for it to react. The AgAb complexes are larger than at antigen excess ($Ag_1 Ab_{4,5,6(n)}$) but usually soluble.
The number of antibody molecules bound per antigen molecule at great antibody excess allows an estimate of the antigen valency.

bound to one single antigen molecule gives a rough indication of the *valency* of
the antigen. At great antigen excess, the binding sites of the antibody molecule
will be saturated by different antigen molecules, and not much cross-linking will
take place. The number of epitopes bound by a single antibody molecule corresponds to the valency of the antibody. Monomeric antibodies are bivalent;
the valency of polymeric antibodies is equal to twice the number of monomeric
subunits, although the functional valency of IgM is usually one-half the theoretical valency, because of the spatial closeness of the antibody binding sites of
each monomeric subunit.

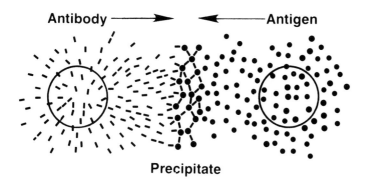

Precipitate

FIGURE 8.7 Diagrammatic representation of a reaction of double immunodiffusion. Antigen and antibody are placed in opposite wells carved in a semisolid medium (e.g., agarose gel). Both antigen and antibody diffuse in all directions and towards each other, reacting and eventually reaching equivalence, at which point a linear precipitate appears between the antigen and antibody wells.

B. Precipitation in Gel

Semisolid supports, such as agar gel, in which a carbohydrate matrix functions as a container for buffer that fills the interstitial spaces left by the matrix, have been widely used for the study of antigen-antibody reactions. Antigen and antibody are placed in wells carved in the semisolid agar and allowed to diffuse passively. The diffusion of antigen and antibody is unrestricted, and in the area that separates antigen from antibody the two reactants will mix in a gradient of concentrations. When the optimal proportions for Ag-Ab binding are reached, a precipitate will be formed, appearing as a sharp, linear opacity (Fig. 8.7).

This reaction is particularly useful in the study of cross-reactions between antigens. When a given antibody reacts with an identical antigen or with two antigens sharing one identical determinant, a reaction of total identity is obtained, characterized by total fusion of contiguous precipitation lines. If an antiserum containing antibodies to two different antigens is used to test each antigen separately, the precipitin lines obtained cross each other, in a reaction of nonidentity. Finally, if an antiserum containing antibodies to two different determinants is used to test two antigens, one of them carrying only one of these two determinants, two precipitin lines are seen, one stopping at their intersection point and the other prolonged beyond that point. This prolongation of "spur" points towards the deficient antigen, and the reaction is designated as of partial identity (Fig. 8.8).

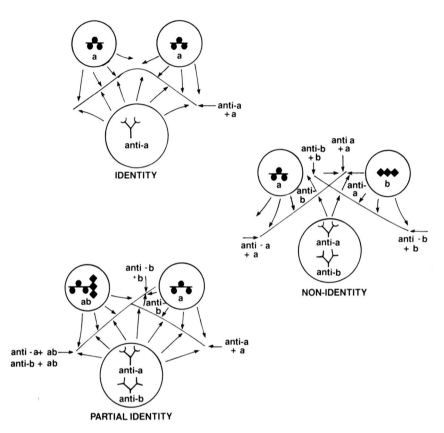

FIGURE 8.8 Diagrammatic representation of the general principles for analytical interpretation of precipitin reactions according to Ouchterlony. When two identical antigens and the corresponding antibody are reacted, the precipitin lines corresponding to the two antigens will grow towards each other and fuse (reaction of identity). If two different antigens (a and b) are reacted against an antiserum containing antibodies to both a and b, the corresponding precipitin lines will grow towards each other and cross, because the unrelated antibodies can diffuse across a precipitate (reaction of nonidentity). Finally, if two related antigens (ab and a) are reacted with an antiserum containing antibodies to both determinants of the more complex antigen, the precipitin lines will show a partial fusion, with a spur growing toward the simpler antigen (reaction of partial identity).

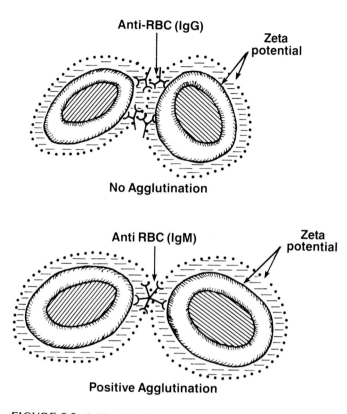

Anti-RBC (IgG)

Zeta potential

No Agglutination

Anti RBC (IgM)

Zeta potential

Positive Agglutination

FIGURE 8.9 IgM antibodies are more efficient in inducing red cell agglutination. Red cells remain at the same distance from each other because of their identical electrical charge (zeta potential). IgG antibodies are not large enough to bridge the space between two red cells, but IgM antibodies, because of their polymeric nature and size, can induce red blood cell agglutination with considerable ease.

VII. AGGLUTINATION REACTIONS

When bacteria, cells, or large particles in suspension are mixed with antibodies directed to their surface determinants, one will observe the formation of large clumps; this is termed as an *agglutination reaction*. Agglutination reactions result from the cross-linkage of cells and insoluble particles by specific antibodies. Due to the relatively short distance between the two Fab fragments, 7S antibodies (such as IgG) are usually unable to bridge the gap between two cells, each of them surfounded by an electronic cloud of identical charge, that will

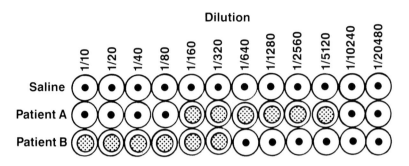

FIGURE 8.10 Diagrammatic representation of a hemagglutination reaction performed in a microtiter plate. The objective of the study is to determine the existence and titer of hemagglutinating antibodies in three different samples. In the first step, each sample is sequentially diluted from 1/10 to 1/20,480 in a separate row of wells. In a second step, a fixed amount of red cells is added to each serum dilution. In the saline row no agglutination can be seen, and the sample is considered negative. In row A the first four dilutions do not show agglutination (prozone), but the next dilutions, up to 1/5120, are positive; this sample is positive, and the titer is 5120. In row B the agglutination is positive until the 1/320 dilution; the titer of the sample is 320.

tend to keep them apart. The IgM antibodies, on the other hand, are considerably more efficient in inducing cellular agglutination (Fig. 8.9).

The visualization of agglutination reactions differs according to the technique used for their study. In slide tests, the nonagglutinated cell or particulate antigen appears as a homogeneous suspension, while the agglutinated antigen will appear irregularly clumped. If antibodies and cells are mixed in a test tube, the cross-linking of cells and antibodies will result in the diffuse deposition of cell clumps in the bottom and walls of the test tube, while the nonagglutinated red cells will sediment in a very regular fashion, forming a compact red button on the bottom of the tube.

Agglutination reactions follow the same basic rules of the precipitation reaction. When cells and antibody are mixed at very high antibody concentrations (low dilutions of antigens), antibody excess may result; no significant cross-linking of the cells is seen, and therefore the agglutination reaction may appear to be negative. Those dilutions at which antibody excess prevents agglutination constitute the *prozone*. At higher dilutions, cross-linking occurs, and very fine clumps cover the walls of the test tube or microtitration wells. When equivalence is approached, larger clumps of cells can be distinguished. At still higher dilutions, when the concentration of antibody is very much reduced, the zone of antigen excess is reached and agglutination is no longer seen (Fig. 8.10).

VIII. COMPLEMENT FIXATION

One of the most important consequences of antigen-antibody interactions is the activation (or fixation) of the complement system. In the case of antigen-antibody interactions, complement is activated by the classical pathway, starting with the binding of C1q to receptors in the Fc region of the immunoglobulin molecule. These receptors are exposed only after binding to antigen, and apparently the binding of C1q requires the spatial contiguity of at least two such receptors. This means that when IgG antibodies are involved, relatively large concentrations are required, so that antibody molecules coat the antigen in very close apposition, allowing C1q to be fixed by IgG duplets. On the other hand, IgM molecules, by containing five closely spaced monomeric subunits, can fix complement at much lower concentrations. One IgM molecule bound by two of its subunits to a given antigen will constitute a complement-binding duplet. After binding of C1q, a cascade reaction takes place, resulting in the successive activation of different complement components. The terminal complement components bind to cell membranes, where they polymerize, forming transmembrane channels and eventually inducing cell lysis. These reactions have great biological significance and have been adapted to a variety of serological tests for diagnosis of infectious diseases, as will be discussed in Chapter 14.

SELF-EVALUATION

Questions

Choose the one best answer.

8.1 At the equivalence point in a precipitation reaction,
   A. Neither antigen nor antibody can be measured in the supernatant.
   B. Only antigen can be measured in the supernatant.
   C. The number of antibody molecules equals the number of antigen molecules.
   D. The number of antibody sites is twice the number of antigen sites.
   E. The concentrations of antigens and antibody are identical.

8.2 Antigen-antibody binding involves
   A. Covalent interactions.
   B. Stabilization by the Fc fragment.
   C. Stabilization by C2-C4.
   D. Hydrophobic and electrostatic interactions.
   E. All of the above.

For Questions 8.3-8.4 refer to the following double immunodiffusion study.

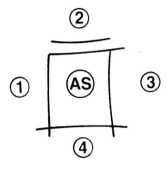

8.3   Immunologically identical antigens are present in wells
      A. 1 and 2.
      B. 2 and 3.
      C. 1 and 3.
      D. 3 and 4.
      E. 1 and 4.

8.4   From the reaction pattern seen, we can assume that the antiserum was
      prepared against antigens in well(s)
      A. (1).
      B. (2).
      C. (3).
      D. (4).
      E. (3) and (4).

8.5   Consider the following Ouchterlony immunodiffusion study using anti-
      serum against human IgG. Well 1 contains Fab separated from human
      IgG. What immunoglobulin or fragment do you expect to have in well 4?

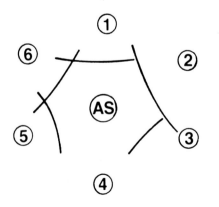

A. IgA.
B. IgM.
C. Fc of IgG.
D. Fab of IgA.
E. Fc of IgM.

8.6. Which of the following statements about the precipitin curve shown below
      is true?

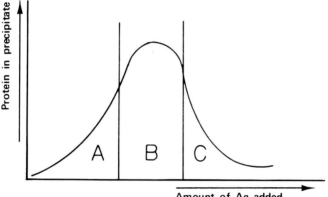

A. A corresponds to antigen excess.
B. A has unreacted antigen in the supernatant.
C. B corresponds to antigen excess.
D. C corresponds to equivalence.
E. C has unreacted antigen in the supernatant.

8.7   Which of the following hypotheses would sufficiently explain the non-
      precipitation of an antigen-antibody system?
      A. The antigen has only two determinants.
      B. The antigen has multiple, closely repeated determinants.
      C. The antibody has been cleaved with papain.
      D. The antibody has been cleaved with pepsin.
      E. Both C and D are correct.

For Questions 8.8–8.10, consider an animal immunized with DNP-ovalbumin
and match the expected result with the corresponding antigen-antibody mixture:
(A) moderate precipitaton (+); (B) heavy precipitation (+++); (C) no precipitation.

8.8   Anti-DNP-ovalbumin + DNP.

8.9   Anti DNP-ovalbumin + DNP-ovalbumin.

8.10 Anti DNP-ovalbumin + DNP-gammaglobulin.

Answers

8.1   (A)

8.2   (D)

8.3   (A)   Although well 2 has two antigens (as reflected by two separate precipitin lines), it contains one antigen identical to that diffusing out of well 1.

8.4   (B)   Well 2 is the only one that contains two antigens.

8.5   (E)   This antiserum to human IgG contains antibodies to light chains and to gamma heavy chains as shown by the reactivity with wells 1 (Fab) and 2, which must contain undigested IgG. It cross-reacts with IgA and IgM, because the light chains are shared by all immunoglobulins. It reacts with the Fc of IgG that contains the immunodominant heavy chain determinants of that isotype. It reacts with the Fab of IgA because this fragment contains light chains. It does not react with the Fc of IgM, which is antigenically different from the Fc of IgG. (The constant regions of the heavy chains are antigenically distinct from isotype to isotype.)

8.6   (C)   A corresponds to antibody excess, B to equivalence, and C to antigen excess.

8.7   (C)   Papain digestion breaks the IgG molecule (which can cross-link multivalent antigen molecules to produce precipitation reactions) into one Fc and two Fab fragments. The Fab fragments have one single binding site and cannot cross-link antigens and cause precipitation. The F(ab')$_2$ fragment obtained with pepsin, on the contrary, is bivalent, able to cross-link multivalent antigens, forming large lattices and precipitates.

8.8   (C)   The soluble DNP hapten, although able to bind to bivalent anti-DNP, will do so without forming a precipitate, because DNP has one single binding site in its soluble form and cannot bind to more than one antibody molecule to cross-link and form a precipitate.

8.9   (B)

8.10 (A)   It is expected that some precipitation will occur if anti-DNP is mixed with a different DNP-carrier combination than the one used for immunization, because each carrier molecule will express several

DNP groups, and cross-linking of the hapten-carrier conjugate can occur through anti-DNP antibodies. However, the amount of precipitate observed should be smaller than when anti-DNP-OVA is mixed with DNP-OVA, in which case both anti-DNP and anti-OVA antibodies will participate in precipitate formation.

BIBLIOGRAPHY

Atassi, M.-Z., van Oss, C. J., and Absolom, D. R. *Molecular Immunology*. Marcel Dekker, New York, 1984.

Berzofsky, J. A. and Berkower, I. J. Antigen-antibody interaction. In *Fundamental Immunology*, W. E. Paul (Ed.). Raven Press, New York, 1984.

Carpenter, P. L. *Immunology and Serology*, 3rd Ed. W. B. Saunders, Co. Philadelphia, 1975. (Includes a good overview of antigen-antibody reactions.)

Eisen, H. N. *Immunology*, 2nd. Ed. Harper & Row, New York, 1980. (Includes a clear and detailed section on antigen-antibody reactions.)

Glynn, L. E. and Steward, M. W. (Eds.). *Immunochemistry: An Advanced Textbook*. John Wiley & Sons, New York, 1977. (Includes the section "Affinity of the Antibody-Antigen Reaction and its Biological Significance.)

Landsteiner, K. *The Specificity of Serological Reactions*. Dover, New York, 1962. (A classic reference for the studies with haptens by one of the masters.)

Steward, M. W. Introduction to methods used to study antibody-antigen reactions. In *Handbook of Experimental Immunology*, Vol. 1, *Immunochemistry*, 3rd Ed. D. M. Weir (Ed.). Blackwell Scientific Publications, Oxford, 1978, p. 16.1.

9

The Complement System

ROBERT J. BOACKLE

As a consequence of antigen-antibody reactions, important changes occur in the physical state of the antibodies. They react with antigens, form aggregates, and undergo conformational changes. These events are responsible for changes in the spatial orientation and exposure of biologically active domains or segments located on the Fc region of the antibodies. These domains on the Fc region of antigen-bound IgG or IgM are able to bind and activate the first component of a series of extremely powerful and rapidly acting plasma glycoproteins, termed the *complement system*. This system includes several proenzymes and components (classically named C1 through C9) that exist in a nonactive state in blood serum. When these complement components are activated, a sequential, rapid, cascading pattern ensues, similar to that of the blood clotting system.

The greatest proportion of the complement glycoproteins are synthesized by liver cells, but macrophages are also a source of various complement components. All normal individuals always have complement components in their blood. The synthetic rates for the various complement glycoproteins appear to be under seveal regulatory mechanisms, such as the type and presence of immune complexes, the extent of complement activation (depletion), and the level of complement catabolic products.

In addition to antigen-antibody complexes, several other substances activate complement components. Nonspecific direct activators include various proteolytic enzymes released either from microbes or from host cells. In addition, membranes and cell walls of microbial organisms are potent complement activators; they activate the complement system starting at C3 via the *alternative pathway* to be discussed in the second half of this chapter.

I. THE CLASSICAL COMPLEMENT PATHWAY

Our discussion will begin with the activation of the *classical complement pathway*, C1 through C9, by antigen-antibody complexes. Immunoglobulins and native complement components are normally found in the blood and in the lymph, but these molecules do not interact with each other until the antibody reacts with its corresponding antigen and undergoes the necessary aggregational and conformational changes. These conformational changes are the basis for specific activation of the *classical complement pathway*. *Native, uncomplexed* immunoglobulin does not activate the complement system (Fig. 9.1). A single native IgG molecule will not bind and activate the first component in the complement pathway (termed C1). However, if antibodies of the IgG class are aggregated by antigen binding, this will result in C1 fixation and activation. The IgG subclasses vary with regard to their efficiency in activating C1 with IgG3 > IgG1 > IgG2. IgG4 does not effectively activate the classical pathway. An activated component on complex of components with enzymatic activity is designated by a bar placed over the symbol, i.e., $\overline{C1}$. The concentration of antibody of the IgG class must be such that at least two IgG molecules are adjacent on the antigenic surface. Adjacent IgG molecules would also require that the specific antigenic determinants with which they react be in close proximity. For IgM, which is a pentamer, these logistic problems are of lesser importance.

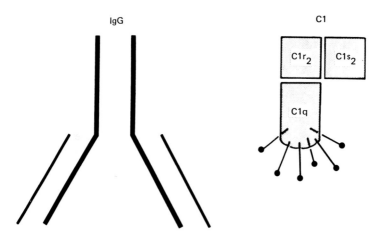

FIGURE 9.1 Lack of interaction between native, soluble IgG and C1.

A. The Early Stages: C1 to C3

The exposed aggregated Fc regions of the IgG molecule have binding sites (on the C_H2 domain) for an umbrella-like molecular portion of C1, called C1q (Fig. 9.1). Detailed chemical studies have revealed that C1 actually is a complex of three different types of molecules (C1q, C1r, and C1s), held loosely together through noncovalent bonds. In plasma, the subcomponents of C1 exist in conformations, which partially limits their degree of association. Normal physiological levels of calcium and normal ionic strength are essential to stabilize the proper associations within the C1 macromolecular complex and prevent spontaneous activation. One part of the C1 complex is C1q, which contains a collagen-like stem and an umbrella-shaped cluster of globular regions that strongly bind to the aggregated Fc region of antibodies. In addition, C1 contains two C1r molecules and two C1s molecules. Together this macromolecular complex is simply referred to as C1. Upon contact with immune complexes, the C1q, $C1r_2$-$C1s_2$ subcomponents, which were in a loose association in the fluid phase (plasma), overcome the stabilizing effects of Ca^{2+} and ionic strength and become more tightly associated. As a consequence, C1q undergoes a conformational change that facilitates the cleavage and activation of the two C1r proenzymes by one another to form activated $\overline{C1r_2}$ (Fig. 9.2).

The activated $\overline{C1r_2}$ esterolytic (proteolytic) enzymes cleave a peptide bond within the C1s molecules, which in turn become activated. Activated $\overline{C1s}$ molecules are then able to cleave proteolytically and activate the next component in the series, C4. As will become apparent, almost every component in the series is cleaved by and/or bound to a previously activated component or complex of complement components. Also, each component or complex of components, once activated, generally amplifies the series by activating many molecules of the next component in the series.

When a native C4 molecule contacts the activated bound $\overline{C1s}$, a peptide fragment is proteolytically cleaved into a small fragment, which remains soluble (C4a) and a larger, active form termed C4b (b refers to the fragment that can *bind* to a foreign surface, i.e., a heterologous cell membrane; herein the nomenclature rules for complement fragments specify that all fragments released into the fluid phase are designated by the letter *a*, while those fragments that may remain bound to membranes are designated by the letter *b*).

Upon activation, a short-lived and very reactive binding site appears on the activated C4b molecule. Therefore it must quickly form covalent bonds with an adjacent cell membrane (Fig. 9.3). Each $\overline{C1s}$ subcomponent is able to cleave and activate many C4 molecules. The activated C4b molecules bind to the antigenic surface around the areas of the antigen-bound antibody $\overline{C1}$ complexes. Any activated C4b molecules that do not reach the membrane within a few nanoseconds after activation lose their short-lived binding site and become

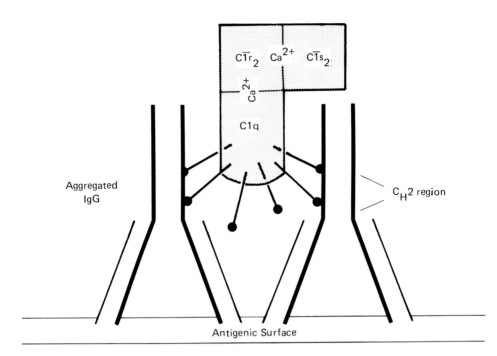

FIGURE 9.2 C1 activation by an antibody duplet formed by binding to the corresponding antigen.

functionally inactive. The loss of the binding site is believed to be due to both the rapid conformational changes occurring in the activated C4b molecules and the irreversible reaction of the active site with H_2O. The rapid loss of activity by the nonbound fluid phase C4b molecules is one very important control mechanism for protecting the nearby membranes of the host's cells from "bystander" attack by C4b. That is, C4b molecules are required to travel only part of the length of the immunoglobulin molecule, to the antigenic surface, in order to accomplish their binding function.

$\overline{C1s}$ is also responsible for the activation of C2, the next component to be activated in the classical pathway. In the presence of magnesium (Mg^{2+}), C2 interacts with antigen-bound C4b and is in turn split by $\overline{C1s}$ into two fragments, termed C2a and C2b. C2a fragments are released into the fluid phase, and C2b binds to C4b (Fig. 9.4).

Thus Ca^{2+} ions are needed for proper C1q-C1r-C1s interactions, and Mg^{2+} ions are required for proper C4b-C2 interactions. In the absence of Ca^{2+} and/or Mg^{2+} (due to the addition of metal chelators), the classical activation pathway is interrupted.

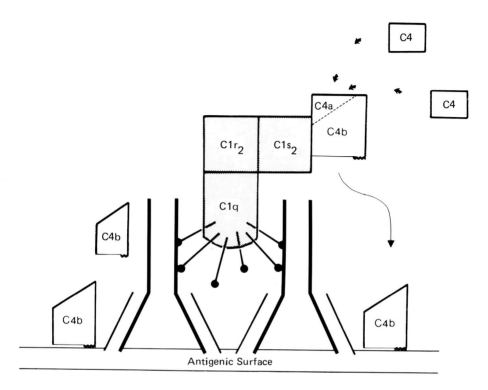

FIGURE 9.3   Binding of C4b to the cell membrane.

It is speculated by some scientists that C2a fragments may directly increase capillary permeability, resulting in edema. However, the C2 fragment with the best defined role is C2b, which contains the active enzyme site for the activation of C3 and C5. For this effect to take place, C$\overline{2b}$ must remain as a stable complex with the activated membrane-bound C4b molecule. The C$\overline{4b2b}$ complex has an enzymatic activity, termed *C3 convertase* because it causes the selective fragmentation and activation of the next component in the series, C3. Again, one must picture a rapid deposition of hundreds of C$\overline{4b2b}$ complexes on the antigenic surface surrounding the immune complex (Fig. 9.4). In general, as each additional component is added, the growing complexes acquire the information needed for binding and activating the next component in the series. The activities expressed at each stage of the sequence are regulated by several specific mechanisms. Included in the regulatory mechanisms is the spontaneous decay of C$\overline{2b}$ activity with time. However, this particular regulatory event

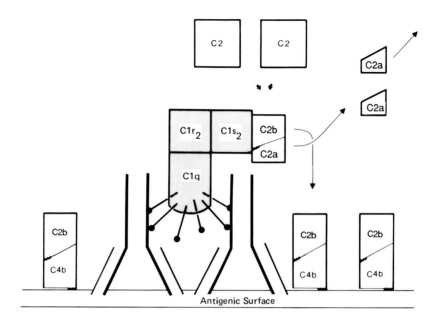

FIGURE 9.4   Formation of C4b2b complexes on cell membranes. Although C1s can cleave any C2 molecule that it encounters, the cleavage of a C2 mole-cule adjacent to membrane-bound C4b increases the probability of generating C4b2b complexes on the cell membrane.

requires several minutes and thus in restricting the range of complement's effects in vivo, may not be as critical as many of the other more rapid specific inhibitory reactions regulating the fast-acting complement system, such as the short-lived active binding sites on activated complement fragments and the effects of the normally occurring serum complement inhibitors. These serum inhibitors are especially effective in inhibiting activated complement compo-nents that fail to bind to the antigen and thus enter the circulation in the free (unbound) state. Normally these serum inhibitors restrict the complement cascade to the surface of the foreign material, prevent bystander damage to the host, and limit unnecessary consumption of complement components.

B. Regulatory Mechanisms of the Early Stages

Recent evidence suggests that as complement proteins (i.e., C4b) deposit on the antigen (and to a limited degree on the Fabγ region of bound IgG), the antibody tends to dissociate from the antigen surface. This partial dissolution of the immune complex results in a favored release of the C1 macromolecule from the immune complex into the fluid phase of the blood. As C1 separates from the immune complex, it tends again to loosely dissociate into its C1q, $\overline{\text{C1r}_2}$-$\overline{\text{C1s}_2}$ subcomponents. Now activated and in a relatively loose association, the unbound $\overline{\text{C1r}_2}$ and $\overline{\text{C1s}_2}$ enzymes are extremely susceptible to irreversible inhibition by a normal serum glycoprotein termed C1 inhibitor. Thus C1, once having performed its function by cleaving substantial amounts of C4 and C2 while bound to the immune complex, is quickly and irreversibly inhibited from activating any more C4 and C2 in its unbound, activated state.

This C1 inhibitor function represents an important regulatory mechanism that restricts the range of activated C1 action and prevents useless consumption of C4 and C2. Some individuals have deficient C1 inhibitor levels or a dysfunctional C1 inhibitor. When C1 inhibitor levels are depleted below a critical level, the activated $\overline{\text{C1r}_2}$-$\overline{\text{C1s}_2}$ are free to circulate in the bloodstream and cause an unrestricted and unregulated systemic complement activation. $\overline{\text{C1r}}$ activates more C1r as well as C1s, and $\overline{\text{C1s}}$ activates C4 and C2 in the fluid phase without substantial activation of the remaining complement sequence. The clinical consequences of this uncontrolled activation of C4 and C2, termed angioneurotic edema, will be discussed in a later section of this chapter.

C. Immune Adherence and Phagocytosis

Prior to its decay or its inactivation, each one of the activated membrane-bound $\overline{\text{C4b2b}}$ enzyme complexes activates thousands of C3 molecules. The normal concentration of serum C3 is about 130 mg/dl, which is relatively high and indicates the importance and central role of this complement component in both the classical and the alternative pathway. C3 is activated through a process, which involves proteolytic cleavage and the release of a small peptide, termed C3a (Fig. 9.5). The larger C3b fragment upon activation behaves very much like the C4b fragment, in that it also has a short-lived, highly reactive binding site for the nearest membrane surface, which is usually the antigen. As shown in Figur 9.6, several C3b molecules (C3b_n) fix to the antigenic membrane and to each $\overline{\text{C4b2b}}$ complex. In addition, there are other exposed parts of the C4b and C3b molecules that extend away from the antigenic membrane. These exposed parts of the activated molecules are biologically important because they contain molecular segments that are able to bind to C3b/C4b receptors (currently designated as CR1) located on host phagocytic cells. In Figure 9.7 an antigenic cell or particle is represented as an oval structure, and the many areas on the foreign cell surface where antibody-mediated complement activation and deposition have occurred are represented as irregular blocks. The activated complement components form clusters around the antibodies bound to the

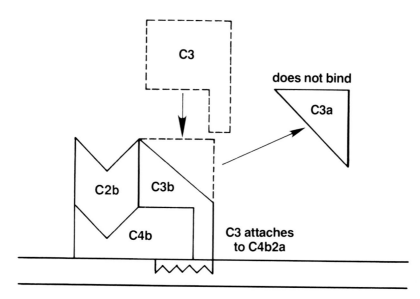

FIGURE 9.5 C3 activation by $\overline{C4b2b}$.

foreign membrane surface. The large cells represent polymorphonuclear leukocytes, which like other phagocytic host cells have a special affinity (immune adherence) for foreign surfaces coated with C3b and C4b. Because of this immune
adherence phenomenon, phagocytosis is greatly enhanced. In this process, the
phagocyte is stimulated by the interaction of C3b and C4b molecules coating
the phagocytic cell more readily engulfs the complement-coated particle. The
polymorphonuclear leukocytes have many intracellular structures, termed lysosomes, which contain a large variety of hydrolytic enzymes. As the foreign
material is phagocytosed, an internal cellular membrane surrounds it, forming a phagosome. The membranes of the lysosomes merge with this membrane, forming a phagolysosome. As a consequence, the lysosomal digestive
enzymes are dumped onto the foreign particle. The phagocytic process is one
of the most important fundamental defense mechanisms because it provides a
direct way for the host to digest foreign substances.

D. The Late Stages: C5 to C9

C5 molecules may be activated by any of the many $\overline{C4b2b3b}_n$ complexes on
the antigenic surface or by alternative pathway enzymes to be discussed later.
As expected, the specific protelytic cleavage of C5 molecules by the antigen-

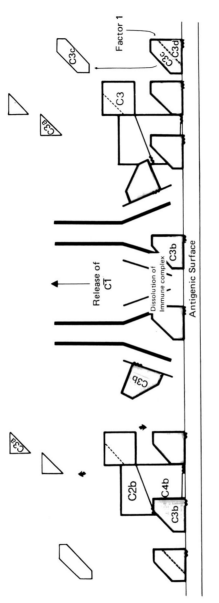
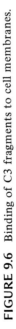

FIGURE 9.6 Binding of C3 fragments to cell membranes.

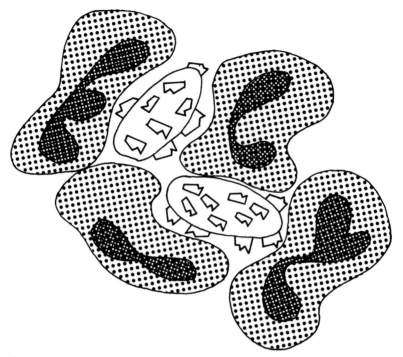

FIGURE 9.7 Opsonization and phagocytosis. On the left, immune adherence
of phagocytic cells to antigenic cells coated with antibody and complement, and
on the right, the ingestion (phagocytosis) of an opsonized cell.

bound $\overline{C4b2b3bn}$ complexes on the foreign cell membrane is required for C5
activation. Each C5 molecule first binds to $\overline{C4b2b3bn}$ and then is split into a
small fragment (C5a), which is released into the fluid phase, and a large fragment (C5b). Unlike other complement fragments previously discussed, C5b
does not bind immediately to the nearest cell membranes. A complex of C5b,
C6, and C7 is first formed as a soluble complex, and it then attaches to the cell
membrane (Fig. 9.8) though hydrophobic amino acid groups of C7 that become exposed as a consequence of the binding of C7 to the C5b-C6 complex.
The membrane-bound C5b-6-7 complex acts as a receptor for C8 and C9. C8,
on binding to the complex, will stabilize the attachment of the complex to the
foreign cell membrane through the transmembrane insertion of its α and β
chains. The C5b-8 complex acts then as a catalyzer for C9, a single chain glycoprotein with a tendency to polymerize spontaneously. The C5b-9 complex is
also known as the membrane attack complex (MAC); this designation is because on binding to C8, C9 molecules undergo polymerization, forming a trans-

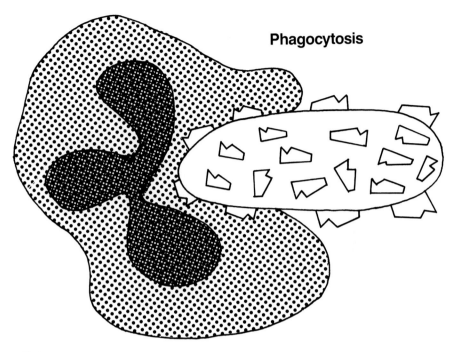

Phagocytosis

FIGURE 9.7 (continued)

membrane channel of 100 Å diameter, whose external wall is believed to be hydrophobic, while the interior wall is believed to be hydrophilic. This transmembrane channel will allow the free exchange of ions between the cell and the surrounding medium. Because of rapid influx of ions into the cell and their association with cytoplasmic proteins, the osmotic pressure rapidly increases inside the cell. This results in an influx of water, swelling of the cell, and, for certain cell types, rupture of the cell membrane and lysis. For many heterologous cell types this may result in immediate lysis. Less than 20 seconds is required for lysis of 1 million sheep erythrocytes coated with excess IgG antibody when they are mixed with one milliliter of fresh undiluted human serum as a source of complement. In contrast, many gram-positive bacteria are not susceptible to damage by the MAC as long as their membrane is covered by an intact cell wall. For these organisms, complement-mediated enhanced phagocytosis is of prime importance.

Normal human cells are generally resistant to lysis by human complement. It is postulated that either human cells quickly endocytose and destroy membrane-bound complement components or they express substances in the mem-

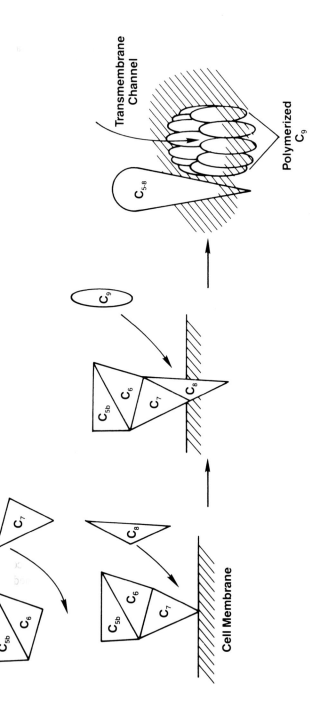

FIGURE 9.8 The membrane attack complex.

brane that inhibit the human complement sequence (the two postulates are not mutually exclusive). Interestingly, one of these substances is the CR1 receptor glycoprotein, which in binding to activated C3b blocks its function in the complement sequence and causes C3b to be more susceptible to irreversible inhibition by a serum enzyme termed factor I. Another complement-inhibitory substance located in a large variety of host cell membranes is a glycoprotein known as decay-accelerating factor (DAF). DAF associates with membrane-bound C4b and C3b and prevents the subsequent interaction with C2 and factor B, respectively. As a consequence, C4b2 and C3bB complexes will not be formed. The existence of these protective mechanisms may explain how a phagocyte approaching a complement activating immune complex is itself resistant to bystander damage initiated by activated complement fragments being formed on and near its surface. A deficiency of DAF in the membrane of host cells has been described. In individuals with such deficiency, a disorder termed paroxysmal nocturnal hemoglobinuria may occur, as discussed later in this chapter.

E. Biologically Active Fragments: C5a and C3a (Anaphylatoxins)

The small complement fragments (particularly C5a), released into the fluid phase, are specifically recognized by phagocytic cells (i.e., polymorphonuclear leukocytes) and stimulate them to migrate in the direction from which these small fragments originated. The term for this chemical attraction is *chemotaxis*. Once the phagocytes arrive, they adhere to the C4b- and C3b-coated antigenic substance via their CR1 receptors (Fig. 9.7) and thereby more easily phagocytize the foreign material. The C5a and C3a fragments also bind to circulating basophils and to mast cells located in subepithelial and submucosal tissues. These cells produce and store large amounts of histamine and heparin, and contact with C3a and C5a causes the release of histamine into the tissues, which results in increased capillary permeability and smooth muscle contraction. Fluid is released into the tissue, causing edema and swelling. There is some evidence that the complement fragments C3a and C5a may also act directly on the cells of the capillary, causing them to be more permeable. The result is similar to the classical anaphylactic reaction that takes place when IgE antibodies, bound to the membranes of mast cells and basophils, react with the corresponding antigens. For this reason, these complement fragments are termed *anaphylatoxins*.

At this point the following important concepts should be stressed. First, complement exists in a stable and nonactivated form, and its classical pathway is activated by aggregated antigen-antibody complexes. Second, complement is a biologically potent system. Once it is activated, edema and contraction of smooth muscle may occur in the area of activation. Third, complement is a fast-acting cascading (amplifying) system, with most effects occurring within a few minutes. Fourth, each step in the complement sequence is tightly regulated and controlled to maximize the damage to foreign substance. Such controls spare the nearby cells of the host and prevent unnecessary consumption of complement components.

II. PROTEOLYTIC ENZYMES AS NONSPECIFIC ACTIVATORS OF INDIVIDUAL COMPLEMENT COMPONENTS

Thus far, we have discussed the classical pathway of complement activation by antigen-antibody complexes. There are other ways in which complement components can be activated. For example, a second group of nonspecific activators includes a variety of proteolytic enzymes, which may be produced by microbes at the site of an infection. Also, various lysosomal proteolytic enzymes are released from host cells in areas of inflammation. For example, polymorphonuclear leukocytes leak proteolytic enzymes into the extracellular fluids during phagocytosis. Also, within inflamed or traumatized tissue, the damaged host cells release lysosomal proteases during their degeneration. Plasmin, a fibrinolytic enzyme, also activates certain complement components. These bacterial and/or host proteases are able to cleave directly and thus generate the active fragments of C1, C3, and C5 and perhaps other components of the complement system. As a consequence of direct cleavage and activation of C3 and C5, biologically active peptides (C3a and C5a) are released into fluid phase, generating a local inflammatory reaction by their direct action and by the products released by polymorphonuclear leukocytes attracted by C5a to the area of tissue damage.

III. THE ALTERNATIVE COMPLEMENT PATHWAY

A third group of activators of the complement system includes many types of aggregated proteins and microbial membranes and cell walls (see Table 9.1). These activators affect the complement sequence via a mechanism termed the *alternative pathway*. The alternative pathway is an alternative to the classical pathway in that this system ultimately enters the classical sequence at C3 and does not absolutely require antibody, C1, C4, or C2 for activation. However, it must be stressed that activation of the classical pathway is always associated with activation of the alternative pathway, which in that case acts as an "amplification loop" generating more activated C3.

Interestingly, aggregated immunoglobulins of all classes and subclasses (including IgG4, IgA, and IgE) will weakly activate this alternative pathway, mediated in part by regions on their aggregated Fab fragments. The complement sequence and its two activation pathways are schematically summarized in Figure 9.9.

TABLE 9.1   Activators of the Alternative Pathway

Bacterial membranes (endotoxic lipopolysaccharides)
Bacterial and yeast cell walls
Classical pathway (via C3b generation)
Proteases (i.e, enhanced C3b generation)
   PMNs
   Bacteria
   Organ failure (pancreatitis)
   Damaged tissue (burns, necrosis, trauma)
   Fibrinolytic system (plasmin)
Aggregated immunoglobulins (including IgA, IgG4, and IgE)
Virus-transformed host cells (limited effects)

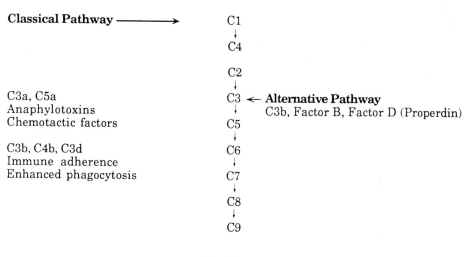

FIGURE 9.9   The sequence of complement activation.

Some of the most powerful activators of the alternative pathway are the endotoxic lipopolysaccharide components in the bacterial membranes from gram-negative bacteria and the peptidoglycans and techoic acids from the cell walls of certain gram-positive organisms. These substances indirectly activate and fix to their surfaces a group of plasma glycoproteins that constitute the initial portion of the alternative pathway sequence. These serum components are termed C3b, factor B, factor D and a stabilizer termed properdin. It is believed that generation of a "protected" (non-degraded) activated-bound form of C3b must first occur for the alternative complement pathway to be initiated. So the alternative pathway begins with at least one protected C3b and ends with cleavage of hundreds of C3 molecules to form C3b and C3a.

A. Sequence of Activation of the Alternative Pathway

C3b is produced (1) during normal C3 turnover in blood, (2) readily in the presence of active host or bacterial proteases, and (3) during classical pathway activation. Once formed, C3b binds via its short-lived labile binding site to the nearest surface. By definition, if the surface is an activator of the alternative pathway, then C3b will not be rapidly inactivated by natural plasma inhibitors and will survive on the activating surface long enough to bind to factor B forming a C3bB complex. The interaction between C3b and Factor B is stabilized by Mg^{2+}, which is the only ion required for functional activation of the alternative pathway. Therefore, tests to discriminate between the two complement activation pathways are often based on the selective chelation of Ca^{2+} (to disrupt $C1q$, $C1r_2$, and $C1s_2$) and addition of sufficient Mg^{2+} to allow activation of the alternative pathway.

Factor B within the C3bB complex is activated by a plasma enzyme, factor $\overline{D}$, to yield activated $\overline{C3bBb}$. $\overline{C3bBb}$ is able to activate more C3 leading to $\overline{C3b_nBb}$' which is capable of activating C5 and the *membrane attack complex*. $\overline{C3b_nBb}$ is stabilized by properdin, a plasma glycoprotein which binds to C3b. Since factor $\overline{D}$ has never been isolated from serum in its proenzyme form, it is generally believed that it is activated upon leaving the hepatocyte where it is synthesized.

C3b binds, regulates to a great extent its reactivity with specific host enzyme inhibitors and inhibitor cofactors which are naturally occurring plasma constituents. It is the interference with the normal regulatory system that allows the alternative complement system to be activated.

If C3b binds to a surface or a molecule that is not an activator of the alternative pathway (i.e., host cells), then C3b is rapidly inactivated. This inactivation of C3b may occur by the action of several different host substances, including DAF, and by the action of several cofactors working with a specific plasma protease inhibitor termed factor I, which cleaves C3b and renders it incapable of

TABLE 9.2 Alternative Pathway Sequence

C3 fragmentation (C3 cleavage via natural turnover, classical pathway, fibrinolytic system, tissue proteases or bacterial proteases)

Deposition of C3b via its labile binding site on a surface that retards its rapid inactivation by factor I and factor I cofactors (factor H or CR1)

Binding of factor B to C3b leading to C3bB

Activation of the bound B by $\overline{D}$ leading to $\overline{C3bBb}$

Binding of properdin to C3b and stabilization of the association of Bb on C3b

$\overline{C3b_nBb}$ activation of C5 (with liberation of C5a); activation of the terminal sequence (i.e., membrane attack complex).

---

properly binding to factor B. At present, two types of factor I cofactors have been identified, the CR1 (C3b/C4b receptor) on host cell membranes and a plasma glycoprotein termed factor H. In the presence of either of these cofactors, Factor I mediated cleavage of C3b renders it incapable of further involvement in either the alternative or the classical pathway. The CR1 cofactor appears to be most effective in binding and regulating C3b that inadvertently binds to bystander host cells, while Factor H appears to bind and inactivate C3b that escapes from the activating surface and enters the fluid phase.

B. Biological Significance of the Alternative Complement Pathway

The biological significance of the alternative pathway can be understood if we consider, as an example, an infection with a hypothetical bacterium. Because all normal individuals have low levels of antibody to most bacteria, some limited classical pathway activation occurs. Theoretically, in the presence of large numbers of bacteria, the relatively low levels of specific antibody may be effectively absorbed from the serum by antigens present on the proliferating bacteria, allowing many uncoated bacteria to escape destruction by the more effective classical pathway. While optimal classical pathway function is awaiting production of specific antibody, C3b molecules are being deposited on the bacteria, initiating the alternative complement sequence. Most bacteria, fungi, and viruses will activate the alernative complement pathway, but with varying efficiencies. That is, there is a large variability in the avidity and degree of interaction with this pathway, depending on the species and strain of microorganism. Perhaps aiding the activation of the alternative pathway are the proteolytic enzymes being produced by the organisms, which spontaneously activate components like C3. If C3 cleavage occurs near the membrane of the organism, C3b is more rapidly formed and subsequently deposited on the foreign surface via its highly reactive binding site, and the alternative complement sequence is more effectively initiated.

The alternative pathway for the activation of complement is important especially during the early phase of the infection, when specific antibody is limited. After antibodies are formed, the classical and alternative pathway work concomitantly, the alternative pathway functioning as an amplification loop of the classical pathway.

IV. ACTIVATION AND INACTIVATION OF C3

Once C3 is activated by $C\overline{4b2b}$ or $C\overline{3bBb}$, fragmentation of C3 into a large fragment C3b and a small fragment C3a occurs (Fig. 9.10). One area of C3b has a highly reactive binding site (an internal thiol ester bond becomes broken during C3 activation to form an acylating group) that binds covalently to either an -OH or an NH_2 group on the nearest molecule. C3b may bind to the antigen, to the antibody (Fab region), or remain in solution and react with H_2O. The efficiency of binding would be represented by the percent of C3b bound to the immune complex or activating substance. Other areas of the C3b molecule also have regions with functional activities that become exposed as a result of C3b deposition, such as the sites that interact with complement receptors (i.e., CR1) located on a variety of host cells, most notably on phagocytes.

The rate at which C3b is cleaved by the factor I system is dependent upon the availability of susceptible sites on C3b. If the C3b short-lived active binding site simply reacts with H_2O, C3b will be very rapidly cleaved in its α chain region by factor I (with factor H or CR1 as cofactors), and C3b will lose irreversibly its ability to participate in the complement sequence. However, the inactivation is slower if C3b is bound to the surface of a foreign substance (Fig. 9.10). The reaction of C3b with factor I and cofactors, inactivates C3b to form iC3b, thereby irreversibly disrupting the sites that bind to other complement components. However, two other sites become exposed when factor I first cleaves the C3b α chain. The newly exposed regions on the α chain react with other host cell surface glycoproteins termed CR2 and CR3. The site that reacts with CR3 is lost as iC3b continues to be degraded by factor I, which actually causes the iC3b to break into two major fragments C3dg and C3c. The C3dg fragment remains bound to the antigen and retains the site that interacts with the cell receptors CR2 and CR4 (Fig. 9.10). After the continued action of plasma or tissue proteases, the major portion of C3dg, termed C3d, remains bound to the antigen and continues to express the site for interaction with CR2 and CR4.

V. COMPLEMENT RECEPTORS IN HOST CELL MEMBRANES

Complement receptor 1 (CR1) (Table 9.3) is a common membrane glycoprotein that can be detected on a large variety of host cells from various tissues and or-

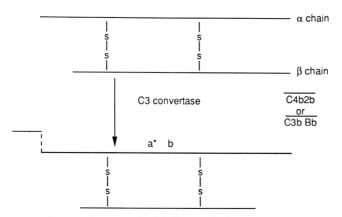

α chain

β chain

C3 convertase

C4b2b
or
C3b Bb

a* b

a. The short-lived highly reactive binding site which is exposed briefly just after C3 activation. This site forms a covalent bond with the antigenic surface.

b. A site appears which binds to the cell surface glycoprotein CR1.

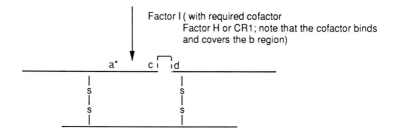

Factor I (with required cofactor Factor H or CR1; note that the cofactor binds and covers the b region)

a*   c ⌐ ⌐d

c. A site appears which binds to the cell surface glycoprotein CR2

d. A site appears which binds to the cell surface glycoprotein CR3

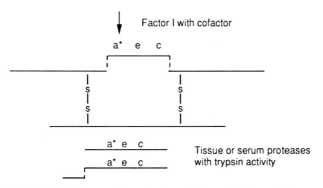

Factor I with cofactor

a*   e   c

a* e c   Tissue or serum proteases
a* e c   with trypsin activity

*a. Note that the C3d fragment remains bound to the antigenic surface.

e. A site appears which binds to the cell surface glycoprotein CR4.

FIGURE 9.10 Diagrammatic summary of the different steps involved in C3 activation and inactivation.

TABLE 9.3 Selected Cell-Surface Glycoprotein Receptors for Complement Fragments on Human Cells

Cell surface glycoprotein	Cellular distribution	Specifically binds
CR1	Erythrocytes Neutrophils Basophils/mast cells Moncytes/macrophages B lymphocytes T lymphocytes Glomerular podocytes	C3b, C4b, "iC3b"*
CR2	B cells Follicular dendritic cells Pharyngeal epithelial cells	The C3d region of C3 (expressed by C3dg, C3d, iC3b and "C3b")
CR3	Neutrophils Monocytes/macrophages NK cells Eosinophils "T lymphocytes" "B lymphocytes"	iC3b (Ca^{2+} is required)
CR4	Neutrophils Platelets	The C3d region of C3 (same as CR2)

gans. CR1 molecules protect these various host cells from complement-mediated bystander damage because they quickly bind to C3b deposited on host cells and act as a cofactor for the serum factor I enzyme that cleaves C3b and inactivates the lytic sequence. CR1 continues to react with C3b until C3b becomes cleaved by factor I. The main biological role of these complement receptors is to enhance the phagocytosis of antigenic substances to which C3b is covalently bound. In addition, complement receptors may serve as regulators of B cell activation. When complement receptors are cross-linked (i.e., by large-sized immune complexes containing multiple C3b, C3dg, and C3d molecules), B cell activation occurs, whereas single C3 molecules (present in small immune complexes, formed at antibody excess) have a suppressive effect on B cells.

Complement receptor 2 (CR2) is another cell surface glycoprotein that has primary binding specificity for a single site on the α chain that is exposed on iC3b, C3dg, and C3d. C3d is the remaining antigen-bound fragment after cleavage of C3dg by plasma proteases. B lymphocytes have CR2 molecules on their surface. Other cells, especially follicular dendritic cells, also express CR2 receptors. The CR2 receptors may be involved in the reception of co-stimulatory signals to B cells, which may have a synergistic effect with other signals, including those delivered by occupancy of antigen receptors and by helper T cell factors.

Complement receptor 3 (CR3) is a cell surface glycoprotein that binds to site(s) exposed only on iC3b; this receptor is expressed on neutrophils, monocytes/macrophages, certain natural killer (NK) cells, and on a low proportion of B and T lymphocytes.

Complement receptor 4 (CR4) is expressed mainly by neutrophils, and, like CR2, it binds to C3dg fragments, which usually remain covalently bound to the antigenic surface.

In addition to the CR1, CR2, CR3, and CR4 glycoproteins, certain host cells also have receptors for C3a and C5a. For example, neutrophils, mast cells, basophils, and certain lymphocyte populations have receptors for C3a and C5a. The binding of C3a and/or C5a to these receptors stimulates several cellular functions, such as release of active mediators, upregulation of C3b receptors (leading to enhanced phagocytosis), etc.

Besides the role in B cell activation mentioned above, complement receptors mediate the cooperation and stimulation of several other arms of the immune system. Antigens coated with antibody and complement (i.e., C4b, C3b, iC3b, and C3dg) adhere strongly to macrophages, neutrophils, and lymphocytes (B lymphocytes and activated T lymphocytes) and cause them to release many biologically active factors, including soluble mediators (cytokines, interleukins, prostaglandins, and/or leukotrienes) that influence immune responses and cause inflammation.

VI. PATHOLOGICAL SITUATIONS ASSOCIATED WITH EXAGGERATED COMPLEMENT ACTIVATION

Once the fast-acting complement cascade is activated, the complement components are under very tight regulation and control. An important aspect of this regulation is the continued presence of plasma inhibitors for the activated complement components. It is speculated that for each type of activated fragment there is at least one inhibitor or inhibitory mechanism. For example, there are serum inhibitors for the biologically active C3a and C5a fragments. The tight regulation and rapid neutralization of the active fragments limit their range of action. In the case of C3a and C5a, one of the inhibitors is believed to be a serum protease which cleaves off the carboxy-terminal arginine residue of the peptides and limits their ability to stimulate polymorphonuclear leukocytes, basophils, and mast cells. The inhibitor for C3b is factor I, a serum protease that requires one of two cofactors, factor H or CR1. C4b is also inhibited by factor I and by a cofactor termed C4 binding protein (C4bp). Factor I cleaves C4b and restricts its function in the complement sequence (i.e., its C2 binding properties). The serum inhibitor for C1 is a serum protein, termed C1 inhibitor (C1 INH), which tends to stabilize the nonactivated C1 macromolecular complex, preventing spontaneous activation. More importantly, C1 INH also binds covalently to activated $\overline{C1}$, in or near the active site of $\overline{C1r}$ and $\overline{C1s}$. As a consequence, activated C1r and C1s bind irreversibly to C1 INH, and these inactivated complexes are released into the circulation. If a deficiency of any of these complement inhibitors or cofactors exists within an individual, an imbalance in complement regulation occurs and disease may ensue.

A. Hereditary Angioneurotic Edema

In the case of genetically inherited C1 INH deficiency, patients have been reported with normal levels of C1 INH protein, but 75% of the molecules are dysfunctional, i.e., they will not inhibit $\overline{C1r}$ or $\overline{C1s}$. In such cases, functional tests are required for detection. In the majority of cases, the genetic inheritance of a silent gene results in a low level of C1 inhibitor. A similar deficiency can be induced in certain malignant diseases. Individuals with hereditary C1 INH deficiency may suffer from hereditary angioneurotic edema, having spontaneous swelling of the face, neck, genitalia, and extremities, often associated with abdominal cramps and vomiting. Their clinical symptoms can be life-threatening if the airway is compromised by laryngeal edema, and tracheotomy may be a life-saving measure. This anaphylactoid reaction is due not to IgE-mediated reactions but rather to spontaneous uncontrolled activation of the complement system by C1. The reaction is usually self-limiting and will cease after all C4 and C2 have been consumed. Since most of the spontaneous attacks in patients with C1 INH deficiency occur after surgical trauma, particularly after dental surgery, or after severe stress, it is tentatively postulated that C1 (C1r and C1s) may become activated not only by antigen-antibody complexes but also indirectly by other serum enzymes with protease activity, such as the Hageman factor, kallikrein, or plasmin, which may be released and activated under circumstances of trauma or severe stress. It is notable that activated Hageman factor, kallikrein, and plasmin are also controlled by binding to C1 INH. Such binding further depletes the available C1 INH towards a noneffective concentration with regard to its regulation of fluid phase C1 activity. In the absence of sufficient C1 INH, spontaneous activation of a limited number of C1 molecules will gradually accentuate the depeltion of C1 inhibitor and further the unrestricted autocatalytic $\overline{C1r}$-mediated activation of more C1 and more of the other enzymes controlled by C1 INH. $\overline{C1r}$ will activate C1s in the fluid phase. In turn, the continued presence of activated, uninhibited fluid phase $\overline{C1s}$ will cause spontaneous and continuous activation of the next two components in the sequence, C4 and C2, until their complete consumption. Low C4 levels are considered diagnostic of C1 INH deficiency, and they remain low even when the patients are not experiencing an attack, probably because of a continuously exaggerated C4 catabolism by activated $\overline{C1}$. The responsible angioedema-producing peptide has been suggested to be a fragment of C2 liberated by the action of C1 on C2 followed by the cleavage of C2 by plasmin. This theory has developed because it is generally accepted that serum C3 levels are not significantly altered during attacks of angioedema. However, in vitro evidence has shown that if appropriate levels of antibody to human C1 inhibitor are added to whole human serum, 100% C3 activation occurs. This complete C3 conversion can only be achieved when the function of C1 INH is blocked. Thus, the participation of low levels of C3a in angioneurotic edema cannot be ruled out when local C1 inhibitor levels approach zero.

B. Paroxysmal Nocturnal Hemoglobinuria

Paroxysmal nocturnal hemoglobinuria (PNH) is an acquired disorder of the hemopoietic cells and erythrocytes. The patients develop anemia associated with the intermittent passage of dark urine (due to the elimination of hemoglobin), which usually is more accentuated at night. The hemoglobinuria is due to an increased susceptibility of an abnormal population of erythrocytes to complement-mediated lysis. The erythrocytes are not responsible for the activation of the complement system; rather, they are lysed as innocent bystanders when complement is activated. Detailed studies of the circulating erythrocytes in PNH patients have demonstrated the existence of three subpopulations (PNH erythrocytes types I to III), with varying degrees of sensitivity to complement (minimal for type I, maximal for type III). It has also become clear that this is an acquired disease with clonal proliferation of the abnormal erythrocyte precursors.

The molecular basis of PNH has been recently elucidated. Several membrane proteins are attached to cell membranes through phosphatydil inositol anchors. The red cell membrane contains two such proteins: the decay accelerating factor (DAF), whose controlling effect on the formation of $\overline{C4b2b}$ and $\overline{C3bBb}$ we have previously discussed, and a C8-binding protein (C8bp), which prevents the proper assembly of the membrane attack complex. These two proteins, together with CR1, have an important protective role for the bystander erythrocytes in controlling the rate of complement activation on the erythrocyte membrane. The deficiency of the phosphatydil inositol anchoring system is reflected be deficiencies of DAF and C8bp. Type I PHN red cells have normal or slightly lowered levels of these two proteins and usually show normal resistance to complement-mediated hemolysis; type III PHN red cells lack both proteins and are very sensitive to hemolysis; type II PHN red cells lack DAF and have intermediate sensitivity to hemolysis.

Phosphatydil inositol is involved in the membrane binding of other proteins, such as LFA-3 molecules (see Chapter 11) and the predominant type of Fc receptor in the neutrophil. In PNH patients the expression of DAF is also deficient in platelets and other cells. Similarly, in these patients LFA-3 is deficient in a variety of cell types, and neutrophils are deficient in both DAF and Fc receptors. These deficiencies seem to be the basis of other abnormalities seen in PNH patients: thrombotic complications, attributed to increased complement-induced platelet aggregation, and bacterial infections and persistence of immune complexes in the circulation, attributed to a lack of Fc-mediated phagocytosis.

C. Pulmonary Vascular Leukostasis as a Side Effect of Hemodialysis

Recent evidence indicates that passage of heparinized blood over a variety of filter materials (i.e., artificial hemodialysis membranes and nylon fiber substances used in the heart-lung machine) causes varying degrees of complement activation. Rapid generation of C5a causes a transient leukopenia with a short-term reversible accumulation and aggregation of PMNs in the blood capillaries of the lungs, with PMN release of superoxide. As a result, repeated hemodialysis may lead to chronic fibrosis of the lung. When fresh serum is passed over filters such as those used in hemodialysis, complement activation via both pathways may occur. The classical pathway may be activated by interfacially (solid-liquid or air-liquid) aggregated immunoglobulin or by direct binding of C1q. Alternatively, membrane filter-bound C3b may mediate activation of the alternative pathway. In vivo, a blood anticoagulant such as heparin or citrate must be used, which not only alters blood clotting but also affects the complement system and alters its normal activation. Citrate, by chealting Ca^{2+}, partially restricts C1 activation because it disrupts C1q binding to C1r and C1s. At low concentrations, non-bound heparin has a limited direct inhibitory effect on C1 activity but its major effect is to bind (and potentiate) C1 INH and factor H. In vitro, heparinized blood appears to generate more C3a and C5a fragments than citrated blood when passing across artificial filtration membranes.

D. Pancreatitis, Severe Trauma, and Pulmonary Distress Syndrome

Any mechanism that causes a rapid release of high levels of C5a peptides into the blood may cause massive PMN aggregation and consequent *pulmonary distress syndrome*. For example, when large amounts of proteases are released into the blood (i.e., pancreatitis or severe tissue trauma), pulmonary distress syndrome and sometimes temporary blindness occurs due to blockage of small blood vessels with aggregated PMN. Similarly, in myocardial infarction, blockage of critical heart capillaries with PMN may extend cardiac damage. Steroids that prevent and reverse the PMN aggregation have been used to retard such damage in experimental animals.

VII. COMPLEMENT METABOLISM LEVELS IN DISEASE

The complement proteins have one of the highest turnover rates of any of the plasma components. At any one time the level of a complement component is a direct function of its catabolic and synthetic rates. The catabolic rates of the complement system are a function of the extent of complement activation by the classical pathway, the alternative pathway, or direct proteolytic cleavage. Complement catabolic fragments are rapidly cleared from the circulation. Synthetic rates of the complement proteins (which are produced mainly by the liver) are controlled by ill-defined mechanisms but probably involve such variables as the levels of complement activators (i.e., immune complexes), the class and subclass of immunoglobulin within the immune complexes, the rate of complement activation, the steady-state level of complement fragments in the blood, and in cases of certain chronic inflammatory diseases the level of autoantibody to complement components. Therefore it is not surprising that the synthetic rates of complement glycoproteins vary widely in disease states and during the course of a given disease. At any one time the level of a complement component is a function of its metabolic rate (consumption versus synthesis) and the type and course of the infection, which itself is dependent on the nature of the host's immunological response. Elevated levels of a given complement component in a disease state probably means that there is both a rapid catabolic and a rapid synthetic rate. Low levels mean that consumption is greater than synthesis.

A. Hypocomplementemia and Clearance of Immune Complexes

Individuals with immune complex diseases often suffer from the inability properly to eliminate the immune complexes from the kidney and/or from the basement membrane of dermal tissues. As previously mentioned in our discussion of the classical pathway, activation of a normal complement system by immune complexes will eventually lead to dissolution of the immune complex. This phenomenon is due to the deposition of large complement fragments such as C4b and C3b on the antigen and on the Fab region of the antibody, which interrupts the antigen-antibody binding reaction (Fig. 9.6). If a deficiency in the early complement components exists, there will likely be a corresponding defect in the production and binding of C4b and C3b to the immune complex. As a result the rate of formation of new immune complexes surpasses the inefficient rate of immune complex dissolution. The reasons for the lower levels of early complement components (i.e., C1q, C4, and/or C2) are multiple and include not only genetic factors but also a variety of metabolic control mechanisms mentioned above.

In patients with systemic lupus erythematosus, a reduction in the levels of erythrocyte C3b receptors (CR1) has been reported. The effect of a partial deficiency in this important complement regulatory protein may affect the clearance of complement fragments, which in turn may play a role in regulating complement metabolism. Also, the binding of complement-coated immune complexes to host erythrocytes is believed to be an important physiological mechanism of immune complex removal from circulation. Erythrocyte-bound immune complexes are efficiently stripped from the red cell surface by phagocytic cells, particularly in the liver and spleen. Although human erythrocytes can adsorb immune complexes in the absence of complement, binding through CR1 may be important in stabilizing the interaction. Small- to medium-sized immune complexes are not taken up as efficiently by CR1 and tend to persist longer in circulation. If the number of CR1 receptors in red cells decreases, even large-sized immune complexes may persist for longer periods in circulation and may have a greater opportunity to be deposited in organs and tissues and cause inflammation.

B. Complement Deficiencies

Deficiencies of several of the components of the complement system have been reported by different groups. Basically these deficiencies are associated with two types of clinical situations: chronic infections, often by *Neisseria* species (usually associated with deficiencies of components of the terminal complement sequence), and autoimmune disease, mimicking systemic lupus erythematosus (usually associated with deficiencies in components of the earlier part of the complement sequence). Complement deficiencies and that associated pathology will be discussed in greater detail in later chapters.

SELF-EVALUATION

Questions

Choose the one best answer.

9.1   Complement is responsible for
      A. Agglutination reactions.
      B. Antibody-dependent cell-mediated cytotoxicity (ADCC).
      C. Neutralization reactions.
      D. Cytolytic reactions.
      E. Precipitation reactions.

9.2   Which of the following is not observed when complement is activated solely by the alternative complement pathway?
      A. Breakdown of C3 into C3a and C3b.
      B. Breakdown of C4 into C4a and C4b.
      C. Breakdown of C5 into C5a and C5b.

D. Activation of the membrane attack complex.

E. Generation of anaphylatoxins.

9.3   The proper sequence in which the individual complement components
       are activated and fixed through the classical complement pathway is

A. C123456789.

B. 124536789.

C. C145236789.

D. C142356789.

E. C124356789.

9.4   Histamine is released from mast cells stimulated by

A. C1q.

B. C2a.

C. C4b.

D. C5a.

E. C3b.

9.5   The alternative pathway is activated by

A. Antigen-antibody complexes.

B. C1.

C. Bacterial peptidoglycan.

D. $C\gamma_2$ domain of IgG.

E. Mg.

9.6   CR1 receptors on phagocytic cells have greatest affinity for

A. C3b.

B. iC3b.

C. C3dg.

D. C3d.

E. C3a.

9.7   In hereditary angioneurotic edema,

A. There is an excessive synthesis of C3a and C5a.

B. C1 INH is deficient, quantitatively or functionally.

C. Patients have very high levels of IgE.

D. The levels of C2 and C4 are usually within normal limits.

E. Reactions are usually precipitated by inhalation of sensitizing agents.

9.8   Neutrophil aggregation as a consequence of hemodialysis is believed to
       result most directly from

A. Activation of the alternative pathway by heparin.

B. Release of C3b.

C. Excessive amounts of calcium.

D. Generation of C5a.

E. Retention of antigen-antibody complexes in the dialysis membrane and activation of the classical pathway.

9.9 A deficiency of erythrocyte CR1 receptors is associated with

A. Increased deposition of antigen-antibody complexes in tissues.

B. Increased incidence of angioneurotic edema.

C. Release of massive amounts of histamine.

D. Accumulation of C3dg and C3d in circulation.

E. Proxysmal nocturnal hemoglobinuria.

9.10 The "membrane attack complex" is formed by

A. $C4b2b3b_n$.

B. C56789.

C. C4bC3b.

D. C3bBb.

E. C4b2b.

Answers

9.1 (D)

9.2 (B) C4 is only activated through the classical pathway.

9.3 (D)

9.4 (D) C3a and C5a are the biologically active complement components able to trigger the release of histamine from mast cells (anaphylatoxins).

9.5 (C) Magnesium ions are essential requirements for alternative pathway activation (classical pathway activation, in contrast, requires both Ca^{2+} and Mg^{2+}), but it is not an activator by itself.

9.6 (A)

9.7 (B) The symptoms of hereditary angioneurotic edema are believed to be caused by C2 fragments. Limited breakdown of C3, leading to the generation of C3a, may take place, but there is no increased synthesis of those fragments or of their precursors. C4 and C2 levels are usually low, because they are consumed as a consequence of the excessive activity of C1, while C3 levels tend to be less affected.

9.8 (D) Cellophane membranes used for hemodialysis are able to activate the alternative pathway, leading to the generation of C5a, which causes neutrophil aggregation.

9.9   (A)   Soluble antigen-antibody complexes with attached C3b can be removed from the plasma through adsorption to the CR1 receptor
on red cells; if those receptors are reduced in number, soluble antigen-antibody complexes will persist in circulation for longer periods
and will be more likely to be eventually trapped in tissues and cause
inflammation.

9.10 (B)

BIBLIOGRAPHY

DiScipio, R. G. Late-acting components of complement: Their molecular
biochemistry, role in host defense, and involvement in pathology (A review). *Pathology & Immunology Research* 6:343, 1987.

Hansch, G. M., Weller, P. F., and Nicholson-Weller, A. Release of C8 binding
protein from the cell membrane by phosphatidylinositoll-specific phospholipase C. *Blood 72*:1089, 1988.

Immunology Letters *14*:175-259, 1986-1987. (A series of reviews on the complement system.)

Laurell, A. B. C1 inhibitor dysfunction and complement activation in hereditary
angioneurotic edema. *Pseudo-Allergic Reactions. Involvement of Drugs and
Chemicals 4*:13, 1985.

Reid, K. B. M. The complement system. In *Molecular Immunology—Frontiers
in Molecular Biology*, B. D. Hames and D. M. Glover (Eds.). IRL Press,
Oxford, 1988.

Ross, G. D. (Ed.). *The Immunobiology of the Complement System.* Academic
Press, New York, 1986.

10

Lymphocyte Ontogeny and Membrane Markers

JEAN-MICHEL GOUST

The functional diversity of the immune system is generated during embryonic life by differentiation of cell populations with defined functions. The steps leading to this differentiation are the consequence of two processes; the *disappearance* of characteristics found on embryonic cells, and the *appearance* of new and previously nonexpressed characteristics.

These changes reflect the intense activity of genes undergoing rearrangements leading to sequential changes in the expression of the corresponding gene products as the cells progressively differentiate.

T and B cells start to develop during the genesis of the hematopoietic system from a common stem cell, but early in fetal life they start to differentiate into separate cell lineages (Fig. 10.1). In humans, the embryonic yolk sac of the developing embryo is the first structure that forms stem cells that develop into leukocytes, erythrocytes, and thrombocytes. The fetal liver receives stem cells from the yolk sac at the 6th week of gestation and begins hematopoietic activity. On the 12th week, a minor contribution is made to the production of blood cells by the spleen. At 20 weeks of gestation, thymus, lymph node, and bone marrow begin hematopoietic activity, and at that time the two major types of lymphocytes are already identifiable. The bone marrow becomes the sole hematopoietic center after 38 weeks. At that time, differentiated T cells and B cells are present in circulation.

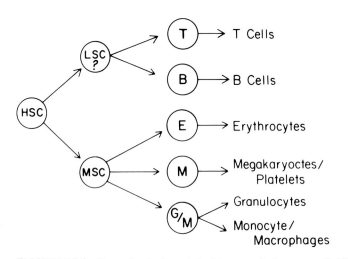

FIGURE 10.1 Hypothetical model of hemopoietic stem cell differentiation. Multipotential hemopoietic stem cells (HSC) may give rise to more restricted progenitor cells with self-renewal capacity. Thus lymphocyte-committed stem cells (LSC) give rise to T and B cells. Another group of hemopoietic cells, for which the immediate progenitor is a more differentiated myeloid stem cell (MSC), includes erythrocytes, megakaryocytes, and platelets as well as the granulocyte, monocyte/macrophage series. (Reproduced with permission from Cooper, M. D., Kearney, J., and Scher I. B lymphocytes. In *Fundamental Immunology*, W. E. Paul (Ed.). Raven Press, New York, 1984.)

I. B-LYMPHOCYTE ONTOGENY

As mentioned in Chapter 2, B lymphocytes received this designation because in birds a specialized organ, the bursa of Fabricius, is responsible for their final differentiation. Removal of this organ, at or before hatching, is associated with the lack of differentiation of B lymphocytes and inability to produce antibodies. B lymphocytes are relatively eary to individualize; their antigen-specific receptor exists in the form of membrane-bound immunoglobulins, which can be easily visualized with fluorescein-labeled antibodies. After adequate stimulation, B lymphocytes differentiate into plasma cells that secrete large quantities of immunoglobulins. It has been shown that the antibody-binding sites of membrane and secreted immunoglobulins are identical (within a single cell or a clone of cells), so studies of the genetic control of immunoglobulin synthesis and of the mechanisms responsible for the generation of binding site diversity have been relatively easy (see Chapter 7).

A. DNA Rearrangements and Expression of the Immunoglobulin Genes

It is now known that the synthesis of antibodies by B lymphocytes is preceded by rearrangements of the genomic DNA during embryonic life. Such rarrangements occur in a defined sequence that brings together noncontiguous coding segments and deletes intervening noncoding segments. This sequence starts early in differentiation (Fig. 10.2); the first rearrangement involves the DNA segment coding for the synthesis of the heavy chain of IgM (the Cμ gene). After this gene complex is rarranged, the embryonic lymphocyte is able to synthesize and store μ chains in its cytoplasm where they can be detected by immunofluores-

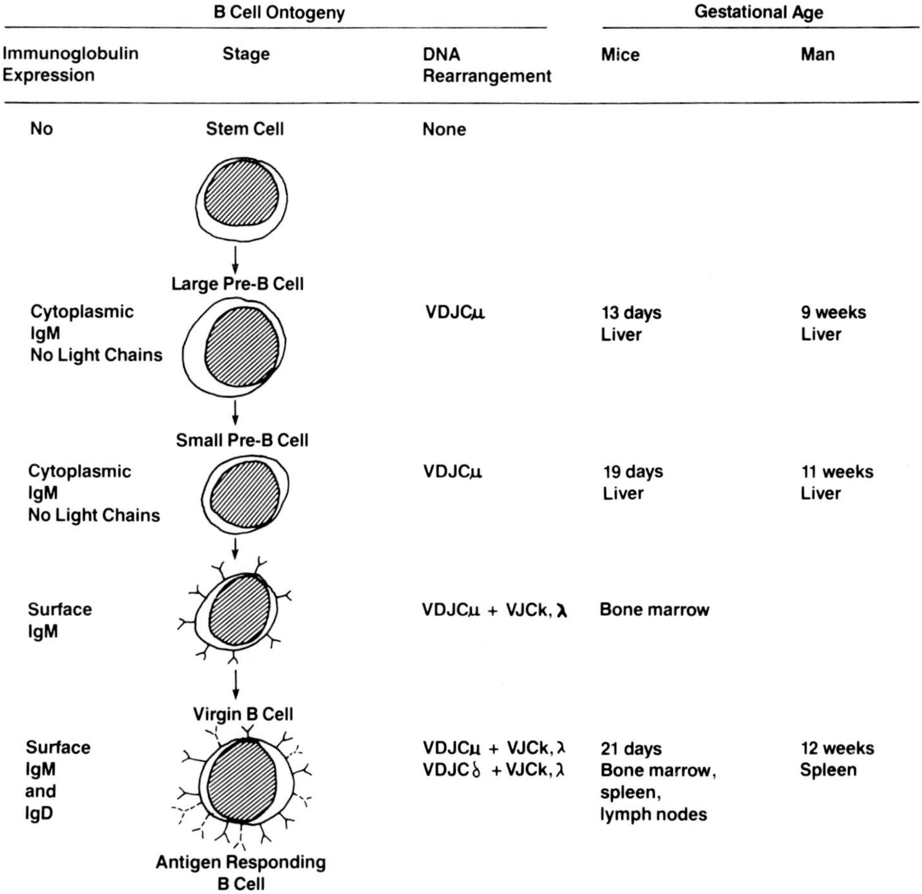

B Cell Ontogeny			Gestational Age	
Immunoglobulin Expression	Stage	DNA Rearrangement	Mice	Man
No	Stem Cell	None		
Cytoplasmic IgM No Light Chains	Large Pre-B Cell	VDJCμ	13 days Liver	9 weeks Liver
Cytoplasmic IgM No Light Chains	Small Pre-B Cell	VDJCμ	19 days Liver	11 weeks Liver
Surface IgM		VDJCμ + VJCk, λ	Bone marrow	
Surface IgM and IgD	Virgin B Cell	VDJCμ + VJCk, λ VDJCδ + VJCk, λ	21 days Bone marrow, spleen, lymph nodes	12 weeks Spleen
	Antigen Responding B Cell			

FIGURE 10.2 Diagrammatic representation of the early steps in B-cell ontogeny.

cence. This "large pre-B cell" proliferates very rapidly. In the next differentiation step, the rate of cell proliferation is slower, and further rearrangements of the germ line DNA take place. The rearrangement of the Cκ or Cλ genes if followed by light chain synthesis. At this point, association of the heavy and light chains yields complete IgM molecules that are transported from the cytoplasm and inserted into the cell membrane. During these rearrangements of the heavy and light chain genes, most of the antigen specific B-cell clones are generated. It follows that if antibody diversity is generated (at least in part) during B-cell ontogeny, any B-cell clone emerging by this process of random rearrangement with the capacity to produce antibody reactive with self-antigens (autoreactive clone) must be eliminated or turned off. This process of elimination or down-regulation of autoreactive clones is thought to represent one of the mechanisms of tolerance.

Around birth, "virgin" B cells will coexpress IgM and IgD on their membranes, subsequent to the rearrangement of the Cδ genomic DNA. On individual B-cell clones, the coexpressed IgM and IgD have the same variable regions and antigenic specificity. These mature B cells subsequently home to peripheral lymphoid organs, where upon antigenic challenge they lose membrane IgD and undergo further gene rearrangements to switch to the production of a different immunoglobulin isotype (IgG, IgE, or IgA). These immunoglobulins are then found on the membrane of nonoverlapping B-cell subsets, in association or not with membrane IgM. After birth, B cells are exclusively produced in the bone marrow at the rate of approximately 10^6/day. A newborn infant, though having differentiated B cells, will not be able to produce antibodies for the first two to three months of life. During that period, the newborn is protected by placentally transferred maternal IgG, which starts to cross the placenta at the 12th week of gestation. By the 3rd month of age, IgM antibodies produced by the newborn are usually detectable (although in cases of intrauterine infection, fetal IgM production obviously can take place). The circulating concentration of IgM reaches adult levels by 1 year of age, while IgG and IgA reach adult levels at 6-7 years of age.

B. Other B-Cell Markers

As B lymphocytes develop, other markers of functional significance appear on their surface, as shown in Table 10.1. Both classes of MHC are prominently and abundantly expressed on B lymphocytes, a correlate of their ability to distinguish self from nonself.

Receptors for complement fragments (CR1 and CR2) are detectable on mature human B cells; the CR2 receptor appears to be associated with (or represent a part of) the receptor for the Epstein-Barr virus. This virus, after binding to this receptor, will penetrate the B cell and become integrated into its genome in

TABLE 10.1 Nonimmunoglobulin Markers Found on B Cells

Receptors for
  Interleukin 2
  Fc fragment of IgG and IgM
  C3b and C3d[a] fragments (CR1 and CR2)
  Epstein-Barr virus[a]

MHC antigens
  Class I (HLA, A,B,C)
  Class II (HLA D/DR)

Differentiation antigens
  Mice: Lyb 2, 3, and 5
  Humans: CD19 (B4), CD20 (B1)

Leukocyte function antigen 3 (LFA-3)[b]

[a]Specific for human B cells, the receptor for C3d is part of the EBV receptor.
[b]Present in most nucleated cells.

more than 90% of infected adults. Other B-cell markers have been described in mice (Lyb system) and humans (CD19, CD20), but their functional significance is undefined.

II. T-LYMPHOCYTE ONTOGENY

The vital importance of the T lymphocytes is well reflected by the fact that the removal of the thymus at birth in mice (or its congenital absence in humans) is incompatible with prolonged survival. The thymus is the organ responsible for the differentiation of the second major subpopulation of lymphocytes and exists in all mammals. The lymphocytes homing and differentiating in the thymus are thus designated T lymphocytes.

It has been much more difficult, however, to unravel the sequence of events during T-cell ontogeny. T cells are activated through the recognition of cell-associted antigens; soluble and extracellular antigens are unable to stimulate them. Also, in contrast to B cells, T cells do not secrete their antigen-specific receptor, depriving investigators of an easy approach to establish the structure of the genes involved in determining antigen-binding specificity.

Experiments using thymectomized and reconstituted animals have demonstrated that mature antigen-specific and antigen-responding T cells differentiate intrathymically from precursor cells originating in the bone marrow. Once they reach the thymus, the T-cell precursor stem cells proliferate very rapidly, but only 1% of the progeny survives. The magnitude of this precursor-cell proliferation suggested a very important role for DNA rearrangements in T-cell differen-

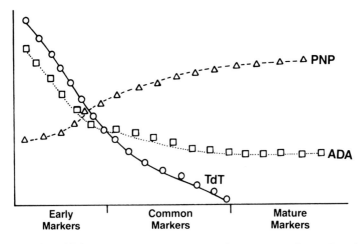

FIGURE 10.3   Longitudinal changes in the concentrations of purine nucleoside phosphorilase (PNP), adenosine deaminase (ADA), and terminal nucleotidyl transferase (TdT).

tiation. This intuitive notion was reinforced when it was observed that maturing thymocytes expressed several enzymes of the purine salvage pathway such as adenosine deaminase (ADA), purine nucleoside phosphorylase (PNP), and terminal deoxyribonucleotidyl transferase (TdT) (Fig. 10.3). The crucial role of ADA can be inferred from the severe immunodeficiency associated to its genetically determined absence (see Chapter 30). The "messages" received by differentiating thymocytes from their environment are poorly known. The thymic hormone designated as *thymosin* seems to have a major influence in T-cell differentiation. After exposure to this hormone, the content of TdT in lymphocytes starts to drop, coinciding with other changes associated with T-cell maturation. However, the study of the variations in the intracellular levels of purine salvage pathway enzymes did not offer more than a very crude indication that maturing T cells rearranged their DNA. Progress started to be swifter when membrane markers identifying distinct T-cell subsets were identified with the help of monoclonal antibodies (see the Appendix, Section VI of this chapter).

A. Membrane Markers

As mentioned in Chapters 1 and 2, it was established by functional studies that the T lymphocyte population includes several subpopulations with defined functions. The major subsets are the helper T cells and the suppressor T cells. The helper T cells are endowed with two distinct roles: they assist in the activation of B lymphocytes, and they induce the two other T-lymphocyte subpopulations (suppressor T cells and cytotoxic T cells) to become effector cells. The suppressor T cells probably play a dual role: they maintain a state of tolerance to self (discussed in Chapter 23), and they provide a negative feedback mechanism to avoid unnecessary continuation of a response after the antigen has been eliminated (see Chapter 12). The cytotoxic T cells lyse virus-infected cells and cells bearing MHC antigens different from those of the host.

The interactions between these different T-cell subpopulations are integrated in a functional loop in which helper/inducer T cells participate at different levels in the sequence of events that leads to the differentiation of antibody-producing B cells, cytotoxic T cells, and delayed hypersensitivity effector cells. Suppressor T cells, on the opposite side of the loop, represent the negative feedback mechanism that will turn off the helper/inducer circuit when the antigenic stimulus has been eliminated (Fig. 10.4). Further progess in this area remained very slow, because for many years the only known T-cell marker was the T cell's ability to form rosettes with sheep red blood cells (SRBC). This marker identified most of the T cells but gave no major clue concerning their function. With the development of monoclonal antibodies specific for T cells and their subsets in mice and humans, our whole understanding of T-cell heterogeneity improved considerably. The number and source of monoclonal antibodies identifying different membrane markers on human T cells has grown very rapidly, and this is an area of considerable complexity at present. Not only has a variety of different markers been identified, but each differentiation marker is a complex antigen expressing many different determinants or epitopes so that monoclonal antibodies raised in different laboratories often recognize slightly different forms of the same molecule. In an attempt to standardize the nomenclature, scientists meeting in a series of World Health Organization workshops agreed to designate all different epitopes of a given-T cell marker molecule by the initials CD for cluster of differentiation markers. For instance, the designation CD1 applies to the CD1 molecule and the designation $CD1^+$ to a T cell expressing this molecule on its membrane, as recognized by any monoclonal antibody directed against any of the known epitopes of CD1. It also became clear that T-cell subset markers were similar in all mammals, and it has become commonly accepted to designate helper cells at $CD4^+$ and cytotoxic/suppressor T cells as $CD8^+$, regardless of the mammalian species in which they are found. These markers have allowed not only the identification of T-cell subsets but also the study of T-cell ontogeny.

B. Membrane Markers in T-Cell Ontogeny

The ontogenic differentiation of T-cell subpopulations is associated with important changes in the distribution of membrane markers (summarized in Figure 10.5 for human intrathymic differentiation).

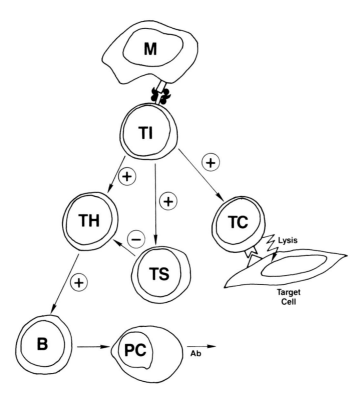

FIGURE 10.4 The T-cell functional loop. The macrophage (M) presents to the T-cell receptor a complex constituted by a class II MHC antigen and processed antigen (associative recognition unit). The inducer T (TI) cell stimulates the proliferation and differentiation of helper T cells (TH), which in turn assist the proliferation and differentiation of B cells into antibody-producing plasma cells (PC), cytotoxic T cells (TC), which can directly lyse a nonself target, and suppressor T cells (TS), which provide a down-regulating signal to the T helper cells.

FIGURE 10.5 Diagrammatic representation of the antigenic changes that take place during the different steps of intrathymic differentiation of human T cells. The earliest T-cell precursor detected in the thymus originates in the bone marrow and expressed both CD1 and Tdt. These two markers disappear as the cell moves to the next stage of differentiation (state II) at which class I HLA antigens and the CD2 molecule become permanently expressed on the T cell membrane. The β chain also starts being synthesized at this stage, but it remains intracytoplasmic. To undergo the following differentiation stage (stage III) the T-cell precursors need to establish intimate contact with the thymic epithelium (which expresses both class I and class II MHC). The CD4 molecule is retained by T-cell precursors establishing contact with MHC II molecules, and CD8 is retained by T-cell precursors establishing contact with MHC-I molecules. In this stage the α chain of the T-cell receptor begins to be synthesized, and the T-cell-receptor-CD3 complex is expressed on the T-cell precursors membrane.

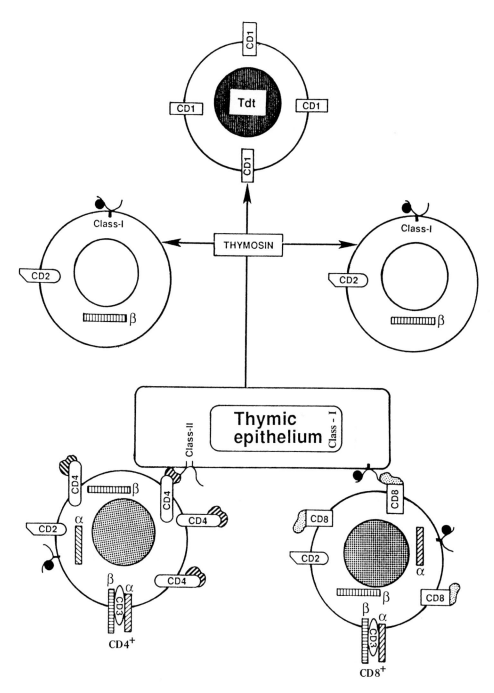

1. *Some markers disappear*: Markers are found on precursor thymocytes, which are abundant in the cortical area of the thymus but absent from most of the thymocytes that have matured and reached the medullary area. The specific markers for precursor thymocytes include the TL (thymus-leukemia) antigen in mice, equivalent to CD1 (previously named T6) in humans, and the nuclear enzyme TdT. Neither CD1-T6 nor TdT are expressed in normal adult differentiated cells but they may be detected again on leukemic cells. In other words, the genes coding for these markers are not deleted from the genome, but their expression is repressed in normal mature T cells.

2. *Other markers appear* when the thymocyte reaches further stages of differentiation and will henceforth be found on a large proportion of maturing T lymphocytes. The CD2 marker appears first. It belongs to a group of molecules playing important functions in cell-cell interactions, which for that reason are named immune cell adherence molecules or *ICAMs*. These behave as complementary molecules, which, through receptor-ligand types of interactions, allow cells to interact. The ligand to which CD2 binds is the LFA3 molecule present on many cells: antigen-presenting cells, B cells, erythrocytes, and endothelial cells. The binding between CD2 and an LFA3-like molecule present on sheep erythrocytes is the basis for rosette formation. As the T-lymphocyte precursors approach maturation, they start expressing the gene products of the major histocompatibility complex (MHC). The differentiated T cells that leave the thymus express only class I MHC antigens, but some subpopulations of T cells express class II MHC antigens after activation.

3. *Divergence of markers to nonoverlapping T-cell subsets*: A turning point in ontogeny is the appearance of the CD4 and CD8 molecules on cells that did not express them previously. The intimate contact established by the developing T cells and the MHC molecules expressed by thymic endothelium is believed to be the driving force for the selective expression of these molecules on certain cells and not on others. Experiments performed in mice have shown that if the expression of class I MHC antigens is blocked by monoclonal antibodies injected during pregnancy, the newborn animal will fail to express CD8$^+$ cells but will express an increased percentage of CD4$^+$ cells. Conversely, if class II antigens are blocked with monoclonal antibodies, the newborns are deficient in CD4$^+$ cells but show an increased percentage of CD8$^+$ cells. These experiments indicate that contact with MHC class II expressing thymic cells is necessary for the differentiation of CD4$^+$ cells and that contact with MHC class I expressing cells is necessary for the development of CD8$^+$ cells. This reflects the basic function of the CD4 and CD8 molecules expressed by mature T cells, which seems to be to allow interactions with other cells expressing MHC antigens. Therefore, the CD4 and CD8 molecules can be considered as ICAMs specific for MHC molecules. Intrathymically, many lymphocyte precursors coexpress CD4 and CD8, but most of those cells seem to die in situ. Eventually, two nonoverlapping sub-

populations emerge, one expressing CD4 and the other CD8, which correspond, in broad terms, to helper T cells (CD4$^+$) and cytotoxic/suppressor T cells (CD8$^+$). The maturation of these two subsets is complete only when the CD3 molecule is expressed. As we shall discuss later in this chapter, the CD3 molecule is an essential component of the antigen receptor on T lymphocytes.

III. THE ANTIGEN-SPECIFIC T-CELL RECEPTOR

A. The Nature of the T-Cell Receptor

Considerable research has been concentrated on determining which structure is used by T cells to recognize antigens, why the antigens recognized by T cells have to be *cell-associated*, and how the very large number of T-cell clones with receptors of different specifities necessary to respond to any antigenic challenge is generated. According to the clonal selection theory, at birth or shortly thereafter every individual has a full implement of immunocytes able to respond to any and all antigens. In the case of antigen-recognition by T cells, it has been established that it takes place only when the antigens are associated to class I MHC molecules expressed on the membrane of target cells or to class II MHC molecules expressed on the membrane of antigen-presenting cells. As it became technically possible to isolate the antigen-specific portion of the T-cell receptor, it became obvious that it was constituted by a heterodimer with two unequal chains, designated as α (acidic) and β (basic), covalently linked to the CD3 molecule. There is good experimental evidence suggesting that the CD3 molecule is part of a transducing system without which the binding of antigen to the corresponding binding sites of the T-cell receptor does not result in T-cell stimulation.

Using strategies similar to those developed in the studies of the molecular genetics of immunoglobulin genes, the genes coding for the α and β chains of the T-cell receptor (TcR) were identified. It became obvious that although the immunoglobulin genes and the TcR genes are extremely different in their structure, the same basic mechanisms are used to generate the diversity of binding sites necessary in the two types of molecules. Similarly to immunoglobulin genes, TcR genes undergo rearrangements though deletions of noncoding sequences and joining of segments of noncontiguous DNA, resulting eventually in the assembly of a functional receptor. The intense proliferation and DNA synthesis that takes place in the thymus is likely to reflect the extensive DNA rearrangements leading to the expression of a full array of T-cell receptor molecules. Like the genes coding for the heavy and light chains of immunoglobulin molecules, the genes coding for the two polypeptide chains that constitute the T-cell receptor are not even on the same chromosome. The genes coding the α chain are located on chromosome 14, whereas those coding for the

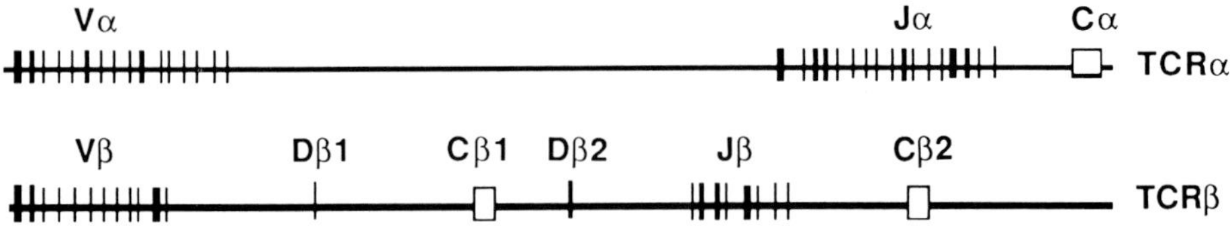

FIGURE 10.6   Genomic organization of the T-cell receptor genes. In their genomic configuration the segments constituting the α and β genes are located in noncontiguous areas, which are brought together during the differentiation process. The most significant difference between them is that the β genes include two constant regions (Cβ1 and Cβ2) and a D region, whereas the genes coding for the α chain lack a D region and have a single C region.

β chain are on chromosome 7. In their germ-line configuration, the genes coding for the β chain are distributed in four noncontiguous domains that must be brought together by chromosomal rearrangements in order to allow their expression as a constant region (Fig. 10.6). The nomenclature of the T-cell receptor genes follows similar rules to that of the immunoglobulin genes. The four coding genes are designated as constant (C), diversity (D), joining (J), and variable (V); a Greek letter (α or β) is added to the capital letters designating each gene to identify the chain coded by each particular gene.

B.   Ontogeny of the T-Cell Receptor

During embryonic differentiation, the β chain genes are rearranged first. The process is initiated by an incomplete rearrangement that brings together the Cβ and Dβ genes. This is rapidly followed by DβJβ rearrangements, and eventually the Vβ gene is brought together with the rearranged CβDβJβ. At this time, complete β chains can be detected in the T-cell cytoplasm. The prothymocyte expressing cytoplasmic β chains is homologous to a pre-B cell expressing only cytoplasmic μ chains. The genes coding for the α chain are rearranged later; the most significant difference between the genes coding for the α and β chains is that there is no D region for the α chain.

In a particular T-cell clone specific for a given epitope, the DNA sequence of the variable region of the TcR is unique. Calculations similar to those made to estimate the diversity of immunoglobulin genes were made to assess the potential diversity of the T-cell repertoire, and similar conclusions were reached. The number of recombinations between different V and DJ segments indicates that T cells should be able to recognize at least 1×10^8 different antigens. Therefore, a mature individual would possess at least that many different T-cell clones. Proof that the TcR genes contain the information necessary to generate antigen recognition sites was provided by experiments in which completely rearranged α and β chain genes were transfected into nonlymphoid cells. The transfected genes were normally expressed, and the cell expressing their products became able to be stimulated by the proper antigen-MHC complex. This type of experiment also provided that the T-cell receptor does not recognize self-MHC unless the MHC molecule has been modified by the binding of a processed or endogenous antigen.

Given the random nature of the DNA rearrangements occurring during intrathymic proliferation, it can be assumed that self-reactive T cells will emerge carrying receptors that bind to their own unmodified HLA molecules. These cells are not expressed after ontogenic differentiation, and therefore a mechanism ensuring their elimination from the T-cell repertoire or their functional suppression must exist. In other words, the organism considers the rearrangements leading to autoreactive antigen receptors as nonproductive, and the clones expressing them are aborted or suppressed; in contrast, clones that do not respond to unmodified self HLA are considered useful and conserved. The mechanisms responsible for this selection are unknown, but direct contact of the differentiating T cell with thymic interstitial cells appears to play a crucial role.

C. The Mature T-Cell Receptor

Once both α and β genes have been rearranged, the first major step necessary for the expression of their products on the cell membrane has been accomplished. However, a second essential step needs to take place to allow expression of the α/β heterodimer on the T-cell membrane. The α/β heterodimer has to become covalently linked to the CD3 molecule by disulfide bridges joining the two molecules. The importance of this association is well illustrated by the fact that genetic defects in the expression of the CD3 molecule are associated with T-cell deficiencies caused by lack of expression of functional heterodimers.

Figure 10.7 illustrates the structure of the antigen-specific T-cell receptor on a CD8[+] cytotoxic T cell and a hypothetical view of the interactions that take place between the T-cell receptor and the MHC-antigen complex of (for example) a virus-infected cell. According to the concept illustrated in this figure, the α/β heterodimer interacts with the complex formed by the viral antigen and the groove of an HLA molecule. A similar interaction is believed to occur between CD4[+] lymphocytes and antigen-presenting cells, involving processed antigen complexed with a class II MHC molecule. The interaction between the T-cell receptor and the MHC-associated antigen is unstable and needs to be strengthened by other interactions with accessory molecules.

These secondary interactions with accessory molecules are not antigen-specific and involve proteins present on both T-cell subsets and their ligands expressed on target cells and APC. The complex interactions established between these molecules bring the cells in close contact and appear to be required for the

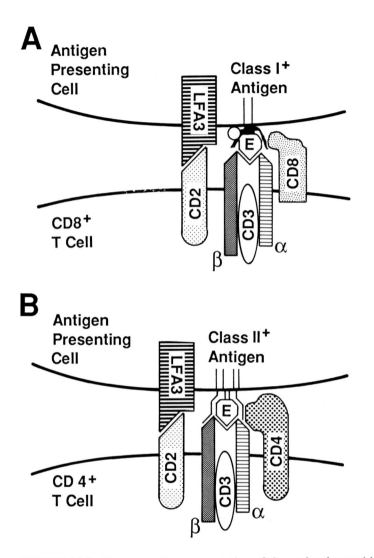

FIGURE 10.7 Diagrammatic representation of the molecules used by CD8[+] (A) and CD4[+] (B) T cells in their interactions with target cells and with antigen-presenting cells. In both situations the epitope (E) of a processed antigen is presented after it has become associated to MHC I (association recognized by CD8[+] cells) or to MHC II (association recognized by CD4[+] cells). The association of processed antigen and MHC interacts with the TcR heterodimer-CD3 complex. At that point the affinity of the interaction between CD2 and LFA3 increases, resulting in an additional activating signal to the T cell.

proper antigenic stimulation of T cells as well as for T-cell-mediated cytotoxicity. In most cases the interactions stabilize the cell-to-cell contact while other molecules are involved in signaling. For example, the CD2 molecule expressed by all T cells seems to play a crucial role in T-cell stimulation. The natural ligand for CD2 is the LFA3 molecule widely expressed by many cells including APC, but the interaction between CD2 and LFA3 is strong only when the TcR-CD3 complex is already engaged in an interaction with the antigen-HLA complex. At that point the CD2-LFA3 interaction delivers a second activating signal to the T cell that synergizes with the one provided by the engagement of the TcR-CD3 complex.

IV. MATURE T-CELL SUBSETS

All mature resting T lymphocytes carry the CD3-associated α/β heterodimer, the CD2 marker, class I MHC, and either CD4 or CD8. In a normal adult, CD4$^+$ lymphocytes represent about 50 to 60% of the mononuclear cells circulating in the peripheral blood, 10 to 25% of the rest being CD8$^+$ lymphocytes. The remaining 10 to 20% of circulating mononuclear cells includes B lymphocytes, monocytes, and natural killer cells (Fig. 10.8).

The T-cell populations carrying the CD4 and CD8 antigens are heterogeneous. Among CD8$^+$ cells, cytotoxic and suppressor T cells are functionally distinct subsets. The CD4$^+$ cells can now be subdivided by monoclonal antibodies into two subsets, each one bearing a specific marker in addition to the CD4 molecule. One of the CD4 subsets is in charge of assisting the differentiation of cytotoxic and suppressor T cells (designated as the *suppressor inducer* CD4 subset). The second subset is in charge of assisting the differentiation of helper T cells, which in turn will assist B cells to produce immunoglobulins (designated as the *helper inducer* CD4 subset).

V. MONOCYTES

Very little is known concerning the differentiation pathway of the monocytes. They are continuously produced in the bone marrow and enter the peripheral circulation, where they are identifiable by (1) the presence on their membrane of large numbers of Fcγ receptors as well as of class I and class II MHC antigens, (2) their ability to adhere to plastic and glass surfaces, and (3) the presence in their cytoplasm of lysosomal granules that allow them to digest engulfed bacteria and to process antigens.

The capacity to adhere to plastic and glass surfaces is paralleled in vivo by the ability of monocytes to adhere to endothelial cells. This enables the monocytes to exit the capillaries and enter the tissues where they reach their final differentiation stage. Indeed, it is believed that circulating monocytes eventually

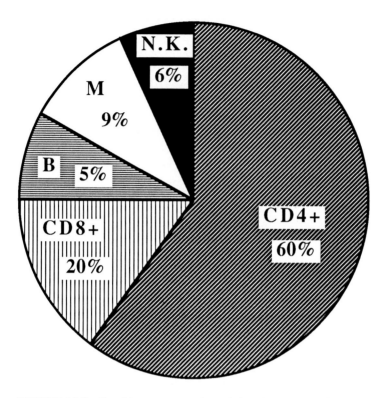

FIGURE 10.8 Graphic representation of the distribution of cell populations among peripheral blood mononuclear cells.

home into various organs to become tissue-bound macrophages and antigen-presenting cells in virtually every organ and tissue of the body: dendritic cells in the spleen and lymph nodes, Langerhans cells in the skin, Kupfer cells in the liver, microglial cells in the central nervous system.

The phagocytic ability of most antigen-presenting cells is rather limited, compared to that of neutrophils, but they are capable of receptor-mediated endocytosis and can process antigen in the acid endosomal compartment. The endocytosis process is associated with a marked increase in the expression of MHC I and MHC II molecules, to which the processed antigen becomes associated.

Most antigen-presenting cells express a molecule very similar to CD4, slightly smaller in size than the T lymphocyte CD4 molecule, but similar enough to be recognized by the same monoclonal antibodies. The density of CD4 molecules on APC is about 1/30th of the density in CD4[+] T cells. The significance of this low-level expression of CD4 on monocytes and APC is unknown, but this feature, shared with helper T cells, makes both cell populations susceptible to HIV infection, because the virus uses the CD4 molecule as receptor (see Chapter 30).

VI. NATURAL KILLER CELLS

Natural killer or NK cells, whose function will be discussed in Chapter 11, have a still controversial ontogeny because they express both monocytic and T-cell membrane markers (the CD8 molecule). It is also possible that more than one cell subpopulation may function as NK, therefore confusing even more any attempts to establish their ontogeny. Although the mechanism of target recognition by NK cells is not antigen-specific, recent data suggests that they express a membrane heterodimer similar to the TcR. The significance of this unique type of TcR-like molecule is unknown.

VII. APPENDIX

A. The Development of Monoclonal Antibodies

The surface of each of the various subpopulations or subsets of cells that participate in the immune response is the site where particular membrane glycoproteins (immunological markers) will be found, indicating that a particular cell (1) has reached a distinct stage in *differentiation*, and (2) has a specific *function*. These markers behave as antigens in a species different from that in which they are found. For example, membrane antigens of human lymphocytes are immunogeneic in other mammals. Early studies of T-lymphocyte ontogeny in humans suggested a marked heterogeneity among the otherwise homogeneous small T-lymphocyte population. Progress in this field was very slow; only a few laboratories in the world raised polyclonal antihuman T-cell antibodies of defined specificity.

In 1975 Kohler and Milstein published a fundamental report showing that by fusing a malignant cell with a non-antibody-producing B lymphocyte, they could form a hybrid cell (hybridoma) that would constantly proliferate, like a malignant cell, but at the same time would conserve the antibody-producing ability of the single B cell involved in the fusion. As shown in Fig. 10.9, this was possible because the malignant cell, a plasmocytoma variant, had lost both its immunoglobulin-secreting ability and an enzyme, the hypoxanthine guanine phosphoribosyltransferase (HGPRT) that allows cells to synthesize purines from hypoxanthine. A normal mouse injected with an extract of human T-cell membranes will produce antibodies against the very heterogeneous mixture of antigens present in those cell membranes. A very large number of B-cell clones will appear, each clone producing a single antibody against one of the antigens, but

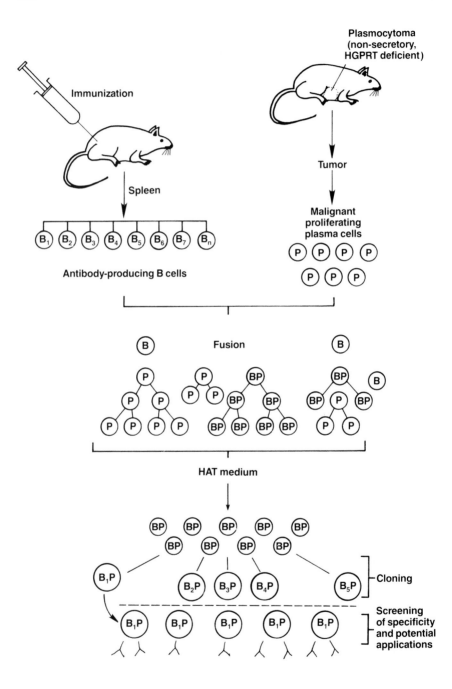

they will survive in culture only a few days unless they are fused with malignant nonsecretory and HGPRT-deficient plasmacytoma cells; this can be achieved in several different ways, the most popular being the use of polyethylene glycol to promote cell fusion. The fused B cell will provide the hybridoma with the capacity to produce a specific antibody and the capacity to produce HGPRT, the fused plasmocytoma cell will provide the hybridoma with the capacity to proliferate indefinitely. The nonfused malignant plasmocytoma cells, still HGPRT deficient, are easily killed by growing them in a medium (HAT) containing hypoxanthine (which these cells cannot utilize to synthesize purines) and aminopterine (which blocks the remaining intracellular pathways for the synthesis of purines). The nonfused B cells will be unable to survive after a few rounds of proliferation. Then a lengthy screening process begins whose aim is to select from the large number of hybrids produced by fusion those clones that produce antibody against antigens of interest. This cloning process involves the preparation of limiting dilutions that will ensure that single cells are seeded into individual receptacles containing tissue culture medium and allowed to grow into clones producing antibody of a single specificity (monoclonal antibody). Large quantities of the monoclonal antibodies generated in this fashion can be obtained, tested, and eventually used for diagnostic purposes and in some experimental therapeutic protocols.

SELF-EVALUATION

Questions

Choose the one best answer.

10.1 The earliest marker of B-cell differentiation is
      A. DNA rearrangement.
      B. Cytoplasmic IgM.
      C. Membrane IgD.
      D. Membrane IgM.
      E. The synthesis of light chains.

FIGURE 10.9 Schematic representation of the major steps involved in hybridoma production. First, antibody-producing lymphocytes are fused with nonsecretory malignant plasma cells, deficient in hypoxantine guanine phosphorybosil transferase (HGPRT). Nonfused lymphocytes will not proliferate, and nonfused plasma cells will die in a hipoxantine-rich medium (HAT). The HGPRT-deficient plasma cells cannot detoxify hypoxantine, while the hybrid cells have HGPRT provided by the antibody-producing B lymphocytes. The surviving hybrids are cloned by limiting dilution, and the resulting clones are tested for the specificity and potential value of the antibodies produced.

10.2 Human suppressor/cytotoxic T cells are identified by monoclonal anti-
bodies against the cluster of differentiation antigens designated as
A. CD8.
B. CD4.
C. CD3.
D. CD2.
E. CD1.

10.3 A fully differentiated T cell will be negative in a test to detect
A. Adenosine deaminase (ADA).
B. Terminal deoxyribonucleotidyl transferase (TdT).
C. Purine nucleoside phosphorylase (PNP).
D. Class I HLA antigens.
E. Ligands for LFA-3.

10.4 In hybridoma production, the specificity of a monoclonal antibody is
ensured by
A. Careful purification of the antigen.
B. Careful selection of the cells to be fused.
C. Incubation in HAT medium.
D. Preparation of limiting dilutions to ensure clonal proliferation.
E. Antigenic stimulation of the cells grown in tissue culture medium.

10.5 The α/β heterodimer of the T-cell receptor
A. Is covalently associated to class I MHC molecules.
B. Interacts with the CD2 molecule.
C. Is covalently associated to the CD3 molecule.
D. Is the first mature T-cell marker expressed on differentiating T cells.
E. Has a considerably lesser degree of heterogeneity than the B cells' mem-
brane immunoglobulins.

10.6 B cells do not express
A. CD2.
B. Class I MHC antigens.
C. Class II MHC antigens.
D. CR2.
E. LFA-3.

10.7 The CD4 molecule
A. Is expressed by antigen-presenting cells.
B. Is a functional marker of cytotoxic cells.
C. Is the receptor for the Epstein-Barr virus.
D. Is coexpressed with the CD8 molecule in about 10% of peripheral blood
lymphocytes in a normal adult.
E. Interacts with class I MHC molecules.

10.8 The first synthetic product of a B cell is
   A. IgM.
   B. IgD.
   C. μ chains.
   D. κ chains.
   E. J chains.

10.9 After birth, human B-lymphocyte differentiation takes place in the
   A. Bone marrow.
   B. Liver.
   C. Gut-associated lymphoid tissue.
   D. Spleen germinal center.
   E. Peyer's patches.

10.10 As a consequence of thymosin action, T cells
   A. Become $CD1^-, CD4^+$.
   B. Express the CD2 antigen.
   C. Become ADA-positive.
   D. Rearrange their chromosomal DNA.
   E. Become TdT-negative.

Answers

10.1 (A) DNA is rearranged to bring together a VDJ unit ready to be trans-
           scribed and processed into an mRNA coding the synthesis of μ
           chains.

10.2 (A)

10.3 (B) All other markers listed are found in normal, fully differentiated T
           cells.

10.4 (D) No matter how purified the antigen is, many different clones of anti-
           body-producing cells will be stimulated by the wide variety of epi-
           topes contained by the antigen. After fusion and elimination of
           nonfused cells, limiting dilutions are used to separate single cells
           and allow them to proliferate into antibody-producing clones,
           which, by deriving from a single cell, synthesize molecules of a single
           specificity.

10.5 (C) The T-cell receptor for antigen is constituted by the α/β heterodimer
           covalently linked to the CD3 molecule. The variable regions in-
           volved in antigen-binding are located in the α/β heterodimer, while
           the CD3 molecule seems to transduce the signals generated on the
           antigen-binding site to the cytoplasm.

10.6 (A) The CD2 molecule, which is the natural ligand for LFA-3, is expressed by T cells but not by B cells.

10.7 (A) The CD4 molecule, which identifies the helper-T-cell subpopulation, is never coexpressed with CD8 in differentiated lymphocytes, but it is also expressed by antigen-presenting cells.

10.8 (C) Before IgM is found on the cell membrane, intracytoplasmic μ chains can be detected in B-cell precursors.

10.9 (A) Plasma cells apparently can differentiate in the germinal centers of lymphoid organs, but resting B cells differentiate in the bone marrow.

10.10(E).

BIBLIOGRAPHY

Allison, J. P. and Lanier, L. L. Structure, function, and serology of the T-cell antigen receptor complex. *Ann. Rev. Immunol. 5*:503, 1987.
Bierer, B. E. and Burakoff, S. J. T cell adhesion molecules. *FASEB J 2*:2584, 1988.
Boyse, E. A. and Cantor, H. Surface characteristics of T-lymphocyte subpopulations. In *The Biology of Immunologic Disease*, F. J. Dixon and D. W. Fisher (Eds.). Sinauer, Sunderland, Massachusetts, 1983.
Hood, L. E., Weissman, I. L., Wood, W. B., and Wilson, J. H. *Immunology*, 2nd Ed. Benjamin/Cummings Publishing Co., Menlo Park, California, 1984. (Includes the section "Development of the Immune System," in which both ontogeny and cell markers are discussed.)
Scharff, M. D., Roberts, S., and Thammana, P. Hybridomas as source of antibodies. In *The Biology of Immunologic Disease*, F. J. Dixon and D. W. Fisher (Eds.). Sinauer, Sunderland, Massachusetts, 1983.
Paul, W. E. (Ed.). *Fundamental Immunology*. Raven Press, New York, 1984. (Contains the section "The Cells of the Immune System," in which ontogeny and membrane markers are discussed in detail.)

11

Cell-Mediated Immunity

JEAN-MICHEL GOUST

We have seen in previous chapters that lymphocytes are organized into several subpopulations with different attributes that collaborate in complex regulatory and effector circuits. From studies with experimental animals and from clinical observations with immunodeficient patients, it became obvious that immune responses can be broadly subdivided into humoral (antibody-mediated) and cellular (cell-mediated). As a rule, humoral mechanisms are prevalent in the elimination of soluble antigens and the destruction of extracellular microorganisms, while cell-mediated immunity is more efficient when the elimination of intracellular organisms (such as viruses) is the objective of the immune response. This dichotomy obviously oversimplifies the facts, by ignoring that in many instances the humoral response depends on the help of T lymphocytes and that some types of effector cells depend on antibodies for target selection. But with these reservations in mind, the division of immune mechanisms and responses into cellular and humoral has persisted, partly because of its broad practical application, partly because of its didactic usefulness. In the next two chapters we shall discuss the main features of these two types of immune phenomenon: those primarily mediated by T lymphocytes and those primarily mediated by antibody-producing cells.

I. DELAYED HYPERSENSITIVITY

During the mid-1960s, the existence of an immune response independent of circulating antibodies was firmly established by experiments investigating the nature of Koch's phenomenon described 70 years earlier: guinea pigs immunized with heat-killed tubercle bacilli were reinjected subcutaneously with bacterial culture supernatants from the same bacilli and showed, 24-48 h later, an area of redness and induration that in highly sensitized animals often became necrotic (delayed hypersensitivity reaction). The delay between antigenic challenge and skin changes contrasted with the immediate wheal and flare observed with substances that cause the immediate hypersensitivity reactions (such as hives and hay fever). Histologic examination of a delayed hypersensitivity lesion shows a perivenular infiltration of lymphocytes and monocytes, forming a perivascular cuff associated with local edema. The abundant cellular infiltrate explains why a delayed hypersensitivity lesion in the skin is characteristically indurated. In contrast, immediate hypersensitivity lesions are red, warm, painful, but soft to the touch, and histologically they show periarteriolar accumulation of granulocytes and extracellular edema. Experimental studies demonstrated that while immediate hypersensitivity reactions could be elicited in unsensitized animals after injection of serum from a sensitized animal, delayed hypersensitivity reactions could not be transferred with serum but only with live lymphocytes from the sensitized animal. These observations first identified a specific type of immune response that was mediated by T lymphocytes. With time, it became obvious that T lymphocytes play a key role not only as effector cells of hypersensitivity but also as inducers of both cellular and humoral immune responses and as major effector cells in the destruction of virus-infected cells.

II. ANTIGEN PRESENTATION AND THE ONSET OF THE IMMUNE RESPONSE

Early observations showed that T cells cannot respond to soluble, unmodified antigens to which the B-cell system obviously responds, because antibodies binding to the native antigens can easily be demonstrated after immunization. This difference between T and B cells remained puzzling for a very long time but is now explained by the fact that T cells recognize only antigens associated to self MHC molecules; most soluble antigens cannot bind to MHC molecules until they are processed by monocytes/macrophages. After the antigen is processed, its tertiary structure is profoundly modified (to the point that any resemblance with the tertiary structure of the native antigen may be totally lost), and the processed antigenic fragments become associated with self MHC II molecules expressed by all antigen-presenting cells (APC). It is this association that, as discussed in Chapter 10, will be recognized by the T-cell receptor and deliver the specific signal necessary to stimulate the T lymphocyte. The T lymphocyte, therefore, recognizes processed antigens whose structure is totally different from that on the native antigen.

The ingestion and processing of antigens are associated with the activation of several functions in APCs. One of the effects of this activation is the secretion of the first of the interleukins that participate in the induction of the immune response; the first interleukin released by APCs is designated as interleukin 1 (IL1). This small protein (MW 12,000-17,000) is produced during the early phase of infections and will contribute significantly to the mobilization of a series of components of what is known as the acute phase response.

A. Biological Activity of IL1

Interleukin 1 diffuses freely through the blood brain barrier and rapidly exerts a number of effects on the central nervous system. By interacting with cells of a group of nuclei in the anterior hypothalamus, IL1 causes an increase in body temperature (fever) and sleep as well as an increased production of ACTH. IL1 also contributes to the leukocytosis associated with most bacterial infections by acting as growth factor on the bone marrow. It is also a chemotactic factor on neutrophils and induces the release of their enzymatic contents. IL1 has many other general metabolic effects, many of them shared with another cytokine, produced by the same antigen-presenting cells, known as *cachectin* or *tumor necrosis factor* α (TNFα) (see later in this chapter).

B. IL1 and the Immune Response

From a biological perspective, the immunologic role of IL1 appears less important than its role as a promoter of the acute phase reaction. IL1 is the first of a series of second signals necessary but not sufficient to induce proliferation of antigen-primed murine and human T and B lymphocytes. All interleukins that act on T cells, including IL1, act as cofactors in T-cell activation; by themselves they are unable to activate T cells. This is another example of the complex system of checks and balances controlling the activation of the immune system. If IL1 alone could activate T cells, any inflammation would trigger unneeded T-cell proliferation.

C. Role of CD4$^+$ Lymphocytes at the Onset of the Immune Response

The essential role of CD4$^+$lymphocytes in assisting the induction of immune responses has been dramatically demonstrated in AIDS patients whose CD4$^+$ cells are numerically depleted and functionally impaired as a consequence of infection by the human immunodeficiency virus (HIV). As a consequence of the lack of functional $CD4^+$ (helper) T cells, HIV-infected patients become eventually unable to mount both cellular and humoral immune responses (see Chapter 30).

The CD4 molecule, which, as stated earlier, is expressed by the helper-T-cell population, plays a crucial role in the normal immune response, helping to establish stable interactions between the $CD4^+$ T cells and the antigen-presenting cells. The $CD4^+$ cells use their antigen-specific receptor to recognize processed antigen associated with class II HLA molecules on the surface of the antigen-presenting cells. The specificity of the recognition lies with the CD3-associated α/β heterodimer; at the same time the nonpolymorphic area of the class II MHC molecule also interacts with the T-cell receptor. The interactions between helper T cell and APC are further strengthened by CD2 binding to LFA-3. In addition, this interacton delivers an activation signal to the T cell, synergistic with the signal provided by antigen-TcR interaction.

It is important to stress that the contact between a $CD4^+$ lymphocyte and an APC will not lead to T-cell activation unless the lymphocyte receives other activating signals. In other words, it is a rule without exception that T cells require more than one signal to proliferate. The first change triggered by the contact of the processed antigen with the T-cell receptor is a sharp rise in intracellular calcium concentration because of the opening of a CD3-associated calcium channel. However, unless additional signals are delivered to the T cell at this stage the response will not progress. These signals are mainly delivered by the soluble molecules known as interleukins; these molecules deliver signals that allow the antigen-stimulated T cell to progress towards mitosis. Interleukin 1 complements the activating effect of the binding of antigen to the T-cell receptor, but it is only after the release of a second interleukin, interleukin 2 (IL2), that T cells start to proliferate.

D. Interleukin 2

Interleukin 2 was initially known as T-cell growth factor (TCGF), a designation that underlines its main biological effect. It is a small glycoprotein (MW 15,000) with two disulfide bridges whose integrity is essential for the binding to its specific receptor on T cells. The best documented property of IL2 is to function in an autocrine loop that amplifies T-cell proliferation. $CD4^+$ cells, in the simultaneous presence of IL1 and antigenic stimulus, will, after a few hours, express two new genes that were silent before activation: the IL2 and the IL2 receptor (IL2 R) genes. Therefore, IL2 is released by and binds to the very same T-cell population. On binding IL2, the $CD4^+$ cell increases the synthesis and expression of IL2 receptors, and these receptors show an increased affinity for their ligand. DNA synthesis, proliferation, and clonal expansion of antigen-specific $CD4^+$ cells takes place as a consequence of the activation of this autocrine loop.

CELL TYPE: **CYTOKINE:** **PRINCIPAL ACTIVITY:**

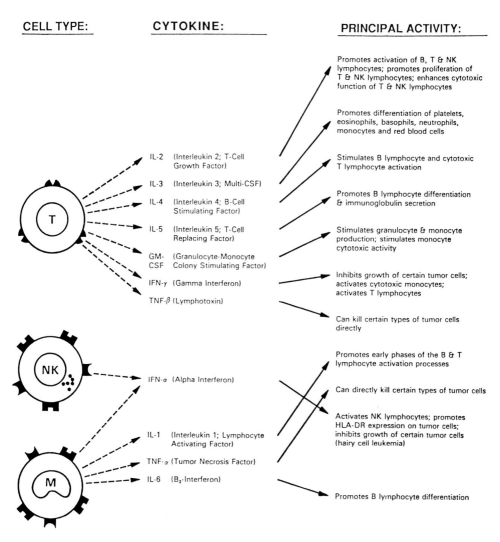

FIGURE 11.1 Diagrammatic representation of the cellular source and principal activities of the main cytokines released by lymphocytes and accessory cells.

It should be noticed that the signal provided by IL2 is not antigen-specific, but the responding T cells were originally stimulated by cell-to-cell interactions that included an antigen-specific signal. Therefore, the overall response is antigen-specific.

However, clonal expansion of CD4$^+$ cells is not the only consequence of T-cell activation: a cascade of other events ensues, reflecting the activation and expression of many other genes. Their best characterized products, interleukins 3, 4, 5, and 6 (Fig. 11.1), play very important roles in many other areas of the immune and inflammatory responses.

III. T-CELL-MEDIATED CYTOTOXICITY AGAINST VIRUS-INFECTED CELLS

The essential function of cell-mediated immunity is the defense against intracellular infectious agents, most specifically viruses. The understanding of the mechanisms used to achieve this goal has been based mainly on experimental models. The first model to provide insights was the study of cell-mediated cytotoxicity against virus-infected cells.

A. Target Cell Destruction

Splenic T lymphocytes isolated from mice that have survived an infection with lymphocytic choriomeningitis (LCM) virus destroy fibroblasts infected with this virus in 2 to 3 hours. To detect the cytotoxic effect virus-infected fibroblasts are labeled with chromium^{51} (^{51}Cr). This isotope diffuses across the membrane into viable cells and remains in the cytoplasm until the cell membrane is altered. If the cell is damaged by a cytotoxic reaction, the cell membrane becomes more permeable and ^{51}Cr diffuses back into the extracellular medium where it can be detected and measured. The steps leading to the target cell death are very well known (Fig. 11.2): CD8$^+$ effector T lymphocytes strongly adhere to their target, which disintegrates 30 min to 4 h later. The cytotoxic T cell, still viable after this first hit, moves on to destroy other targets. As these studies developed, a very puzzling fact emerged: to achieve optimal efficiency, target and effector CD8$^+$ T cells had to express identical MHC antigens (Table 11.1).

B. CD8 Binding is MHC-Restricted

The above-described results compelled immunologists to create a series of designations such as "associative recognition," "MHC restriction," and "cognate interaction" to indicate that cytotoxic T cells recognize the association of a histocompatibility antigen and a viral antigen on the virally altered target cell.

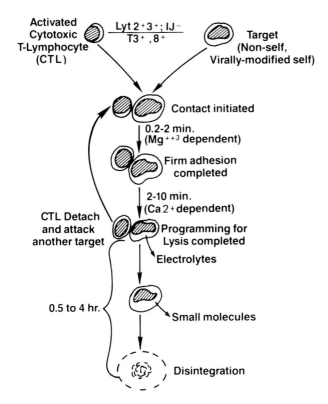

FIGURE 11.2 Mechanism of T-cell-mediated cytotoxicity. Notice that an activated cytotoxic $(CD8^+)$ T cell is able to kill several targets.

TABLE 11.1 Influence of MHC Background on Antigen-Specific Cytotoxicity

MHC type of infected target cells	MHC type of cytotoxic T cell	$\%\ ^{51}Cr$ release
k	k	64
d	k	3
b	k	4

Source: Modified from Zinkernagel, R. M. and Doherty, P. C., *Nature 251*: 547, 1974.

Although not all the steps involved in associative recognition are known, particularly in humans, the molecular mechanisms involved in this process have been recently clarified. Intracellular infectious agents are characterized by their ability to reproduce inside host cells. This is particularly true in the case of viruses, which use the cell's synthetic machinery to synthesize their own proteins and enzymes. During viral replication antigenic oligopeptides (as small as 7 or 8 amino acids in length) are generated and released into the endoplasmic reticulum, where they encounter newly synthesized HLA class-I antigens in the process of reaching the cell membrane. A complex is formed between these small epitopes and HLA class I, which is eventually inserted in the infected cell's membrane. In the case of nonreplicating antigens that are engulfed and processed by APC, it is believed that small peptides generated in the phagosomes bind to MHC II molecules already expressed in the phagosome membrane and later transported in association with the class II molecule into the cell membrane. Crystallographic studies of human HLA-A2 antigen (see Chapter 3) suggest that these antigenic oligopeptides probably bind in the groove seen in the most polymorphic area of the HLA-A molecule (Fig. 3.3). A similar binding groove is believed to exist in MHC class II antigens.

Because of the extensive genetic polymorphism of MHC molecules, the number of potential binding sites for epitopes is relatively large, but a given individual will express only those markers that he inherited from his parents. Considering the allotypic MHC specificities only, a heterozygous individual could, at best, express twelve different antigens (2 for each class I locus and 2 for each class II locus). Even if additional loci are discovered, the repertoire of MHC binding sites defined by MHC alloantigens will remain always numerically restricted. However, many MHC specificities (the so-called "public" or "shared" specificities) are shared by large proportions of the population. It has been postulated that these public specificities of the HLA system provide binding sites for the "aggretopes" of common antigens, so that most individuals would be able to initiate protective immune responses against common infectious agents. The affinity of the binding of aggretopes to HLA molecules may be the molecular basis for high versus low responsiveness to a given antigen. In high responders, the fit of a particular aggretope with self HLA would be of high affinity, while low responders may not express the HLA antigen with the best fit for that particular aggretope.

Once this self + X complex is expressed on the infected cell's membrane, it is recognized by the antigen specific receptor of the CD8[+] cells, which is as exquisitely specific as the immunoglobulin binding sites. Indeed, a CD8[+] cell sensitized to a specific virus subtype will not kill a target cell infected with a virus whose antigenic proteins differ from those of the sensitizing virus by as few as 2 amino acids. This is why efficient vaccination against viruses expressing many different serotypes or mutating very rapidly is so difficult, because each different subtype needs to be recognized independently by different T- and B-cell clones.

The interaction between virus-infected cells and T cells is complicated in that cells behave as moving spheres in a liquid environment and are unlikely to remain in close contact unless held by multiple bonds. However, in vitro experiments showed that once a CD8$^+$ T cell was attached to its target, the binding is so strong that the cells literally had to be torn apart to be separated. The self + X complex is rather small, and if the CD8$^+$ T cell is attached to the target by this single small area, the link between the two cells would be very unstable. Two more connections are needed to achieve strong binding: (1) the CD8$^+$ molecule itself interacts with the nonpolymorphic part of the MHC class I molecule, and (2) the CD2 molecule present on all T cells interacts with the LFA3 molecules present on most cells. Any resting T cell can interact with LFA3-expressing cells, but this interaction *by itself* is also weak and does not lead to cell activation. There is evidence suggesting that after T cells are activated via the CD3-associated antigen receptor, the CD2 molecules is somewhat modified and the binding affinity towards LFA3 increases. In any case, a cytotoxic reaction cannot take place unless both MHC + Ag/TcR and CD2/LFA-3 interactions take place simultaneously. Once the attachment of the CD8$^+$ cell to its target is firm, the granules present in cytotoxic T cells will move toward the binding site, fuse with the cytoplasmic membrane, and empty their contents in the space between the cytotoxic T cells and target cells. These granules contain proteins with enzymatic activity (mostly esterases) that cross-react immunologically with the C9 component of the complement (see Chapter 9). Known as perforins, these proteins polymerize as soon as they are released, forming polyperforins, which in turn are inserted into the cell membrane. The membrane-inserted polyperforins constitute transmembrane channels through which intracellular ions are lost to the extracellular environment, resulting in cell death.

C. Amplification of Preexisting Clones

Antigen-specific T cells exist before antigenic exposure. When the immune system is at rest, cytotoxic T cells are just inactive precursors, and the number of cells able to respond to any given antigen is low ($<1/10^5$). Proliferation and differentiation are absolutely needed to generate a sufficient number of fully active effector CD8$^+$ T cells. When it became possible to separate CD8$^+$ cells from the other T cells it was observed that contact between a CD8$^+$ cell and either a virus-infected target or a cell bearing a different MHC antigen does not trigger CD8$^+$ proliferation or differentiation. The differentiation and proliferation of cytotoxic T cells requires collaboration from helper T cells and their products, particularly interleukin 2 and interferon γ.

IV. NATURAL KILLER CELLS

Although CD8$^+$ T cells may start proliferating early during the incubation phase of a viral infection, an efficient antiviral response may take one to two weeks to develop. During this time the host would be defenseless if it were not for several first lines of defense against viruses. A crucial factor is the production of interferons, which is initiated as soon as the virus starts replicating. Interferons α and β, released by infected cells, induce a state of resistance in noninfected cells and in this way curtail viral replication. Also, interferon β activates natural killer (NK) cells, which specialize in the elimination of malignant or virus-infected cells. This interferon release is like a first distress call from virus-infected cells, initiating the fight against viral infection *before* the differentiation of cytotoxic T lymphocytes. NK cells are further activated by IL2, which is released as soon as CD4$^+$ T cells are stimulated. In the case of NK cells, IL2 can induce the activated state by itself; the NK cell-recognition mechanism is not antigen-specific, and perhaps because of this difference NK cell activation does not follow the rules of T-cell activation. As mentioned in Chapter 2, IL2-activated NK cells are known as lymphokine activated killer cells (LAK cells).

V. MONOCYTES

A third type of interferon, which is predominantly released by T lymphocytes, is interferon γ (IFNγ). IFNγ activates resting monocytes by itself; therefore it constitutes the second exception to the rule that T-cell products act as cofactors whose effectiveness depends on other stimuli. It is interesting to note that both exceptions apply to interleukins acting on cells that are not intrinsically endowed with specific antigen-recognition mechanisms.

IFNγ-activated monocytes rapidly become very aggressive and efficient predators. Several major changes occur in activated monocytes: (1) the number of cytoplasmic microvilli increases by a factor of ten, resulting in a considerable increase in phagocytic capacities; (2) there is also a parallel increase in the number of class II MHC antigens and Fcγ receptors per cell; the increase in the expression of HLA class II antigens enhances the efficiency of monocytes as antigen-presenting cells; (3) there is an increased production of proteolytic enzymes; as a result, engulfed cells or proteins are rapidly digested in the phagolysosomes, filled up with cathepsin B, phospholipases, collagenase, and many other proteolytic enzymes; (4) stimulated monocytes and macrophages produce high levels of tumor necrosis factor α (TNFα) and of products from both the cyclooxygenase (PGE2 and PGF2 among others) and lipooxygenase (leukotrienes) pathways of arachidonic acid. Of this last series of mediators PGE2 is particularly interesting, because of its down-regulating effects on T lymphocytes. While monocyte-released IL1 contributes to the induction of IL2 production by T lymphocytes, PGE2, secreted by the same activated monocytes, suppresses IL2 production.

Excessive and protracted production of IFNγ may have adverse effects on monocytes. Hyperstimulated monocytes tend to fuse together and form multinucleated giant cells, similar to those seen in the granulomas of tuberculosis, leprosy, sarcoidosis, and other conditions. IFNγ also induces stimulated macrophages to become exceedingly cytotoxic, and their unbridled cytotoxicity may exceed the range of the beneficial. For example, in autoimmune diseases, overactivated macrophages may mediate tissue damage.

VI. MEDIATORS ACTING ON NONLYMPHOID CELLS

The fight against a life-threatening infection is an all-out battle that mobilizes all the resources of the organism in a concerted effort in which the immune system will be a main participant. Given the significant role played by leukocytes in a variety of defense mechanisms, one of the most striking manifestations of the host response is a general mobilization of leukocytes, which is objectively reflected by peripheral blood leukocytosis. This results from the release of IL1 and IL3, which act at the bone marrow level, inducing release of leukocytes into peripheral blood. IL3, also known as multicolony stimulating factor, is produced by activated T cells. At the same time, IL1 is acting at other levels (particularly in the liver) and inducing the synthesis of a variety of proteins known as acute phase reactants. A negative protein balance will result from this intense synthetic activity. However, IL1 is not the only molecule contributing to these important metabolic changes. Activated monocytes produce two other biologically active molecules known as tumor necrosis factor α and β. TNFα is also known as cachectin, and it has many effects similar to those of IL1, contributing to establish the negative protein balance associated with infectious processes. The synergistic effects of IL1 and TNFα on protein metabolism will result in significant weight loss in a patient with a protracted infection. TNFβ, also known as lymphotoxin, is a T-cell product, a cytotoxin that contributes to the elimination of abnormal cells. As shown in Fig. 11.1, all these products are tightly linked in a complex network of mediators whose main effects are related to the elimination of infectious agents and infected or altered cells.

VII. T-CELL HELP AND THE HUMORAL IMMUNE RESPONSE

A. T-Cell Help in Antibody Production

Helper T cell function was first recognized in studies of the antibody response to sheep erythrocytes (SRBC). Mice whose immune systems had been totally ablated by exposure to sublethal x-radiation were reconstituted with either puri-

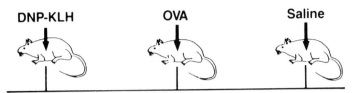

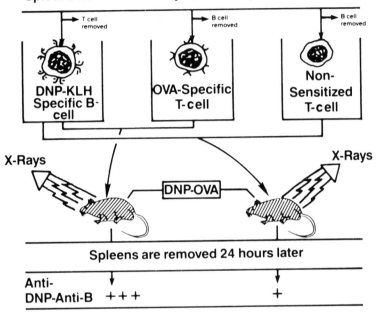

FIGURE 11.3   Helper T cells in response to DNP. Help is provided by T cells specific for the carrier molecule (which may be different from the one inducing the primary B-cell response, provided the T cells are sensitized to it).

fied B cells or purified T cells. The reconstituted mice failed to produce antibody upon immunization with SRBC. However, if the mice were reconstituted with both B and T lymphocytes they would mount an excellent anti-SRBC antibody response. The role of T cells in this antibody response was inferred to be helping the stimulation of B cells by antigen.

This type of experiment was taken a step further by measuring antibody responses to haptenic groups such as the dinitrophenyl (DNP) radical. For example, one group of mice was immunized with DNP-keyhole limpet hemocyanin (DNP-KLH), a second group with ovalbumin (OVA), and a third group (the control) received only saline (see Fig. 11.3). From these immunized animals, one would then purify T cells and B cells using a variety of techniques. If both DNP-primed B cells and OVA-primed T cells were transferred to a sublethally irradiated recipient, that animal would be able to produce anti-DNP antibody upon challenge with DNP-OVA. If the T cells were derived from a donor that had not been immunized with OVA, only a meager anti-DNP antibody response was obtained after immunization with DNP-OVA. This indicated that the antigenic specificity of the helper T lymphocyte is carrier-directed and that helper T lymphocytes exert their function best when stimulated by an antigen-carrier complex that includes a carrier to which they were previously sensitized. Furthermore, for efficient collaboration between T and B cells to occur, the antigenic determinants for which each cell type is specific must be on the same molecule. Thus an irradiated mouse reconstituted with DNP-specific B cells and OVA-specific T cells will make an anti-DNP antibody response upon challenge with DNP-OVA but will not produce anti-DNP antibodies in response to a conjugate of DNP with another protein such as bovine gamma globulin, even if unconjugated OVA is injected at the same time. This indicates that the helper effect is most efficient if the collaborating B and T cells are brought into intimate contact, as should be achieved when each cell reacts with distinct determinants on the same molecule. To demonstrate T-B cell cooperation in this type of experiment, it is essential that the T and B cells used in the reconstitution of irradiated animals are MHC identical. The easiest way to explain the collaboration of T and B lymphocytes in this model is to assume that the B cell reacts with epitopes expressed by the native antigen, including the DNP radical, while the T cell recognizes small peptides resulting from the processing of the carrier. B cells are able to process antigen, express it in association to MHC class II antigens, and release IL1. The $CD4^+$ helper/inducer T cells would then interact with the MHC II antigen complexes expressed on B cell membranes and, in turn, assist the B-cell response by releasing B-cell growth and differentiation factors (Fig. 11.4).

B. B-Cell Growth Factors (BSF-I/IL4 and BCGF-II/IL5)

Similarly to T lymphocytes, B lymphocytes require second signals in addition to the reaction with a specific antigen to undergo clonal expansion and differentiation. These additional signals are provided by interleukins, which have complex effects. Both IL4 and IL5 are physiologically released by activated T lymphocytes. The genes coding for these interleukins have been cloned, allowing their production by recombinant DNA technology. Consequently, detailed studies of the function of these interleukins have been carried out. A significant finding has been that when recombinant IL4 is added to a B-cell culture stimulated with antibodies directed to their membrane immunoglobulins (cross-linking of membrane immunoglobulins with antibodies results in the same type of

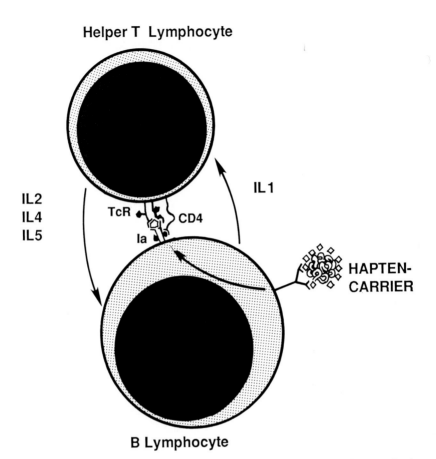

FIGURE 11.4   The interaction between B cells and T helper cells in antibody production involves a hapten-specific B cell and a carrier-specific T cell. The B cell can recognize the haptenic determinants, engulf and process the hapten-carrier complex, and present processed carrier fragments to the helper T cell. The activation of the T cell is favored by the simultaneous interaction between class II MHC antigens on the B cell and the CD4 molecule on the helper T cell. Each cell assists the other's differentiation through the release of interleukins.

cell stimulation as reaction with a polyvalent antigen), one can observe a proliferative response, and the proliferating B cells secrete mainly IgE. A second factor (BCGF-II or IL5) appears to be able to increase B-cell proliferation and selectively to induce differentiation of IgA-producing plasmablasts and plasmocytes. Therefore IL4 and IL5 act both as growth and as differentiation factors.

This differentiation involves DNA rearrangements, responsible for immuno-globulin class and subclass switching. The newly rearranged DNA segments code for different constant regions; in contrast, the genes coding for the variable regions do not undergo rearrangements as a consequence of antigenic stimulation. As a consequence of the rearrangement of the constant-region genes, the B cells will switch the isotype of immunoglobulin they produce during differentiation and proliferation, while at the same time keeping their original antigenic specificity.

C. BSF-II/IL6

Interleukin 6 is produced by antigen-presenting cells and induces the final switch from IgM to IgG secretion (Fig. 11.1). The biological effects of IL6 are not limited to B cells, but the discussion of its other effects is out of the scope of this chapter.

D. B-Cell Responses to T-Independent Antigens

Experimental studies using thymic deficient mice, lacking a functional T-cell system, proved that some antigens can induce antibody responses without T-cell help. Those T-independent antigens are usually composed of repeating units of a simple molecule; chemically, most T-independent antigens are polysaccharides. By being constituted by multiple copies of a few different sugars, the polysaccharide molecules present periodically repeated epitopes in close proximity and can induce extensive cross-linking of the membrane immunoglobulin to which they specifically bind. This type of membrane immunoglobulin cross-linking results (at least in mice) in the stimulation of a particular subset of B lymphocytes that does not require T-cell products to proliferate and differentiate into antibody-producing cells. The steps leading to full differentiation of this subset are not clear. Because immunological memory is greatly determined by T-cell help, and because the immune response to T-independent antigens does not last, the antibodies are almost exclusively of the IgM class, and there is no evidence of memory when the mice are reimmunized.

   Although the evidence for the existence of T-independent antigens in humans is not as clear-cut as it is in mice, it is known that vaccination with polysaccharides meets with considerable difficulties. This certainly can be attributed to the lack of inducement of efficient T-cell help. Antibody production against T-independent antigens is terminated by clonal exhaustion of the B cells, a process that does not secure the differentiation of long-lived memory cells.

VIII. THE ROLE OF HELPER T CELLS IN DELAYED HYPERSENSITIVITY RESPONSES

As we have previously described, it is possible to transfer delayed hypersensitivity reactions manifested in the skin by transferring spleen cells from a sensitized animal to an MHC-identical nonimmune recipient. In this system, the cells primarily involved are CD4$^+$ helper lymphocytes. Through the release of various lymphokines active on lymphoid and nonlymphoid cells, they will lead to the formation of a cellular infiltrate around the area where the T cells are reacting with the antigen. These cellular infiltrates are usually rich in lymphocytes and monocytes and are characteristic of delayed hypersensitivity reactions. The induction of delayed hypersensitivity reactions by intradermal injection of adequate antigens is a common approach to the functional testing of the T-cell system. Patients with severe deficiencies of the CD4$^+$ subset of T lymphocytes usually will not react in this type of skin test.

IX. SUPPRESSOR CELLS IN THE IMMUNE RESPONSE

The appreciation that lymphocytes can specifically terminate antibody responses was one of the most important new immunological principles introduced in the last decade. A particularly cogent example of specific suppression was obtained in studies on the regulation of the immune response of mice to keyhole limpet hemocyanin (KLH). If mice primed with KLH are later boosted with the same antigen, two weeks after the boost it is possible to separate from the mice a population of T lymphocytes that markedly suppresses the IgG anti-DNP response of genetically identical mice primed with DNP-KLH. However, this population will not suppress anti-DNP antibody production in animals immunized with DNP conjugated with a different carrier, such as bovine gamma globulin (BGG). This carrier specificity of the suppressive effect suggests that it is mediated exclusively at the T-cell level. Many other studies in mice have confirmed the existence of antigen-specific suppressor cells and suggested several possible mechanisms of action.

One of the current theories postulates that during an immune response B cell clones able to recognize the hypervariable regions of the specific antibodies are stimulated, producing anti-idiotypic antibodies. These in turn would cross-react with the antigen-binding portion of the T-cell receptor and stimulate CD8$^+$ suppressor-precursors. However, there have been so far no experiments that would suggest that this mechanism may be operational in humans. On the other hand, this theory agrees with the most commonly accepted view of T-cell suppression, which holds that suppression is a negative feedback directly exerted by activated suppressor T cells on helper T cells.

A. Induction of Suppressor Cells

In humans, our only definite knowledge is that suppression is mediated by a subset of CD8$^+$ T cells different from the cytotoxic CD8$^+$ subset. Also, the observation in AIDS patients that efficient suppressor cell activity cannot be generated even though they usually have normal percentages of suppressor cells suggests that the differentiation of suppressor T cells requires the assistance of a special subpopulation of CD4$^+$ T cells usually named the *suppressor inducer CD4$^+$ T cell.* This subset is antigenically different from the subset that assists antibody production. Therefore, at the onset of the immune response, two CD4 subsets differentiate. One is involved in helping antibody production and the second, constituted by the suppressor inducer CD4$^+$ T cells, produces IL2 and activates the suppressor CD8 cells. The activated CD8 cells express class II MHC antigens and become able to interact with CD4$^+$ helper cells. This type of contact between class II MHC molecules, expressed by the activated CD8$^+$ cells, and the CD4 molecule takes place independently of antigenic stimulation, and it is believed to down-regulate the helper T cells.

Physiologically, suppressor T cells appear at late stages of the immune response, after the antigen has been eliminated and memory lymphocytes generated. In the absence of antigen, and once long-living clones of memory T and B cells have been generated, B-cell proliferation is no longer desirable. At that point, the mobilization of suppressor T cells will serve the purpose of down-regulating the humoral response, which is no longer serving a biological purpose.

B. Suppression of Delayed Hypersensitivity Responses

The late appearance of suppressor cells has been observed also in studies of the transfer of delayed hypersensitivity reactions with live cells from immunized mice. In those experiments timing is crucial: if the donor's cells are taken 2 weeks instead of 5 days after the priming challenge, the injected recipient mice fail to acquire delayed hypersensitivity. However, if T cells are depleted before the transfer of donor cells taken after 2 weeks, the recipient mice will develop adaptive delayed hypersensitivity. This experiment is interpreted as demonstrating that two weeks after challenge the animal has developed a large population of suppressor T cells, and only after their elimination was it possible to observe the passive transfer of delayed hypersensitivity.

It has also been proven that non-antigen-specific suppressor T cells can be activated by incubation with a nonspecific mitogen, concanavalin A (ConA). These suppressor cells will prevent the activation of helper T cells by any type of antigen. The supernatant of these cultures contains a substance named the soluble immune response suppressor or SIRS, which suppresses DTH as well as humoral immune responses. Similar molecules have been described in humans, but their precise structure is not known.

SELF-EVALUATION

Questions

Choose the one best answer.

11.1 Interleukin 1
   A. Is produced by T lymphocytes.
   B. Promotes T-lymphocyte proliferation without need for another stimulus.
   C. Can be released as a result of nonspecific stimulation of the producing cell.
   D. Can act only on cells sharing identical MHC antigen with the producing cells.
   E. Is analogous to T-cell growth factor.

11.2 The effect of B-cell differentiation factor(s) on B cells is associated with
   A. Clonal expansion.
   B. DNA rearrangements.
   C. Loss of membrane immunoglobulin.
   D. Release of IL2.
   E. Permanent B-cell proliferation.

11.3 The main effect of suppressor T cells controlling the humoral immune response appears to be
   A. Suppression of the activity of $CD4^+$ cells.
   B. Suppression of IL1 release.
   C. Suppression of B-cell proliferation.
   D. Blocking of IL-2 receptors.
   E. Cytotoxic elimination of $CD4^+$ cells.

11.4 Mice from stain A, expressing antigen H2-K on their lymphocytes, were immunized with influenza virus. Seven days later, T lymphocytes from these animals were mixed with ^{51}Cr-labeled, influenza-virus-infected fibroblasts from H2-d mice. You expect to find
   A. Significant ^{51}Cr release after 5 min of incubation.
   B. Significant proliferation.
   C. Significant ^{51}Cr release after adding IL2 to the system.
   D. Significant ^{51}Cr release after adding interferon γ to the system.
   E. No significant release of ^{51}Cr after 4 h of incubation.

11.5 The cytotoxicity reaction mediated by T lymphocytes
   A. Depends upon soluble factors, not requiring cell-to-cell contact.
   B. Has a lag time of a few minutes between recognition and killing.
   C. Is characterized by death of both target and cytotoxic cells.

D. Cannot occur in the presence of EDTA.

E. Is mediated by soluble factors released by $T4^+$ cells.

11.6 Receptors for IL2 are found in

A. Activated macrophages.

B. Resting T lymphocytes.

C. Resting inducer T lymphocytes.

D. Activated inducer T lymphocytes.

E. All of the above.

11.7 Killing by NK cells is enhanced by

A. HLA compatibility between target and killer cells.

B. Previous specific sensitization of the NK cell.

C. Release of interferon β.

D. Macrophage-activating factor.

E. Ca^{2+} and Mg^{2+}.

11.8 All of the listed effects can be the consequence of the release of interferon except increased

A. Phagocytic capacity.

B. Intracytoplasmic contents of proteolytic enzymes.

C. Production of interleukin 1.

D. Expression of class I MHC antigens in the cell membrane.

E. Production of prostaglandins and leukotrienes.

11.9 If a sublethally irradiated mouse is reconstituted with T cells from syngeneic mice previously sensitized to ovalbumin (OVA), and with B cells from syngeneic mice immunized with DNP, and challenged with DNP-BGG after reconstitution, then 7 days after challenge you expect to detect antibodies to

A. BGG.

B. DNP.

C. OVA.

D. BGG and DNP.

E. OVA, BGG, and DNP.

11.10 A severe depression of the $CD4^+$ subset in man is likely to result in

A. Severe depression of humoral immune responses.

B. Lack of development of skin delayed hypersensitivity reactions.

C. Both A and B.

D. Neither A nor B.

E. Is mediated by soluble factors released by T4.

Answers

11.1 (C)   Interleukin 1 is released by monocytes/macrophages and probably
by other antigen-presenting cells, as a result of nonspecific stimulation with a variety of substances, many of which are also antigenic.
Its effect on T lymphocytes is that of a cofactor leading to cell proliferation and differentiation, but it has no effect by itself.

11.2 (B)   The BCDFs are believed to induce the DNA rearrangements necessary for production of different isotypes of immunoglobulins.

11.3 (A)   The action of suppressor T cells appears to be indirect, mediated by
the inactivation (functional, not cytotoxic) of helper T cells, which
carry the CD4 antigen.

11.4 (E)   The T lymphocytes from H2-K mice will not be able to kill virally
infected T lymphocytes from an H2-d strain.

11.5 (D)   The cytotoxic reaction mediated by T lymphocytes is a relatively
slow process that may take from 30 min to 5 hr. It requires cell-to-
cell contact, is not characterized by death of the T lymphocyte, but
requires Ca^{2+} and Mg^{2+}. EDTA will inhibit the reaction by chelating
Ca^{2+} and Mg^{2+}.

11.6 (D)

11.7 (C)   Interferon β increases the activity of NK cells; Ca^{2+} and Mg^{2+} are
required for the reaction, but these ions do *not* enhance the reac-
tion.

11.8 (D)   Macrophages/monocytes express both class I and class II MHC antigens, but only the expression of class II is increased.

11.9 (D)   The priming of T cells with OVA is inconsequential when the animal is immunized with DNP-BGG; basically, the animal will develop
a primary immune response to the hapten-carrier conjugate.

11.10(C)   Different subsets of $CD4^+$ (helper) cells are essential for the adequate development of both humoral and cellular responses to T-
dependent antigens. In their absence, antibody production is depressed and skin delayed hypersensitivity reactions fail to develop.

BIBLIOGRAPHY

Beutler, B. and Cerami, A. Cachectin/tumor necrosis factor: An endogenous
mediator of shock and inflammation. *Immunol. Res.* 5:281, 1986.

Dinarello, C. A. Biology of interluekin 1. *FASEB Journal 2*:108-115, 1988.

Dixon, F. J. and Fisher, D. W. (Eds.). *The Biology of Immunologic Disease.* Sinauer, Sunderland, Massachusetts, 1983. (Includes several well-illustrated chapters on topics related to cellular immunity.)

Golub, E. S. *Immunology: A Synthesis.* Sinauer, Sunderland, Massachusetts, 1987.

Miyajima, A., Miyatake, S., Schreurs, Y., De Vries, J., Arai, N., Yokota, T., and Arai, K. I. Coordinate regulation of immune and inflammatory responses by T-cell-derived lymphokines. *FASEB Journal 2*:2462-2473, 1988.

Smith, K. A. Lymphokine regulation of T-Cell and B-Cell responses. In *Fundamental Immunology*, W. E. Paul (Ed.). Raven Press, New York, 1984, p. 599.

Smith, K. A. Interleukin 2: Inception, impact, and applications. *Science 240*: 1169, 1988.

12

Humoral Immune Response

GABRIEL VIRELLA

The recognition of a foreign cell or substance triggers a complex set of events that results in the acquisition of specific immunity against the corresponding antigen(s). Because the end point of the immune response is the elimination of nonself, effector mechanisms able to neutralize the source of antigenic stimulation developed during evolution. In the previous chapters we discussed extensively the effector mechanisms directly dependent on T lymphocytes, generally designated as *cellular immune responses*. In this chapter we shall discuss the sequence of events that culminates in the production of antibodies specifically directed against exogenous antigen(s), which constitutes the humoral immune response.

I. ROUTE OF PENETRATION OF NATURAL ANTIGENS

Natural antigens penetrate the organism via the skin, the upper respiratory mucosa, and the intestinal mucosa. The healthy animal is constantly stimulated by small amounts of antigenic material penetrating the organism through those routes; this is responsible for keeping a constant level of antibody in circulation. In contrast, animals reared in germ-free conditions synthesize very limited amounts of immunoglobulins.

II. STIMULATION OF B CELLS—ROLE OF
MACROPHAGES AND HELPER T CELLS

It is currently accepted that the triggering of a humoral response to the vast majority of antigens requires the cooperation of B cells, macrophages, and T cells. On the basis of this concept lies the assumption that a B cell requires more than one signal to be activated. One essential activation signal is the recognition of an antigen, as a consequence of the reaction between antigenic determinants and membrane immunoglobulins, but if purified B cells are exposed directly to soluble antigens such as heterologous proteins, there is no detectable immune response without additional signals.

The delineation of the signals necessary for B-cell activation is one of the most complex areas in modern immunology (as discussed in detail in earlier chapters). There is agreement on the need for macrophages and helper T lymphocytes to assist the B cell. It is believed that antigen-processing by the macrophage is essential for T-cell stimulation, as discussed in Chapter 4, and that the response to an infectious agent or a complex protein involves their breakdown and production of antigenic fragments, which are easier to recognize than the original protein or microorganism. Such antigenic fragments are concentrated on the membrane of macrophages and other antigen-presenting cells (APC), complexed with Ia (MHC class II) molecules. In this form, helper-inducer T cells can be stimulated through their antigen receptor, probably receiving two additional signals: one from the interaction between the *CD2* molecule on the lymphocyte and the *LFA-3* molecule on the APC; the other, also provided by the APC, is *interleukin 1*. Furthermore, the APC class II MHC antigen interacts with the CD4 molecule on the helper-inducer T cell, facilitating the cell-to-cell contact that appears essential for the delivery of activating signals to the cell. The synergistic effect of these activating signals is to trigger the differentiation of helper/ inducer T cells, which will in turn release *interleukin 2*. This lymphokine promotes the expansion and maturation of helper T lymphocytes. The B cells, on the other hand, seem to recognize either unprocessed antigen or antigen fragments that conserve the configuration of the native antigen. The role of APC in what concerns B-cell stimulation seems related to the adsorption of antigens and their fragments; once immobilized in the APC membrane, presentation to B cells is more efficient. The second signals necessary for B-cell activation are delivered both by macrophages (IL6 and possibly IL1) and T cells (interleukins 2, 4, 5, and probably other less well defined B cell growth and differentiation factors; see Chapter 4). B cells can also process antigen and present it to T cells complexed with a class II MHC antigen (see Chapter 4).

The precise way whereby T-independent antigens stimulate a humoral immune response in B cells is less well understood. It has been postulated that these antigens can deliver two signals to the B cell, one through specific combination to the antigen receptor, the other representing a nonspecific mitogenic signal. This postulate is supported by experimental evidence obtained in vitro; lymphocytes stimulated with bacterial lipopolysaccharide (a classical T-independent antigen) produce antibodies to totally unrelated antigens such as PPD (protein purified derivative, a component of tuberculin). However, the ability to induce the production of apparently unrelated antibodies is not restricted to the classical T-independent antigens; animals immunized with tobacco mosaic virus show marked postimmunization hypergammaglobulinemia, but only a very small fraction of the gammaglobulin produced seems to be specific antibody. In man, the initial burst of IgE production after first exposure to an allergen seems to be mainly constituted by nonspecific antibodies. These observations can be interpreted in three possible ways not mutually exclusive. First, some T-dependent antigens can also be mitogenic; second, the soluble mediators released by activated T cells may nonspecifically promote the proliferation and differentiation of B cells not directly involved in the immune response; finally, the antibodies produced early in the humoral response are of low avidity and may be missed by the tests for quantitation of specific antibodies, which select antibodies of moderate to high affinity.

III. DELIBERATE IMMUNIZATION—THE ROLE OF ADJUVANTS

In man, immunization is usually carried out by injecting the antigen intradermally, subcutaneously, or intramuscularly, or by administering it by the oral route (attenuated viruses, such as poliovirus) or as an aerosol (some experimental vaccines).

In animals, all these routes can be used, but to promote a better response, antigens are usually mixed with adjuvants. The most widely used adjuvant is complete Freund's adjuvant (CFA), a water-in-oil emulsion containing killed mycobacteria. This adjuvant has two effects. First, it promotes prolonged antigenic stimulation by slowing the reabsorption of the emulsified antigen, and second, it induces an intense inflammation around the site of injection, that also enhances the response (particularly through macrophage activation). This adjuvant has been used in man only in experimental cancer immunotherapy, because it induces strong inflammatory responses that often lead to abscess formation and eventual suppurative ulceration. However, inorganic gels (alum, aluminum hydroxide) can absorb antigens and release them slowly, acting as adjuvants without inducing strong inflammatory responses, and these are commonly used in man as part of killed or component vaccines (e.g., diphtheria-pertussis-tetanus or DPT).

IV. PRIMARY RESPONSE

The first contact with an antigen evokes a primary response characterized by a relatively long lag between the stimulus and the detection of antibodies by current methods (varying between 3 and 4 days after the injection of foreign erythrocytes and 10 to 14 days after the injection of bacterial cells). Part of this variation depends on the sensitivity of antibody detection methods, but it is also a reflection of the potency of the immunogen. Antibody levels rise exponentially for a while, reach a steady state after some days, and then decline (Fig. 12.1). Adjuvant administration will keep the antibody levels high for months. In the primary response the first antibody class to be synthesized is usually IgM.

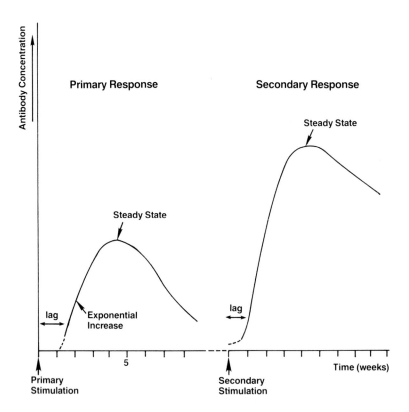

FIGURE 12.1 Diagrammatic representation of the sequence of events during a primary and a secondary immune responses. (Modified from Eisen, N. *Immunology*, 2nd Ed. Harper & Row, Cambridge, Massachusetts, 1980.)

Later in the response, IgG antibodies will predominate over IgM antibodies. This phenomenon is known as IgM-IgG switch. In humans, the differentiation between IgM and IgG antibodies is a useful index for discriminating between recent and past infections, particularly in the case of viral infections such as rubella, where this problem has considerable implications when infection is suspected during the first three months of pregnancy (because of the risk of fetal malformations). The successful triggering of the primary response requires the collaboration and interaction of several cell types, namely macrophages and helper T lymphocytes, as well as a reduced activity of suppressor T cells. The question of how and why suppressor cell activity is relatively low in the early stages of the primary response has been the object of considerable speculation. An appealing possibility is the activation of "contrasuppressor T cells," which have been postulated to induce a suppressor-resistant state in helper T cells. However, further corroboration of the existence and role of contrasuppressor T cells is needed before this additional regulatory loop can be fully accepted.

After the infectious agent (or any other type of antigen) has been eliminated, several regulatory mechanisms will operate in order to turn off antibody production. The elimination of the antigen will remove the most important positive signal. Also, several negative signals are likely to contribute to the down-regulation of B-cell activity in different ways. If the concentrations of IgG increase during the immune response, a general depression of IgG synthesis results from negative feedback regulation. The activity of suppressor cells, on the other hand, appears to predominate after elimination of the antigen. This could be explained by a longer life-span of suppressor cells, as compared to their helper counterparts, by a reduced activity of contrasuppressor T cells, or by the down-regulation of helper T cells by antigen-antibody complexes. Anti-idiotype antibodies, generated during the humoral response, could also play a role in turning off the response by two possible mechanisms: (a) binding to idiotypic regions of the membrane immunoglobulins from antigen-specific B cells carrying the particular idiotype against which the anti-idiotype is directed; this apparently triggers cell proliferation but not antibody production, while at the same time the B cell will not be able to be properly stimulated by antigen because the binding sites of the membrane immunoglobulin are occupied by the anti-idiotypic antibodies (Fig. 12.2); (b) the anti-idiotypic antibodies may stimulate T suppressor/inducer cells carrying antigen receptors with cross-reactive idiotypes, triggering a down-regulating circuit in which the first step is the differentiation and activation of suppressor T cells and the second step is the suppression of the activity of the T helper cells that assist the humoral response to the original antigen (Fig. 12.3).

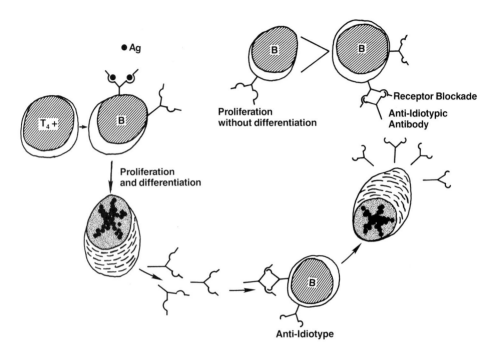

FIGURE 12.2 The role of anti-idiotypic antibodies in down-regulating the humoral immune response (I). From left to right, an antigen-stimulated B cell differentiates into a clone of plasma cells producing specific antibody. A second population of B cells, carrying a membrane immunoglobulin with specificity for the binding site of the first antibody (anti-idiotypic antibody) will be stimulated to proliferate and differentiate into a clone of plasma cells producing anti-idiotypic antibody. This second antibody will be able to bind to the antigen-receptor of the cells involved in the initial responses, which will be stimulated to divide but not to differentiate into plasma cells; the antigen receptor will also be blocked from further reaction with the real antigen.

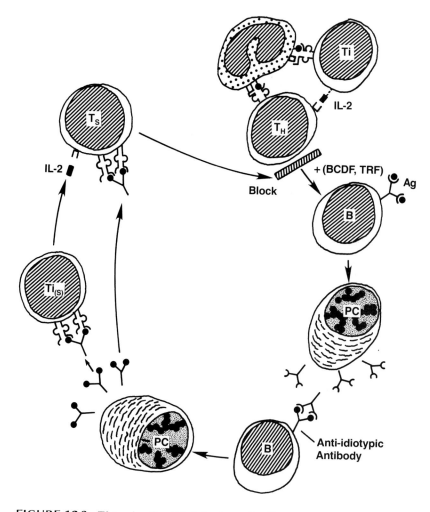

FIGURE 12.3 The role of anti-idiotypic antibodies in down-regulating the humoral immune response (II). The initial stages leading to the production of anti-idiotypic antibodies (right side) are identical to those described in Figure 12.2. However, the anti-idiotypic antibody may be able to interact with the antigen receptor of a T cell which, having the same specificity as the first antibody-producing cells, will share the idiotype of the first antibody. As a consequence of this interaction, T helper/inducer cells able to stimulate the proliferation and differentiation of suppressor cells will be activated, and the resulting suppressor cell population will down-regulate the helper/inducer population assisting the B cells involved in the original immune response.

V. SECONDARY OR ANAMNESTIC RESPONSE

When a previously immunized animal or human being is reexposed to the immunizing antigen, this will result in an enhanced secondary (or anamnestic) response characterized by (1) a lower threshold dose of immunogen; (2) a shorter lag phase; (3) a higher rate and longer persistence of Ab synthesis; (4) higher titers of Ab; and (5) increasing affinity, avidity, and cross-reactivity of antibodies ("maturation" of the immune response) (Fig. 12.1). The antibodies produced are usualy IgG, if the antigen dose is low; B cells with high affinity mIg are preferentially stimulated, and as a consequence a progressive increase in the affinity of secreted antibodies is seen during the secondary response. At the same time, minor determinants are recognized and a wider range of antibodies is produced. This results in increased avidity when the antigens have multiple determinants, but it increases the chances for cross-reactivity based on shared antigenic determinants. The capacity for a secondary immune response can persist for many years, providing long-lasting protection against reinfection. The fact that antibodies might not be detectable does not mean that this capacity is lost. The capacity of having a secondary response depends on the existence of long-lived *memory cells.*

Experimental data obtained mostly in studies carried out with some inbred strains of mice, congenitally or artificially deficient in either B or T cells, has indicated that no memory exists for T-independent antigens. It is believed that both T cells and B cells (particularly those that are mIgG+) can carry immunological memory, but the induction of memory both in T and B cells is T-cell-dependent. The existence of an expanded population of antigen-sensitive or memory cells results in the shortened lag period and in the enhanced response, which basically reflects the proliferation of a larger pool of antigen-specific cells.

VI. THE FATE OF ANTIGENS ON THE PRIMARY
AND SECONDARY RESPONSES

Following intravenous injection of a soluble antigen, its concentration in serum tends to decrease in three phases (Fig. 12.4). First, there is a sharp decrease of brief duration corresponding to the equilibration phase between intra- and extra-vascular spaces. Then, there is a phase of slow metabolic decay. Finally, when antibodies start to be formed, there will be a phase of rapid immune elimination, in which soluble Ag-Ab complexes will be taken up by macrophages. The onset of this phase of immune elimination is shorter in the secondary immune response, and it is virtually immediate if circulating antibody exists previously to the introduction of the antigen. A similar sequence of events, with less distinct equilibration and metabolic decay phases, occurs in the case of particulate antigens. If the antigen is a live, multiplying organism, there might be an initial in-

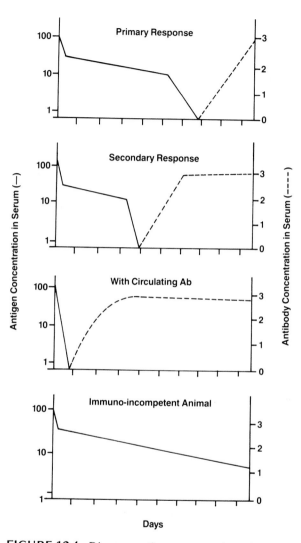

FIGURE 12.4 Diagrammatic representation of the fate of antigen injected (from top to bottom): a) into a nonimmune animal, which will undergo primary immune response; b) into an immune animal, which will show an accelerated, secondary response; c) into an animal with circulating antibodies, which will very rapidly eliminate the corresponding antigen from circulation; and d) into an immunoincompetent animal, which will slowly metabolize the antigen. (Modified from Talmage, D. F., Dixon, F. J., Bukantz, D. S., and Damin, G. J. *J Immunol 67*: 243, 1951.)

crease in the number of circulating or tissue-colonizing organisms, until specific and nonspecific mechanisms start to operate. The role of the humoral immune response will consist in providing complement-fixing antibodies able to induce lysis of the invading organisms, and cytophilic antibodies able to promote the cooperation of lymphocytes, macrophages, neutrophils, or eosinophils, in their destruction.

VII. THE HUMORAL IMMUNE RESPONSE AT THE MUCOSAL LEVEL

As we have previously noted, the gastrointestinal and respiratory mucosa are among the most widely used portals of entry by infectious agents. Consequently, there is considerable interest in studying the specific characteristics of the humoral immune response at the mucosal level and in the ways to induce secretory antibody responses.

The secretory IgA system has been described in previous chapters. It must be stressed at this point that several lines of experimental work, both in animals and in man, have conclusively shown that the induction of secretory antibodies requires direct mucosal stimulation. The investigations of Ogra and coworkers with poliovirus are particularly illustrative of this point: the systemic administration of an attenuated vaccine results in a systemic humoral response, while no secretory antibodies are detected; topical immunization with live, attenuated poliovirus, on the other hand, results in both a secretory IgA response and a systemic IgM-IgG response (Fig. 12.5). These investigations with poliovirus also suggest that the stimulation of a given sector of the mucosal system (GI tract) may result in detectable responses on unstimulated areas (upper respiratory tract). This protection of distant areas is compatible with the unitarian concept of a *mucosal immunologic network* with constant traffic of immune cells from one sector to another (Fig. 12.6). Indeed, supporting evidence has been found experimentally in several animal models, in which gut immunization was followed by detection of antibodies in other secretory areas. It is generally believed that antigen-sensitized cells from the gut-associated lymphoid tissue (GALT) or from the peribronchial lymphoid tissues enter the general circulation via the draining lymphatic vessels and subsequently populate the remaining secretory-associated lymphoid tissues. In addition to the gut and the bronchial tree, the mammary, salivary, and cervical glands of the uterus appear to participate in the recirculation of antigen-stimulated B cells, precursors of the IgA antibody-producing plasma cells that characterize the mucosal immunological network. Therefore all these organs can eventually be populated by plasma cells secreting IgA antibodies to antigens encountered in the or bronchial tree (Fig. 12.6). In some mammalian species, milk-secreted antibodies are actively absorbed in the newborn's gut and constitute the main source of adoptive immunity in the neonate. This usually is observed in species in

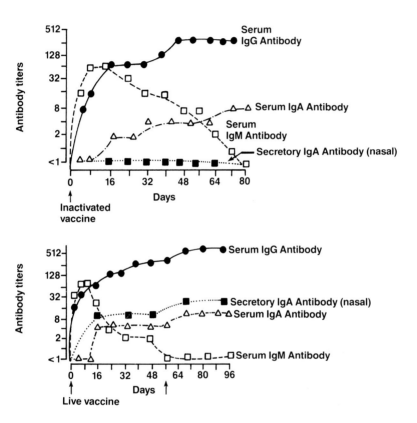

FIGURE 12.5   Comparison of the systemic and mucosal immune responses in human volunteers given killed poliovaccine (top) and live, attenuated poliovaccine (bottom).   Note that secretory antibody was detected only in children immunized with live, attenuated vaccine.   (Modified from Ogra, P. L., Karzon, D. T., Roghthand, F., and MacGillivray, M. *N. Engl. J. Med. 279*: 893, 1968.)

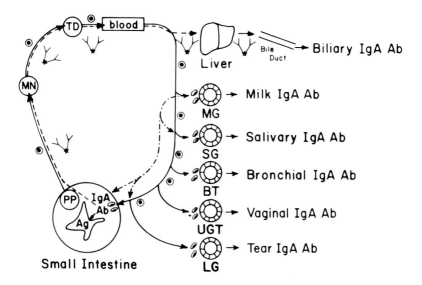

FIGURE 12.6 Diagrammatic representation of the pathways leading to the expression of IgA antibodies after antigenic stimulation of the GALT. IgA immunocytes (●) originating in Peyer's patches (PP) migrate to mesenteric lymph node (MN). Cells leave MN via the thoracic duct (TD) and enter the circulation with subsequent homing to the mammary gland (MG), salivary gland (SG), lacrimal gland (LG), and the lamina propria of the bronchial (BT), intestinal or urogenital tract (UGT) (●). The IgA antibodies are then expressed in milk, saliva, tears, and other secretions. IgA antibodies (⋎) entering circulation (– – –) are selectively removed by the liver and subsequently expressed in bile. Cell traffic between peripheral mocosal sites (–•– MG to SG, LG, and small intestine) is included in this scheme. (Reproduced with permission from Montgomery, P. C., Standera, C. A., and Majumdar, A. S. Evidence for migration of IgA bearing lymphocytes between peripheral mucosal sites. In *Protides of the Biological Fluids*, H. Peeters (Ed.). Pergamon, New York, 1985, p. 43).

which there is limited or no placental transfer of antibodies. In mammalians in which placental transfer of immunoglobulins is very effective (such as humans), the antibodies ingested with maternal milk are not absorbed. This is not to say that such antibodies may not play an important role in gastrointestinal mucosal protection, because the secretory IgA system is not usually developed early in life.

The physiological significance of the mucosal humoral immune response is not entirely clear. In the first place, many IgA-deficient individuals, with very low or absent circulating and secretory IgA, are totally asymptomatic. Second, in the case of the vaccination with attenuated poliovirus there is no conclusive proof that colonization is prevented in an immune individual. Some virologists are of the opinion that the effect of the vaccine is more related to the replacement in the human habitat of wild, virulent poliovirus strains by their attenuated, harmless counterparts. Finally, even accepting that the main immunological function of secretory IgA is to prevent antigen adsorption and microbial adherence to the mucosal epithelia, which usually precedes colonization and systemic invasion, this mechanism may be totally irrelevant in the case of microorganisms that do not depend on mucosal attachment for their pathogenesis. All these doubts and contradictions are due to our incomplete knowledge of the secretory immune system. By concentrating our attention on the parameter easiest to measure (secretory IgA) we may be missing a wide variety of cellular mechanisms of equal or greater physiological significance.

VIII. VACCINATION

The elicitation of immune responses with the aim of inducing protection against the subsequent development of an infectious disease can be historically tracked down to *variolation*, which consisted in the intradermal scarification of powdered small pox scabs in the hope of inducing protection against small pox. This practice, introduced in Europe in the 1700s by Lady Montagu, was followed by the introducton of cowpox vaccination by Jenner in 1796. Jenner observed that milkmaids who had contracted cowpox did not contract smallpox, and he developed an immunization procedure based on the scarificaton of material from cowpox lesions intradermally in children. Eventually, vaccinia virus was characterized as able to induce protective immunity against smallpox. This virus is believed to have been derived from cowpox, although it appears to have acquired unique characteristics in the laboratory that make it different from both cowpox and smallpox viruses.

In the 19th century, Louis Pasteur developed both killed and attenuated vaccines on a considerably more scientific basis. The work with antirabies vaccine contributed enormously to the development of immunoprophylaxis. For example, the discovery of the agent of tuberculosis (*Mycobacterium tuberculosis*) by Robert Koch was followed by the development of a vaccine using an attenuated strain of *Mycobacterium bovis* by Calmette and Guérin (bacillus Calmette-Guérin or BCG). The discovery of bacterial toxins, their chemical attenuation, and immunogenicity in animals resulted in the development of antitoxins and of some of the most effective vaccines available to us, such as diphtheria and tetanus toxoids. In more recent times, the successful introduction of the oral polio vaccine by Sabin demonstrated the possibility of effectively immunizing humans with an attentuated virus by the mucosal route.

A. Types of Vaccines Available

Basically there are three main tpes of vaccines: (1) killed microorganisms; (b) isolated microbial components or products; and (c) attenuated microbes. Most bacterial vaccines are either killed bacteria (e.g., pertussis vaccine prepared with killed *Bordetella pertussis*, the etiologic agent of whooping cough; typhoid vaccine prepared with acetone-inactivated *Salmonella typhi*) or based on the innoculation of bacterial components (e.g., bacterial polysaccharides are used as vaccines for *Streptococcus pneumoniae, Neisseria meningitidis*, and *Haemophilus influenzae* type B, and a new vaccine for typhoid fever made of the Vi capsular polysaccharide is currently being evaluated with promising results) or of bacterial toxoids (e.g., tetanus and diphtheria toxoids, which are basically formalin-inactivated toxins that have lost their active site but maintained their immunogenic determinants and induce antibodies able to neutralize the toxins; recently, *Chlostridium perfringens* type C toxoid has been successfully used to prevent *Chlostridial enteritis*). Some isolated polysaccharide vaccines (e.g., *H. influenzae* polysaccharide) have shown poor immunogenicity, particularly in infants. This problem appears to be eliminated if the polysaccharide is conjugated to a toxoid of known safety and immunogenicity such as diphtheria toxoid. Such "hybrid" vaccines are likely to become popular in the near future.

In contrast, many antiviral vaccines are made of viral strains attenuated in the laboratory (e.g., the oral polio vaccine is a mixture of attenuated strains of the three known types of poliovirus; the measles vaccine, initially killed, has been replaced by attenuated vaccines that are considerably more effective). However, many exceptions to these rules exist: a new bacterial vaccine against typhoid fever is under development based on the use of an attenuated strain of *Salmonella typhi* that grows poorly and is virtually nonpathogenic but induces protective immunity in 90% of the cases, while Salk's polio vaccine is prepared by mixing the three known types of poliovirus after inactivation with formalin. Also, antiviral vaccines based on the immunogenicity of isolated viral constituents have been developed, the best example being the hepatitis vaccine, prepared originally with particles of the hepatitis virus outer coat protein (hepatitis B surface antigen or HBsAg) isolated from chronic carriers, and currently with recombinant HBsAg.

In general, killed vaccines and those based on bacterial products and toxoids are very safe (with notable exceptions, such as the pertussis vaccine), but the efficiency of killed bacteria and killed virus vaccines is often unsatisfactory. Attenuated vaccines, on the other hand, tend to be very efficient but can cause the very disease they are designed to prevent, particularly in immunocompromised individuals.

B. The Vaccines of the Future

1. Recombinant Vaccines

Although some recombinant vaccines are already being used in humans, it is expected that recombinant technologies will be more widely used in the future. Two approaches have been utilized for the production of recombinant vaccines: to use recombinant technology to obtain pure antigens, and to add genetic information to attenuated viruses, creating multivalent vaccination agents.

The best example of the first approach is the production of hepatitis B vaccine by recombinant yeast cells. The gene coding for the hepatitis B surface antigen (HBsAg) was isolated from the hepatitis B virus and inserted into a plasmid. In turn, the plasmid was used to transform yeast cells: inserted in the right position, flanked by promoter and terminator sequences, the gene coding for HBsAg is actively transcribed. HBsAg is obtained from disrupted yeast cells and purified by chromatography.

The same basic approach has been used to produce large amounts of envelope glycoproteins of the AIDS virus (HIV). In this case, *E. coli*, insect cells, and mammalian cell lines have been genetically engineered to produce envelope glycoproteins against which neutralizing antibodies are directed (gp160 or its fragment, gp120). However, HIV-neutralizing antibodies are effective in vitro but do not stop the progression of the disease. It has been shown that the HIV reverse transcriptase is error-prone and induces mutations with high frequency when transcribing RNA into DNA. For unknown reasons the epitopes of gp120 against which neutralizing antibodies are directed are greatly affected by these mutations. As a consequence, the virus can escape the effects of neutralizing antibodies by undergoing serial mutations. This is the main obstacle faced in the development of a vaccine for HIV at this time.

However, this limitation is unique for HIV and should not prevent the successful development of other recombinant vaccines. For example, a recombinant *E.-coli*-produced *Rickettsia rickettsii* antigen has been proposed as a candidate vaccine for Rocky Mountain spotted fever.

Recombinant vaccinia viruses, in which the genetic information coding for relevant antigens of unrelated viruses is added to the genome, have also been developed and used successfully. A recombinant vaccinia virus carrying a retroviral *env* gene protected mice against Friend leukemia virus. Another recombinant vaccinia virus containing the genes coding for the G and N proteins of vesicular stomatitis virus (VSV) has been shown to protect cattle against the diseases caused by VSV. Experimental vaccines for AIDS have been developed by incorporating the *env* gene of HIV into the vaccinia virus genome. There is some data suggesting that recombinant HIV vaccines of this type are more efficient in inducing cell-mediated immunity, which could be a crucial factor in determining the effectiveness of HIV vaccine. Since the genome of vaccinia virus is rather large, recombinants carrying simultaneously the genes for the HBsAg, glycoprotein D for herpes virus, and influenza virus hemagglutinin have been successfully constructed.

2. Anti-Idiotypic Vaccines

The V-region of an antibody molecule (Ab1) has the binding site (paratope) for a specific antigenic determinant (epitope). The configuration of the antibody binding site becomes antigenic (idiotype) as it is expressed, during the immune response, in a large number of molecules, while prior to immunization, it was expressed only by a very small number of molecules, probably at tolerogenic concentrations. As a consequence, antibodies to the idiotype (anti-idiotypic antibodies or Ab2) are formed. Those antibodies, in turn, can elicit a second batch of anti-anti-idiotypic antibodies (Ab3). The anti-anti-idiotypic antibodies cross-react with the original epitope of the immunizing antigen, as shown in Figure 12.7. Therefore, the injection of an anti-idiotypic antibody may induce protective immunity against the original microorganism.

Experimental anti-idiotypic vaccines have successfully protected mice against infection with *Trypanosoma rhodesiense* (one of three etiologic agents of sleep-

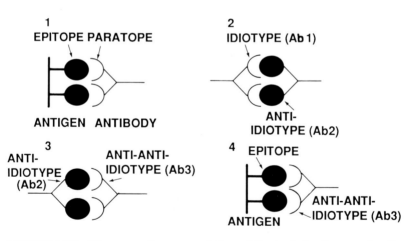

FIGURE 12.7 Diagrammatic representation of the basis for the use of anti-idiotypic antibodies as immunoprophylactic agents. An anti-idiotypic antibody directed to the paratope of an anti-infectious antibody mimicks the configuration of the epitope; therefore, antibodies directed against the idiotype of the anti-idiotypic antibody will cross-react with the epitope of the infectious agent.

ing sickness), *Escherichia coli,* and Sendai virus. This approach appears ideally suited when antigens for immunization may be in short supply or too dangerous (HIV). However, humans would have to be injected with murine anti-idiotypic antibodies that are antigenic; this may lead to the development of serum sickness and/or rapid loss of efficiency. The solution to this problem may be found in the construction of hybrid antibodies, transfecting antibody-producing cells with DNA constructs containing mouse variable region genes corresponding to antibody of a desired specificity and human constant region genes. Such constructs have been successfully produced, but whether they can be scaled up and diversified as needed for the production of the large amounts of defined anti-idiotypic antibodies that would be required for vaccination is not known.

3. Synthetic Peptide Vaccines

The use of synthetic peptides for vaccination has the advantages of easy manufacture and safety. The goal is to reproduce the epitopes recognized by neutralizing antibodies and use them as vaccines. One main problem is the low immunogeneicity of small synthetic peptides. They have been successfully used when injected as conjugates with large proteins (e.g., tetanus toxoid) and emulsified with complete Freund's adjuvant. For human use it may be necessary to develop synthetic carriers, and a less toxic adjuvant will certainly be required.

Experimental work with synthetic peptide vaccines has been carried out with *Plasmodium flaciparum* peptides, influenza hemagglutinin peptides, and coat protein peptides of foot-and-mouth disease virus. The results in a murine malaria model, using a tetanus toxoid *Plasmodium berghei* peptide conjugate, were very encouraging. The rates of protection in immunized mice ranged from 75 to 87%, identical to those observed with a killed vaccine made of the whole parasite.

SELF-EVALUATION

Questions

Choose the one best answer.

12.1 Immunologic memory can be explained on the basis of
A. Increased numbers of antigen-sensitive T and B cells.
B. Increased numbers of IL2-producing T cells.
C. Changes in the amino acid sequence of antibodies formed by individual clones so that the antibodies will fit the antigen more perfectly.
D. Predominant synthesis of IgG antibodies.
E. Predominance of IgG as membrane immunoglobulin of the B-cell population.

12.2 In comparison with primary humoral immune responses, secondary humoral immune responses are characterized by
A. Longer lag phases.
B. A faster decline in antibody concentration after the steady state has been reached.
C. The need for greater doses of stimulating antigen.
D. Increased cross-reactivity of circulating antibodies.
E. Longer persistence of antigen in circulation.

12.3 Antigenic activation of helper T cells
A. Requires interaction with lymphokine-producing macrophages.
B. Requires the recognition of antigen in conjunction with class II MHC antigens displayed by accesssory cells.
C. Is of no consequence as far as the B-cell response is concerned.
D. Cannot take place if processed antigen is presented to the helper T cells by cells other than macrophages.
E. Is essential for the response against polysaccharides.

12.4 The mucosal humoral immune response
A. Can only be elicited by direct antigenic challenge of the mucosa.
B. Is characterized by predominant synthesis of IgG antibodies.
C. Is localized to the mucosal segment that is directly challenged.
D. Is essential for the maintenance of an infection-free state.
E. Leads to complement-dependent killing of many infectious agents.

12.5 The main difference between killed poliovaccine (Salk) and attenuated poliovaccine (Sabin) is that only the later induces
A. Memory.
B. Secretory IgA antibodies.
C. Circulating neutralizing antibiotic.
D. Circulating complement-fixing antibodies.
E. Protection against viral dissemination through the bloodstream.

12.6 The use of bacterial toxoids in vaccines in which a poorly immunogenic peptide or polysaccharide is coupled to a toxoid has as its main advantage the
A. Simultaneous immunization against more than one antigen.
B. Creation of a self-replicating attenuated bacterial strain carrying the genetic information necessary to synthesize epitopes against which protective immunity is directed.
C. Lesser toxicity of the toxoid-peptide or toxic-polysaccharide conjugates..
D. Transformation of poorly immunogenic compounds into integral components of a potent T-dependent immunogen.

E. Adjuvanticity of bacterial toxoids eliminating the need for inorganic adjuvants.

12.7 All of the following events could have a negative feedback effect on antibody production except
A. Elimination of the antigen.
B. Formation of immune complexes.
C. Production of high levels of IgM antibodies.
D. Reaction of anti-idiotype antibodies with mIg on the B-cell membrane.
E. Proliferation of CD8 (T8+) lymphocytes.

12.8 The main characteristic that enables B lymphocytes to function as antigen-presenting cells is their
A. Phagocytic ability.
B. Capacity to secrete large amount of IL2.
C. Expression of class II MHC antigens.
D. Ability to bind antigens specifically through their mIg.
E. Presence in large numbers in the intestinal lymphoid tissues.

12.9 According to the concept of mucosal immunologic network, if an antigen stimulates the peri-intestinal immune system,
A. Secretory antibody production is limited to the intestine.
B. Sensitized B cells migrate from the peri-intestinal tissues to other peri-mucosal lymphoid areas.
C. Secretory IgA diffuses into the systemic circulation and can be excreted in any other mucosal area.
D. Dimeric IgA back-flowing from the intestine through the portal circulation is excreted into the bile.
E. All antibodies formed will belong to the IgA class.

12.10 An antigen infected intravenously into an animal that has free antibody in circulation directed against it will
A. Be eliminated from the circulation very rapidly.
B. Remain in the circulation for a prolonged period as an antigen-antibody aggregate.
C. Cause a new burst of IgM synthesis.
D. Have no effect in the undergoing immune response.
E. Cause immediate release of IgE from circulating basophils.

Answers

12.1 (A) Most authors believe that memory cells include both T and B lymphocytes.

12.2 (D)   In a secondary immune response, the antibody repertoire increases, and as a result the probability of a cross-reaction also increases.

12.3 (B)   The antigenic stimulation of helper T cells is HLA restricted, and the main antigens involved are class II MHC antigens; any cell able to fix processed antigen on its membrane and to express class II antigens can assist a helper T cell to become antigen-sensitized.

12.4 (A)   Many individuals with severely depressed levels of mucosal IgA live free of infections, which raises questions concerning whether IgA is the only, or the main, exponent of the mucosal immune response.

12.5 (A)   Only the attenuated vaccine, given orally, can induce mucosal immunity. However, both vaccines are equivalent in regard to systemic immunity and memory induction.

12.6 (D)   The toxoid-polysaccharide and toxoid-peptide vaccines are not very different from hapten-carrier conjugates. Toxoids, acting as carriers, are recognized by T cells, and the resulting magnitude of the immune response is increased.

12.7 (C)

12.8 (C)

12.9 (B)   Mucosal stimulation is associated both with local and with systemic responses. The response propagates to areas not directly stimulated by the traffic of sensitized B lymphocytes.

12.10(A)   Immediate release of histamine could be possible if the animal had IgE antibodies already bound to basophils. However, it is stated only that the animal has free circulating antibody, which most likely should be IgM or IgG.

REFERENCES

Dixon, F. J. and Fisher, D. W. (Eds.). *The Biology of Immunologic Disease.* Sinauer, Sunderland, Massachusetts, 1983. (Includes the chapter "The development of synthetic vaccines.")

Kennedy, R. C., Melnick, J. L., and Dressman, C. R. Anti-idiotypes and immunity. *Scientific American 255*: 48, 1986.

McGhee, J. R., Mestecky, J., and Babby, J. L. (Eds.). *Secretory Immunity and Infection.* Plenum, New York, 1978.

Mestecky, J. The common mucosal immune system and current strategies for induction of immune responses in external secretions. *J Clin Immunol 7*: 265, 1987.

Moss, B. and Flexner, C. Vaccinia virus expression vectors. *Amer. Rev. Immunol. 5*: 305, 1987.

Paul, W. E. (Ed.). *Fundamental Immunology*. Raven Press, New York, 1984. (Contains several sections discussing the induction and regulation of humoral immunity.)

Plotkin, S. A. and Mortimer, E. A., Jr. (Eds.). *Vaccines*. Saunders, Philadelphia, 1988.

Zuckerman, A. J. The development of novel hepatitis B vaccines. *Bull. World Health Org. 65*: 265, 1987.

13

Immunological Aspects of the Host-Parasite Relationship

GABRIEL VIRELLA

In previous chapters we have discussed in detail the different types of defense mechanisms that humans and most vertebrates have developed. We also have repeatedly stated that the main purpose of those mechanisms is to keep the organism free of nonself material such as pathogenic microorganisms. This chapter attempts to present an integrated perspective of our knowledge about the interplay between immunological defenses and infectious agents; we also discuss some of the reasons why pathogenic agents may eventually prevail and cause disease.

I. THE VERY EARLY MECHANISMS OF DEFENSE: PMN PHAGOCYTOSIS

One of the most common ways to be exposed to pathogenic microorganisms is through superficial wounds. It is hard to imagine an aseptic wound in a normal environment. However, even if left alone, most such wounds will heal without infection, or will show minimal suppuration for a few days and quickly heal. This very early elimination of infecting microorganisms cannot be explained as a result of an active immune response, because it takes at least 3 or 4 days to initiate a detectable secondary response, and by then the infection may have been successfully eliminated. The main mechanism of defense involved is the phagocytosis of infecting microorganisms by polymorphonuclear (PMN) leuko-

240   Virella

A. No Antibody, No Complement

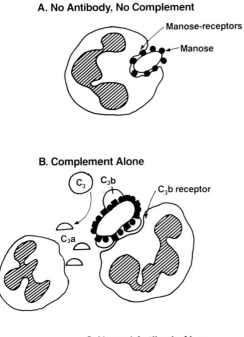

B. Complement Alone

C. Natural Antibody Alone

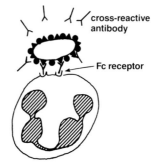

FIGURE 13.1   Diagrammatic representation of three possible pathways for
PMN leukocyte phagocytosis in a nonimmune host: through sugar receptors (a),
through C3b receptors, when the microorganism activates complement by the
alternative pathway (b), and through Fc receptors, whenever natural antibodies
are present in the host (c).

cytes actively attracted to the infected wound. The question that naturally arises then is, what induces active phagocytosis and recruitment of phagocytic cells into the infected area?

A highly significant finding has been the characterization of sugar receptors on the membrane of phagocytic cells, both in rodents and in humans. The human polymorphonuclear leukocyte appears to recognize mannose and is able to engulf organisms actively with mannose-rich capsules such as *Candida albicans* without need for specific antibodies or complement (Fig. 13.1). This could represent a very primitive recognition system, which would allow the phagocytic cells to start ingesting and destroying microorganisms as soon as they penetrate one of our natural barriers.

II. ALTERNATIVE PATHWAY ACTIVATION OF THE COMPLEMENT SYSTEM

One other way to recruit phagocytic cells and induce phagocytosis in the absence of antibody is the activation of complement by the alternative pathway by many microorganisms (bacteria, fungi, viruses, and parasites), e.g., those in Table 13.1. This has been shown, for example, in experiments demonstrating C3 fixation and opsonization of *S. aureus* preincubated with agammaglobulinemic serum (devoid of antibodies) to which a Ca^{2+} chelating agent (EGTA) was added to block complement activation by the classical pathway, while Mg^{2+} was added to allow complement activation by the alternative pathway. Therefore, one can conclude that opsonization and C3 fixation occurs in the absence of antibodies, in conditions that prevent the activation of the classical pathway of complement but that allow complement activation by the alternative pathway. In most cases where adequate studies have been carried out, polysaccharidic structures have been proven to be responsible for the activation of the alternative pathway. This activation will lead to phagocytosis, through the gen-

TABLE 13.1   Some Examples of Infectious Agents Able to Activate the Alternative Pathway of Complement Without Apparent Participation of Specific Antibody

Bacteria	Parasites
H. influenzae type B	*Trypanosoma cyclops*
Streptococcus pneumoniae	*Schistosoma mansoni*
Staphylococcus aureus; S. epidermidis	*Babesia Rodhaini*
Fungi	Viruses
Candida albicans	Vesicular stomatitis virus

eration of C3b, and to chemotaxis, through the release of C3a (Fig. 13.1). Interestingly, direct lysis of bacteria is not observed in the absence of antibody, probably because the alternative pathway of complement activation is not as efficient as the classical pathway triggered by antigen-antibody complexes.

III. NATURAL ANTIBODIES

Early immunologists were greatly impressed by the "spontaneous" appearance of antibodies against antigens to which a host had not been sensitized, which were termed *natural antibodies*. The classical examples were the isoagglutinins of the ABO blood group system, i.e., circulating antibodies that exist in a given individual and that are able to agglutinate erythrocytes carrying alloantigens of the ABO system different from those of the individual himself. The understanding of the origin of the ABO isoagglutinins was clarified by experiments using chickens, which are able to produce agglutinins recognizing the AB alloantigens. The production of such agglutinins, however, takes place only if the birds are fed conventional diets; if sterile diets are used no agglutinins will develop. Anti-A and anti-B agglutinins develop as soon as birds fed sterile diets after birth are placed on conventional diets later in life. In humans, newborn babies do not carry anti-A and anti-B isohemagglutinins at birth but will develop those antibodies (if their blood group is not AB) during the first months of life. The nature of this phenomenon was clarified by the demonstration of structural similarities between the cell wall polysaccharides of several strains of enterobacteriaceae and the A,B oligosaccharides of human erythrocytes.

Cross-reaction, however, does not seem to be the only mehanism that can explain the appearance of natural antibodies. In vitro experiments have shown that substances such as pneumococcal polysaccharides and lipopolysaccharides are able to act as B-cell mitogens and induce the synthesis of several different unrelated antibodies. These mitogenic properties, or, alternatively, the nonspecific stimulatory effects of lymphokines released by antigen-stimulated T lymphocytes, which could activate B cells responding to other antigens, may explain the rise of nonspecific immunoglobulins that is observed in the early stages of the humoral response to many different antigens. It is only a matter of random probability that some of those immunoglobulins may play the role of natural antibodies relative to any given infectious agent, as shown by the experiments summarized in Figure 13.2. Antibodies elicited to *E. coli* K100 cross-react with the polyribophosphate of *Haemophilus influenzae* and can protect experimental animals against infection with the latter organism.

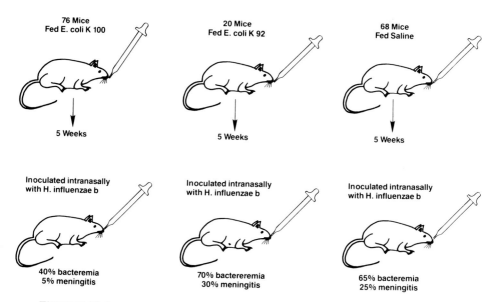

FIGURE 13.2 Diagrammatic representation of an experiment proving the anti-infectious protective role of cross-reactive natural antibodies. Three groups of mice were orally immunized with *E. coli* K100, *E. coli* K92, and saline as a control. Five weeks later all animals were challenged with *H. influenzae* type 6 by the intranasal route. *E. coli* K100 was cross-reactive with *H. influenzae* type 6, but the same is not true for *E. coli* K92. The animals immunized with *E. coli* K100 showed significantly lower rates of bacterial and meningeal infection than the animals immunized with *E. coli* K92 or controls fed with saline. (Modified from Moxon, E. R., and P. Anderson, *J. Inf. Diseases 140*:471, 1979.)

IV. THE HUMORAL IMMUNE RESPONSE

The first lines of immunological defense are not always able to curtail the proliferation of a pathogen. If able to multiply, the pathogen will eventually spread through the blood and lymph and will usually be trapped by macrophages in the lymph nodes and spleen level. In the lymphoid organs, the conditions for stimulating an immune response are ideal. The antigen, processed and presented by macrophages and other antigen-presenting cells, is available for recognition by T and B cells, which are in constant traffic from the peripheral tissues. In this manner both cell-mediated and humoral responses can be triggered. However, the localization of antigen in the lymph node, as well as its processing and presentation to the right cells, are steps that require time. Therefore, there is a lag phase between antigenic challenge and a detectable immune response. This corresponds to the time necessary for the stimulation and proliferation of immuno-component cells until the "critical mass" necessary for the synthesis of detect-able amounts of antibodies is reached, or, in the case of cell-mediated immunity, a clear-cut manifestation of delayed hypersensitivity becomes detectable (in vitro or in vivo). The duration of this lag phase in a primary humoral response is usually 5 to 7 days, but it can be as long as 2 to 3 weeks. In the case of cell-mediated immunity the lag phase appears shorter; evidence for acquired cell-mediated responses (e.g., antigen-induced T-cell proliferation) may be detected 10 days after vaccination, in some cases preceding the detection of circulating antibody.

   Whenever antibodies become available they have a multitude of possible mechanisms for protecting the organism against infection. Antibodies, as we have discussed in other chapters, are very efficient in preventing the binding of toxins to their receptors (neutralization of toxins). If able to fix comple-ment, antibodies can promote the lysis of microorganism or virus-infected cells through the activation of the complete sequence of complement, or by phago-cytosis, mediated by Fc and/or C3b receptors at the surface of the phagocytic cells (IgG antibody alone can induce phagocytosis). Because of their role in promoting opsonization, IgG antibodies and C3b are considered as *opsonins*. Killing through opsonization has been demonstrated for bacteria, fungi, and viruses, while phagocytosis of antibody/complement-coated unicellular para-sites has not been clearly demonstrated.

V. ANTIBODY-DEPENDENT CELL-MEDIATED CYTOTOXICITY

Antibodies and cells can cooperate in the destruction of microorganisms by other mechanisms. For example, antibodies of the right structural charac-teristics (IgG1, IgG3, and IgE antibodies in humans) can elicit the cytotoxic activity of killer cells. In most systems, the killer cells are lymphocytic or monocytic in nature, but in the case of parasitic infections there is substantial proof suggesting that eosinophils may be involved in cytotoxic reactions. For example, as shown in Fig. 13.3, incubation of *Trichinella spiralis* larvae with heat-inactivated immune serum containing antibodies but no active comple-ment and eosinophil-rich peritoneal exudates from nonimmune mice leads to a massive attraction of eosinophils to the parasite, and later to the death of the parasite. This killer-cell role of eosinophils is dependent on the exposure of the parasite to antibody and has been shown for other parasites, such as the larvae of *Schistosoma mansoni*. The mechanism of killing seems to depend on the re-lease of a *major basic protein* by the eosinophil. This protein has been purified and its toxic effects on parasites have been well documented.

   Polymorphs also seem able to lyse virus-infected cells, but in this case the triggering signal for the PMN is given by complement coating the infected cell rather than by antibody.

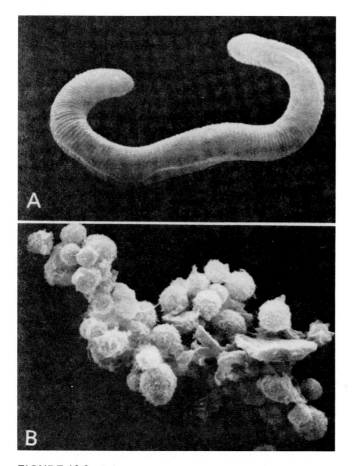

FIGURE 13.3 (A) Scanning electron photomicrograph of a *Trichinella spiralis* larva incubated with eosinophils and complement-depleted normal (nonimmune) mouse serum for 4 hr; (B) Scanning electron photomicrograph of a *Trichinella spiralis* larva incubated with eosinophils and complement-depleted immune serum for 4 hr. Notice that the attachment of eosinophils happened only when eosinophils were added to *T. spiralis* larvae in the presence of immune sera containing antibodies directed against the parasite. (Reproduced with permission from Kazura, J. W. and Aikawa, M. *J. Immunol 124*:355, 1980.)

VI. CELL-MEDIATED IMMUNITY (CMI)

It has been recognized for over a decade that virus-infected cells may be lysed as a consequence of their incubation with immune lymphocytes, obtained from an animal previously exposed to the same virus. This is one of the most classic demonstrations of the development of CMI in infectious diseases. In vivo, there is a correlation between lymphocytic infiltration and viral elimination in infected organs, and in the absence of CMI (as a consequence of primary immunodeficiency or of immunosuppression) viral clearance is delayed.

As discussed in earlier chapters, the cytotoxic T cells appear to recognize a complex constituted by viral antigen and a class I MHC molecule. Recent data suggests that viral antigens, soon after synthesis, become associated to binding sites of broad specificity on the MHC molecules. This complex is recognized as modified self only by cells carrying MHC antigens identical to those of the infected cells, which upon stimulation will differentiate into cytotoxic effector cells, eventually destroying the infected cell.

VII. THE IMMUNE DEFICIENCY SYNDROMES AS MODELS FOR THE STUDY OF THE IMPORTANCE OF IMMUNE DEFENSES AGAINST INFECTIONS IN HUMANS

The main features of clinically evident immune deficiency syndromes are chronic infections with common pathogens and with opportunistic agents, usually not pathogenic in healthy individuals. Most of what we know about the function of human immunocytes has been learned by the sudy of such patients. For example, patients with antibody deficiencies and conserved cell-mediated immunity suffer from repeated and chronic infections with pyogenic bacteria while patients with primary deficiencies of cell-mediated immunity usually suffer from chronic or recurrent fungal, parasitic, and viral infections, the latter sometimes as a result of the administration of live, attenuated, vaccines. Isolated complement component deficiencies have been also characterized, and again, one of the most common presenting symptoms is chronic and repeated infections, mainly bacterial (Table 13.2).

TABLE 13.2 Common Patterns of Infection in Patients With Immunodeficiency

Type of immunodeficiency	Common infections
Combined (cellular and humoral) deficiency	All types of agents, including bacteria, viruses, fungi, and parasites
Humoral (antibody deficiency)	Mostly pyogenic bacteria
Cellular (T-cell deficiency)	Intracellular bacteria, viruses, and parasites; fungi
Complement deficiencies	Pyogenic bacteria (particularly *Neisseria sp.*)

VIII. IMMUNOLOGICAL DEFENSES VERSUS INTRACELLULAR PARASITES

The classical antibody-dependent defenses, involving antibodies, complement, and phagocytic cells, are most effective in the destruction of extracellular parasites. In the case of intracellular parasites, such as most viruses and some bacteria (e.g., *Mycobacterium tuberculosis*), the effectiveness of the immune response depends greatly on the ability either to destroy the infected cells or to activate the intracellular killing mechanisms of the infected cells. The lysis of infected cells can be carried out by cytotoxic T cells recognizing newly expressed determinants on the cell membrane, as discussed above. Antibody-dependent cell-mediated cytotoxicity can also be an effective mechanism, usually more so than direct complement activation by antibodies reacting with newly expressed determinants on the cell membrane. Finally, a variety of microorganisms have developed mechanisms that will allow them to survive in phagocytic cells. Such organisms are able to infect reticuloendothelial cells chronically, unless those cells are activated by lymphokines (such as the macrophage activating factor or IFNγ) released by antigen-stimulated T cells. Such activation is usually followed by intracellular killing of the infectious agent. Therefore, infections with intracellular organisms are prevalent in patients with T-cell deficiency who lack the ability to release the activating lymphokines.

IX. ABNORMAL CONSEQUENCES OF THE IMMUNE RESPONSE

The development of an immune response is no guarantee of efficient protection. A good example is syphilis. In the secondary and tertiary phases the patient produces specific antibodies (used diagnostically in several serological tests), but such antibodies do not appear to lead to the lysis of the spirochete or to promote its phagocytosis. From the biological point of view the immune response to syphilis appears inadequate.

In some types of viral infection it has been shown that viral particles coated with specific antibody may retain infectivity, when usually one would expect viral lysis, or at least the blocking of viral penetration or uncoating in the cell to result from the combination with specific antibody. In human HIV infection, it is believed that one of the mechanisms of infection of macrophages is the phagocytosis of antibody-coated viral particles, which proceed to multiply intracellularly in a nonlytic fashion.

Unexpected twists in the consequences of triggering immune systems can be seen also in responses to parasites. *Babesia rodhaini*, an intraerythrocytic parasite in cows, closely related to human pathogenic parasites, appears able to penetrate the host's cells only after it has bound complement, particularly C3. It appears that binding to the red cells via C3b binding sites might be the first step for the successful penetration.

Blocking factors, so important in cancer immunology, may also play a role in infectious diseases. For example, serum samples collected from army recruits during an epidemic of meningococcal meningitis failed to show bactericidal activity until IgA specific anti-*Neisseria meningitidis* antibodies were removed. It appeared that in such patients, the IgA antibodies acted as a blocking factor. However, it is not clear whether these IgA antibodies were totally unprotective, since they were demonstrated to be able to induce ADCC in vitro. In viral infections, antibodies directed to virus-infected cells may or may not be cytotoxic. If they are not, however, they may block an otherwise efficient response on the part of the killer cells or cytotoxic T cells.

X. EVASION OF THE IMMUNE RESPONSE

Parasites have developed a remarkable capacity to evade the immune response. One of the most interesting mechanisms from the biological point of view is antigenic variation, which has been best characterized in trypanosomes, the agents of African sleeping sickness. The surface coat of these parasites consists mainly of a single glycoprotein (variant-specific glycoprotein or VSG), for which there are about 10^3 genes in the chromosome. At any given time, only one of these genes is expressed, the others remaining silent. Every 10^6 or 10^7 trypanosome divisions a mutation occurs that consists of replacing the active VSG gene on the expression site by a previously silent VSG gene. The previously expressed gene is destroyed, and a new VSG protein is coded, which is now antigenically different. This emergence of a new antigenic coat allows the parasite to multiply unchecked. As antibodies emerge to the new VSG protein, parasitemia will decline, only to emerge again once a new mutation occurs and a new VSG protein is synthesized.

A similar mechanism of bringing a silent gene to an area of gene expression has been characterized in the bacterial genus *Borrelia*, which includes the agent of relapsing fever. *Borrelia* carry genes for at least 26 different variable major proteins (VMP), which are sequentially activated by duplicative transposition to an expression site. The successive waves of bacteremia and fever correspond to the emergence of new mutants which, for a while, can proliferate unchecked until antibodies are formed.

Three totally different mechanisms of evasion have been characterized in vitro using another parasite (*Schistosoma mansoni*) as a model: (a) the stimulation of suppressor cells, (b) the loss of antigens, and (c) the masking of parasitic antigens by adsorption of host proteins.

TABLE 13.3   Tactics by Which Viruses May Escape Immune Defenses and Human Viruses That Exploit These Tactics

Immunodepressive activity	Mumps, measles, HIV[a]
Direct intracellular spread	Herpes simplex, HIV
Intracellular latency with occasional reactivation concurrent with declines in resistance	Herpes simplex, varicella-zoster
Induction of nonneutralizing antibodies that hinder neutralizing ones or facilitate virus entry into cells	Reovirus, dengue, and other arboviruses, HIV
Blocking receptors involved in lymphocyte recognition with soluble viral antigens	Hepatitis B, HIV

[a]HIV = human immunodeficiency virus, the causative agent of the acquired immunodeficiency syndrome (AIDS).
Source: Modified from Bendinelli, M. Mechanisms and significance of immunodepression in viral diseases. *Clin. Immunol. News.* 2:75, 1981.

The stimulation of suppressor monocytes by *Schistosoma* has been demonstrated in studies showing a significant increase in the response of T lymphocytes obtained from infected animals after removal of adherent cells (mostly monocytes). On the other hand, studies with schistosomula (the larval forms of *Schistosoma*) demonstrated that in the few hours after hatching there is a rapid decrease in the surface antigens, as reflected by a progressive decrease in the binding of purified and fluorescein-labeled heterologous antischistosomular antibodies to the parasite membrane. Simultaneously, there is an increased detectability of host proteins in schistosomula recovered from infected animals that led to the theory of antigen-masking. Both phenomena are probably real, since antigen loss can be demonstrated in vitro, with schistosomula cultivated in defined, serum-free media.

Evasion mechanisms are not peculiar to parasitic infections. A variety of mechanisms are believed to be operative in viral infections, as summarized in Table 13.3. Also, in the case of bacteria, several immunosuppressive pathways have been demonstrated, including release of immunosuppressive substances, arrest of bone marrow stem cell maturation, selective activation of suppressor T cells, and activation of monocytes/macrophages with subsequent release of prostaglandins that down-regulate T cells.

XI. IMMUNOSUPPRESSION AS CONSEQUENCE OF A
VIRAL INFECTION

One classical observation in traditional medicine is that a patient in the acute phase of measles or smallpox is more susceptible to bacterial infections such as pneumonia. An experimental proof of the immunodepression often associated with viral infection can be easily obtained by comparing the response to heterologous red cells by two groups of mice, one of them given a live virus simultaneously with the red cells. The second group will produce significantly less antibody. In humans, study of the in vitro response of lymphocytes to unrelated antigens has shown significant depression during the acute phase of measles, with recovery after 4 weeks. Mothers and infants congenitally infected with cytomegalovirus show depressed responses to CMV virus, but normal responses to PHA, suggesting that in some cases the immunosuppression may be antigen-specific, while in others (such as measles) it is obviously nonspecific.

The nature of this immunosuppression has been studied in several ways. In vitro it is possible to show that when virus-infected cells are incubated with normal cells, the responsiveness of the latter is decreased. This can be correlated with the fact that 37 ± 26% of T cells and 7 ± 11% of B cells recovered from pa-

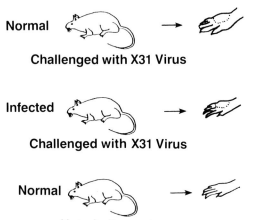

Normal

Challenged with X31 Virus

Infected

Challenged with X31 Virus

Normal

Not challenged

FIGURE 13.4   Diagrammatic representation of an experiment proving that infection with influenza virus Rec 31 induces a depression of the cell-mediated immune response to an antigenically related virus (influenza X31 virus). (Reproduced from Liew, F. Y. and Russell, S. M. *J. Exp. Med. 151*:799, 1980.)

Donor   **Recipient**   **Challenge**
(Immunosuppressed)

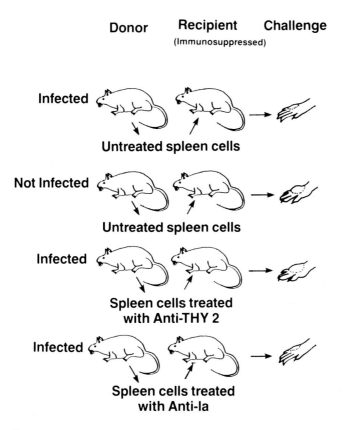

Infected

Untreated spleen cells

Not Infected

Untreated spleen cells

Infected

**Spleen cells treated
with Anti-THY 2**

Infected

**Spleen cells treated
with Anti-Ia**

FIGURE 13.5 Diagrammatic representation of an experiment proving the suppression of delayed hypersensitivity to influenza virus X31 after previous infection with influenza virus Rec 31. Notice that when the immunosuppressed animals were reconstituted with a Thy-2-depleted lymphocyte population they became able to mount a delayed hypersensitivity reaction to X31, while the opposite was true using a B-cell-depleted population (treated with anti-Ia). (Reproduced from Liew, F. Y. and Russell, S. M. *J. Exp. Med. 151*:799, 1980.)

tients in the actue phase of measles can be shown to carry measles antigen. In vivo it can be shown that viral infection with a strain of influenza virus leads to decreased delayed hypersensitivity reactions when the same animal is challenged intradermally with an antigenically related strain of influenza virus (Fig. 13.4). This depression of delayed hypersensitivity can be transferred by spleen cells from an infected animal to an immunosuppressed recipient; if the spleen cells are treated with anti-Ia antisera (that will eliminate B cells), the transfer of suppres-

TABLE 13.4 Immune Cell Alterations Associated with Human Virus Infections

Cell type	Nature of alterations	Virus
Macrophages	Cytotoxicity	Dengue, yellow fever
	Reduced phagocytic activity	Influenza,[a] parainfluenza, Epstein-Barr
	Reduced phagosome/lysosome fusion	Parainfluenza
	Depressed chemotaxis	Influenza, Epstein-Barr, herpes simplex
	Reduced ability to cooperate with T cells in mitogenic responses	Poliomyelitis, influenza
	Reduced ability to cooperate with B cells in antibody responses	Coxsackie B, lymphocytic choriomeningitis
	Augmented suppressive activity	Epstein-Barr
Lymphocytes	Cytotoxicity	Measles, dengue, HIV
	Reduced blastogenic response to antigens and mitogens (T and B)	Measles, influenza, parainfluenza, echo, herpes simplex, reovirus, poxvirus, HIV
	Decreased helper activity (T)	Herpes simplex, HIV
	Augmented "spontaneous" proliferation	Influenza, herpes simplex, Epstein-Barr, measles
	Altered migratory ability	Influenza, parainfluenza
	Increased suppressive activity (T)	Mumps, Epstein-Barr, coxsackie B, dengue, influenza
	Reduced NK activity	Epstein-Barr, HIV

[a]Alveolar macrophages.
Source: Modified from Schaeffer, M. Vaccines and related biologic products: Current assessment of their safety and efficacy. *Clin. Immunol. News.* 2: 80, 1981.

sor activity is unaffected, if, however, the spleen cells are treated with anti-Thy-2 antisera (that will eliminate suppressor T cells), there is no evidence of transfer of suppressor activity, and the recipient animal is able to develop delayed hypersensitivity when challenged (Fig. 13.5). These observations suggest that influenza-virus-stimulated suppressor T cells inhibit the cell-mediated immune responses directed to a cross-reacting virus.

Whether the triggering of suppressor cells is a direct effect of viral infection of T cells is not clear. Several different viruses are known to be able to proliferate in macrophages and lymphocytes. Immune cell alterations are also frequent during human virus infections (Table 13.4), and in the case of HIV infection major alterations in the T-cell population have been demonstrated. The HIV virus infects predominantly $CD4^+$ cells, and the infection usually leads to cyto-toxicity. The exact cause of cell death has not been fully clarified and may be multifactorial. Among the mechanisms that have been suggested to lead to help-er-T-cell depletion are (a) the *formation of syntitia* with concomitant loss of cell identity; (b) the *accumulation of unintegrated viral DNA* in the cytoplasm of infected cells, which seems to be expressed, leading to intense viral proliferation and cell death; and (c) the *antilymphocytic antibodies*, or antibodies directed against viral glycoproteins expressed on the membrane of infected cells, which may also cause cytotoxicity. The numbers of T cells suffer a progressive decline and when their numbers become extremely low (under $300/mm^3$) opportunistic infections become the major clinical problem for the patients. Besides this di-rect cytotoxic effect of HIV, it is possible that the infected cells are affected by several other mechanisms:

1. Viral envelope proteins shed from infected cells may bind to the CD4 molecule (the receptor for HIV in human lymphocytes) and prevent the interaction between CD4 and MHC II antigens, which is believed to play an essential role in the inductive stages of T-cell activation.
2. Immune complexes formed between circulating viral components and the corresponding antibodies may down-regulate the immune response.
3. The reaction against virus-infected lymphocytes may eventually result in the formation of cross-reactive antibodies that may be cytotoxic for unin-fected cells.

Therefore, it appears as if viruses can both prevent the development of immune responses and cause a general depression of the immune system. A variety of mechanisms, which may operate simultaneously or in succession, account for their negative effects in the immune system and reflect an extremely compli-cated biological equilibrium which viruses have developed and that has proven extremely difficult to manipulate therapeutically.

SELF-EVALUATION

Questions

Choose the one best answer.

13.1 Consider the following experiment: 50 mice were injected with ectro-melia virus (murine pox virus, analogue to the vaccinia virus used for vaccination against smallpox); the mice were then subdivided into five groups of 10. Animals in group A were left untreated. Nine died. Animals in group B received intravenously serum collected on day 15 after infection with ectromelia virus in surviving mice of a previous experiment; the serum was injected 2 hours after the virus. All animals survived. Animals in group C received T lymphocytes separated from survivors of a previous experiment; the cells were transferred 2 hours after the virus. Nine animals survived. Animals in group D were treated as those of group B, but the serum was given 24 hours after the virus. Only two animals survived. Animals in group E were treated as those of group C, but the cells were transferred 24 hours after the virus. Eight animals survived. Which of the following conclusions is correct?

A. Humoral immunity has the most important role in protection against ectromelia virus.

B. In the 2 hours after infection, humoral antibody is significantly more efficient in protection than T cells.

C. The virus is accessible to the protective effects of antibody only for a few hours immediately after injection.

D. The protective effect of T lymphocytes depends on the elimination of the virus from circulation in the immediate period following immunization.

13.2 All of the following play a role in the immune defense against intracellular infection, except

A. Sensitization of T cells against surface-expressed determinants on the infected cell.

B. Amplification mechanisms depending on the recognition of the infected cell by a sensitized T cell.

C. Antibody-dependent cell-mediated cytotoxicity.

D. Neutralizing antibodies.

13.3 Antibodies can destroy virus-infected cells by

A. Direct neutralization of intracellular viral particles.

B. Inducing the release of antiviral substances from noninfected T cells.

C. Preventing viral uncoating.

D. Binding to virus-induced antigenic determinants on the cell surface and activating complement.

E. Opsonization followed by phagocytosis.

13.4 The finding of a generalized depression of cellular immunity during the acute phase of measles should be considered as

A. An expected finding, reflecting a transient state of immunosuppression.

B. Evidence of a primary immune deficiency syndrome.

C. A poor prognosis indicator.

D. A very unlikely finding, and all tests should be reordered immediately.

E. The result of a concurrent bacterial infection.

13.5 Non-infected $CD4^+$ T cells may have decreased functional capabilities in HIV infected patients because of

A. Down-regulation of the IL2 gene.

B. Cross-reactivity between anti-gp120 antibodies and the T-cell receptor.

C. Depressed IL1 synthesis by monocytes/macrophages.

D. Excessive proliferation of $CD8^+$ cells.

E. Blocking of CD4/MHC II interactions by gp 120 shed from infected cells.

13.6 An antibody to tetanus toxoid will prevent the deleterious effects of tetanus by

A. Causing the destruction of *Clostridium tetani* before it releases significant amounts of toxin.

B. Forming immune complexes with the toxin that are quickly phagocytized and destroyed.

C. Inhibiting the binding of the toxin to its receptor by binding directly to the toxin active site.

D. Binding to the antigenic portion of the toxin molecule and inhibiting the binding of the toxin to its receptor by steric hindrance.

E. Promoting ADCC reactions against *C. tetani*.

13.7 Herpes virus escapes immune defenses by

A. Causing immunosuppression.

B. Being a very weak immunogen.

C. Producing an excess of soluble antigen that blocks the corresponding antibody.

D. Spreading from cell to cell with minimal exposure to the extracellular environment.

13.8 The ABO isohemagglutinins are synthesized as a result of

A. Genetic predisposition.

B. Blood transfusions with incompatible blood.

C. Cross-immunization with polysaccharide-rich enterobactericeae.

D. Repeated pregnancies.

13.9 In a newborn baby with blood typed as A, Rh positive, the lack of anti-B isoagglutinins is

A. A normal finding.

B. Evidence suggestive of fetal immunoincompetence.

C. Evidence of maternal immunoincompetence.

D. A very exceptional finding, identifying the baby as a nonresponder to blood group B substance.

13.10 The parasite-killing properties of eosinophils are linked to the production and secretion of
A. Leukotrienes.
B. Prostaglandins.
C. Major basic protein.
D. Histamine.

Answers

13.1 (C)   Both cellular and humoral adoptive immunity appear efficient in protecting the animals during the very early stages, but if 24 hr elapse before transfer of adoptive immunity, the protective effect of antibodies is lost, suggesting that at that stage the viremic phase (which is the stage at which neutralizing antibodies can be protective) has already elapsed.

13.2 (D)

13.3 (D)

13.4 (A)   Measles is characteristically associated with a transient depression of cellular immunity during the acute phase; a patient with such immune depression should not be considered as having a primary immune deficiency or as having necessarily a poor prognosis.

13.5 (E)   HIV-infected T cells shed gp 120 molecules, which bind to the CD4 molecule of noninfected cells. The noninfected T cells are not directly affected by the binding of gp120, but their ability to interact with APC is compromised by the binding of viral glycoproteins that, in effect, block the normal interactions between CD4 and MHC II, which are essential for the proper stimulation of helper T cells.

13.6 (D)   An antitetanus toxoid antibody is neither cytotoxic to *Clostridium tetani*, since the toxin in question is an exotoxin, nor able to bind to the active site of the toxin, since the toxoid used for immunization host lost (as a consequence of detoxification) the active site.

13.7 (D)   Herpes virus is a strong immunogen, does not cause immunosuppression, and does not appear to induce the release of large amounts of soluble antigens from infected cells, but its cell-to-cell spread keeps it shielded from all humoral mechanisms of defense.

13.8 (C)

13.9 (A)   Since the newborn's intestine has not been colonized by enterobac-
            teriaceae, the antigenic stimulation for production of isohemagglu-
            tinins has not been received at birth, and negative titers of isohemag-
            glutinins are normal. Maternal isohemagglutinins, being in a large
            majority of cases of the IgM class, do not cross the placenta.

13.10 (C)

BIBLIOGRAPHY

Bendinelli, M. Mechanisms and significance of immunodepression in viral diseases. *Clin. Immunol. News.* 2:75, 1981.

Borst, P. and Graves, D. R. Programmed gene rearrangements altering gene
expression. *Science 235*:658, 1987. (An excellent discussion of the molecular genetic mechanisms responsible for microbial antigenic variation.)

Fauci, A. S. The human immunodeficiency virus: infectivity and mechanisms
of pathogenesis. *Science 239*:617, 1988. (Excellent review on the immune
abnormalities associated with HIV infections.)

Hahn, H. and Kaufman, H. E. The role of cell-mediated immunity in bacterial
infections. *Rev. Infect. Dis. 3*:1221, 1981.

McChesney, M. B. and Oldstone, M. B. A. Viruses perturb lymphocyte functions: selected principles characterizing virus-induced immunosuppression.
Ann. Rev. Immunol. 5:279, 1987.

Moller, G. (Ed.). *Immunological Reviews*, Vol. 61, *Immunoparasitology*. Munks-
gaard, Copenhagen, 1982.

Seyda, M. and Kruger, G. R. F. Complex infectious copathogenesis of AIDS in
HIV-positive individuals. *Clin. Immunol. News. 8*:81, 1987.

Virella, G. and Fudenberg, H. H. Secondary immunodeficiencies. In *The
Pathophysiology of Human Immunologic Disorders*, J. J. Twomey (Ed.).
Urban & Schwarzenberg, Baltimore, 1982. (Contains detailed discussion
of immunodepression caused by infectious agents.)

Zinkernagel, R. M. Major transplantation antigens in host responses to infection.
In *The Biology of Immunologic Disease*, F. J. Dixon and D. W. Fisher (Eds.).
Sinauer, Sunderland, Massachusetts, 1983.

II
Diagnostic Immunology

14

Immunoserology and Diagnostic Immunochemistry

GABRIEL VIRELLA

The exquisite sensitivity and specificity of antigen-antibody reactions has been utilized as the basis for many diagnostic procedures. Depending on the test design, one can detect or quantitate either specific antigens or specific antibodies. Both types of tests have found ample applications in clinical diagnosis. Antigen-detection tests have been applied to the diagnosis of infectious diseases, the monitoring of neoplasia, the quantitation of hormones, drugs, etc. Quantitation of specific antibodies has found wide application in the diagnosis of infectious, allergic, and immunodeficiency diseases.

For detection (or quantitation) of antigen or antibody in body fluids by immunological methods a purified preparation of one of the components of the reaction must be available. For instance, when human serum is tested for antibody to diphtheria toxoid, a purified preparation of the toxoid must be available. Secondly, a method for detecting the specific antigen-antibody reaction must be developed. A wide array of antigen-antibody assays has been applied to diagnosis; in this chapter we review those most widely used, discussing their applications, advantages, and disadvantages.

I. METHODS BASED ON PRECIPITATION

Several of the commonly used serological and immunodiagnostic techniques are based on the detection of antigen-antibody aggregates, either through visualization of precipitates or by measuring the light dispersed by those aggregates.

A. Double Immunodiffusion Method (Ouchterlony's Technique)

In the double diffusion technique wells are punched in a support matrix; antigen and antibody are placed in separate wells and diffuse toward each other and precipitate at the point of antigen-antibody equivalence.

This simple technique is a useful qualitative tool for determining the presence or absence of a given antigen using highly defined antisera, or for determining antibody presence if purified antigen is available. The method's usefulness is limited by its relative lack of sensitivity and by the time required for full development of precipitin patterns—up to 72 to 96 hours of diffusion when either reactant is present in small quantities. Double diffusion in agar is used for the serologic diagnosis of infectious diseases (e.g., candidiasis and echinococcosis), in the investigation of hypersensitivity states, mainly hypersensitive pneumonitis (e.g., pigeon breeder's disease), and in the investigation of precipitating antibodies to food proteins such as milk (Fig. 14.1).

B. Counterimmunoelectrophoresis

Counterimmunoelectrophoresis (CIE) is a sensitive and rapid technique in which antigen and antibody are placed in opposite wells and driven toward each other with an electric current (antibodies move to the cathode while most antigens are strongly negatively charged and move toward the anode). Precipitin lines can be visualized between the antigen and antibody wells. The method is useful for detection of precipitins to *Candida albicans* (Fig. 14.2), anti-DNA antibodies, fungal or bacterial antigens in CSF, etc.

C. Immunoelectrophoresis

Immunoelectrophoresis (IEP) is a two-step technique; first, a small sample of serum is applied in a well and electrophoresed through a support medium, usually agarose. After the electrophoretic step, specific antisera are deposited in a trough cut into the agarose, parallel to the axis of the electrophoretic separation. The electrophoretically separated proteins and the antisera diffuse toward one another, and at the zone of antigen-antibody equivalence, a precipitin pattern in the form of an arc will appear (Fig. 14.3). The qualitative and semi-quantitative interpretation of these precipitin patterns by an experienced interpreter has considerable diagnostic usefulness.

Immunoelectrophoresis is the classical technique for analytical studies in patients suspected of B-cell dyscrasia. In cases of hypergammaglobulinemia, IEP analysis can establish or disprove the monoclonal nature of the immunoglobulin increase through the identification of the immunoglobulin class and light chain type involved. Monoclonal free light chains (Bence-Jones proteins) may be present in the urine of these patients, and IEP of urine is the method most frequently used for their detection.

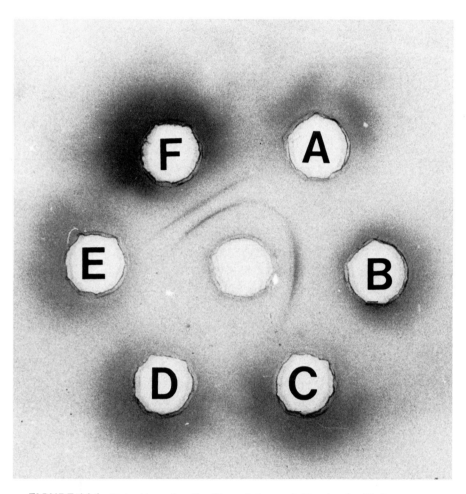

FIGURE 14.1   Detection of anti-milk-protein precipitins by double immunodiffusion. The central well was filled with clarified cow's milk and the peripheral wells were filled with sera from different patients. Patients B and F are
unquestionably positive; patients D and E are negative; patients A and C are
questionable.

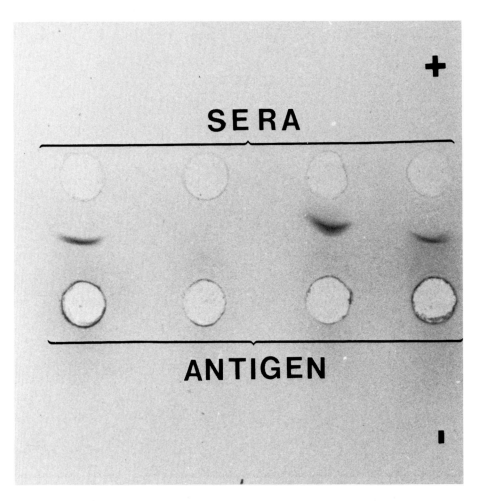

FIGURE 14.2 Detection of anti-*C. albicans* antibodies by counterimmunoelec-trophoresis. The wells on the cathodal side were filled with an antigenic extract of *C. albicans*, and the wells on the anodal side were filled with patient's serum. The appearance of a precipitation line between a given serum well and the anti-gen well directly opposed to it identifies the patients as positive.

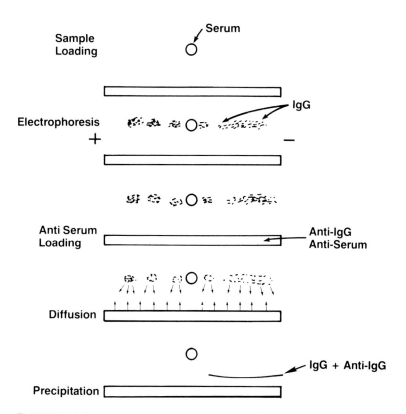

FIGURE 14.3 Diagrammatic representation of the basic steps in immunoelectrophoresis.

D. Immunofixation and Immunoblotting

Immunofixation is a technique that has become progressively more popular as an alternative to immunoelectrophoresis, mainly because the interpretation of results is considerably easier. The principle of the technique is diagrammatically represented in Figure 14.4. In the first step, several aliquots of the patient's serum are simultaneously separated by electrophoresis. One of the separation lanes is stained as reference for the position of the different serum proteins, while paper strips imbedded with different antibodies are laid over the remaining separation lanes. The antibodies diffuse into the agar and react with the corresponding immunoglobulins. After washing unbound immunoglobulins and antibodies off, the lanes where immunofixation takes place are stained, revealing whether the antisera did or did not recognize the proteins they are directed against. In the case illustrated in the diagram a patient's serum was being tested

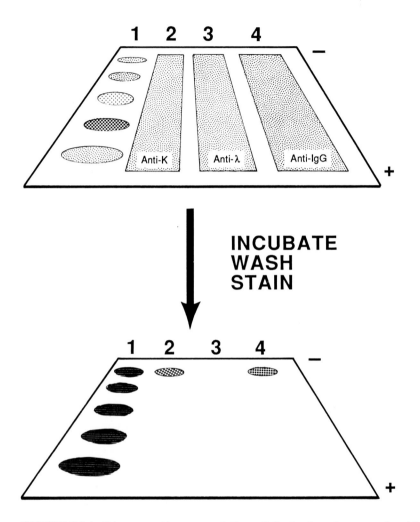

FIGURE 14.4 Diagrammatic representation of the typing of a monoclonal IgG
protein by immunofixation. The top panel illustrates the electrophoretic separation of serum proteins, revealed by staining in lane 1, and the overlay with three
different antisera (anti-κ, anti-λ, and anti-IgG) of lanes 2, 3, and 4, where the
same proteins were separated. After incubation to allow antigens and antibodies
to react, the unreacted proteins and antibodies are washed off and the precipitates formed with the different antibodies stained. In the example illustrated,
precipitates were formed in the cathodal region (where immunoglobulins are
separated by electrophoresis) with anti-IgG and anti-κ, allowing to confirm that
the serum contained a monoclonal protein typed as IgGκ.

for the presence of an IgG monoclonal protein. Such protein, by definition, has to be homogeneous in mobility, and it has to react with anti-IgG antibodies and with either antikappa or antilambda antibodies. In the diagram, the stained precipitates, obtained after all unbound proteins were washed off, correspond to the lanes that were overlaid with anti-IgG and with antikappa light chains. This result would prove that an IgGκ monoclonal protein existed in this patient's serum.

Immunoblotting, originally introduced in research laboratories, has acquired clinical significance since the Western blot was heralded as the confirmatory test in cases of positive serology for the HIV virus. As illustrated in Figure 14.5, the first step in a Western blot is to separate the different viral antigens (gp 160 to p 16) according to their molecular size; the numbers in front on *gp* or *p* refer to the protein mass in kilodaltons (kD). This is achieved by performing electrophoresis in the presence of an anionic detergent (negatively charged) and using a medium that has sieving properties for the separation. After the separation is completed, it is necessary to transfer the proteins to another support, in order to proceed with the remaining steps. This transfer or blotting is easily achieved by forcing the proteins to migrate into a nitrocellulose membrane by a second electrophoresis step (electroblotting). The nitrocellulose membrane to which the viral antigens have been transferred is then impregnated with patient's serum. If antibodies to any or several of these antigens are contained in the serum, the antigen will be precipitated at the point where it was blotted. The following steps are designed to detect precipitates in the cellulose membrane. First, all the unprecipitated antigens and antibodies are washed off; then the protein binding sites still available on the membrane are blocked to prevent false positive reactions; finally, the membrane is overlaid with a labeled antibody to human immunoglobulins. This antibody will react with the precipitates formed by viral antigens and human antibodies and can be later revealed either by adding a color-developing substrate (if the antihuman immunoglobulin is labeled with an enzyme) or by autoradiography (if the antihuman immunoglobulin is labeled with ^{125}I). A positive result, as shown in the diagram, is indicated by the retention of the labeled antibody in the site(s) where viral antigens of known molecular weight have been separated.

E. Radial Immunodiffusion

Radial immunodiffusion (RID), while not as sensitive as some newer techniques and relatively slow, is nonetheless reliable for routine quantitation of many serum proteins. In this method antisera are added to the support matrix and antigen is placed in wells punched into the agar. At antigen-antibody equivalence a precipitin ring forms, and both the area and the diameter of the precipitation ring are porportional to the concentration of the antigen in the sample

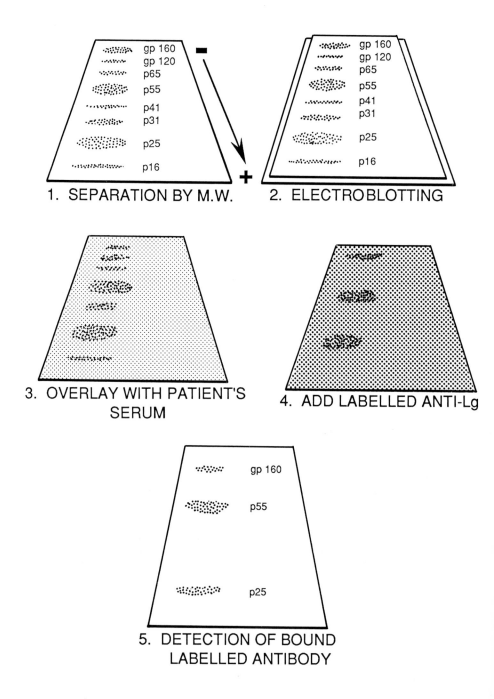

1. SEPARATION BY M.W.

2. ELECTROBLOTTING

3. OVERLAY WITH PATIENT'S SERUM

4. ADD LABELLED ANTI-Lg

5. DETECTION OF BOUND LABELLED ANTIBODY

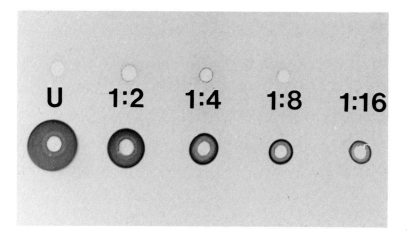

FIGURE 14.6 The principle of radial immunodiffusion: if five wells carved into antibody-containing agar are filled with serial dilutions of the corresponding antigen, the antigen will diffuse and eventually be precipitated in a circular pattern; the diameters or areas of these circular precipitates are directly proportional to the concentration of antigen in each well.

FIGURE 14.5 Diagrammatic representation of a Western blot study to confirm the existence of anti-HIV antibodies. In the first step a mixture of HIV antigens is separated by size (large antigens remain close to the origin where the sample is applied, smaller antigens move deep into the acrylamide gel used for the separation). In the second step the separated antigens are electrophoresced into a permeable nitrocellulose membrane (electroblotting). Next, the patient's serum is spread over the cellulose membrane to which the antigens have been transferred. If antibodies to any of these antigens are present in the serum, a precipitate will be formed at the site where the antigen has been transferred. After washing off the excess of unreacted antigens and serum proteins, a labeled second antibody is overlaid on the membrane; if human antibodies precipitate by reacting with blotted antigens, the second antibody (labeled antihuman immunoglobulin) will react with the immunoglobulins contained in the precipitate. After washing off the excess of unreacted second antibody, its binding to an antigen-antibody precipitate can be detected either by adding a color-developing substrate (if the second antibody is labeled with an enzyme) or by autoradiography (if the second antibody is labeled with an adequate isotope such as ^{125}I).

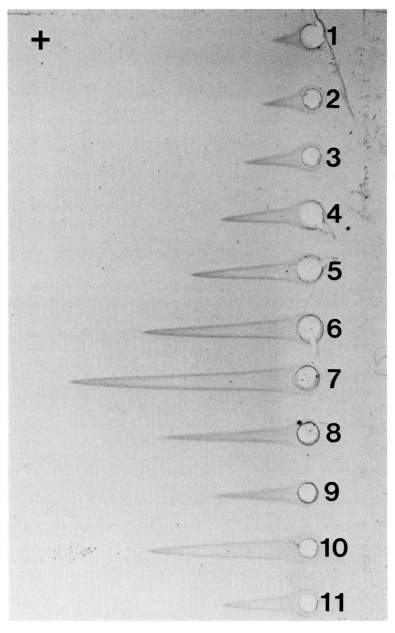

FIGURE 14.7 Quantitative immuno electrophoresis. In this assay, antibody to apolipoprotein B was incorporated into the agar. Reference standards with known concentrations of apolipoprotein B were used to fill wells 1-7; the remaining wells filled with the patients's sera. (Courtesy of Dr. Maria F. Lopes-Virella, VAMC, Charleston, South Carolina.)

(Fig. 14.6). RID is readily applied to the quantitation of immunoglobulins, complement components and, in general, of any antigenic protein that exists in concentrations greater than 5-10 mg/dl.

F. Quantitative Immunoelectrophoresis (Rocket Electrophoresis)

This quantitative adaptation of immunoelectrophoresis is faster and more sensitive than RID, because the antigen is actively driven through an antibody-containing matrix by an electric potential. As the equivalence zone of antigen-antibody reaction is reached, the reaction ceases and elongated precipitin arcs ("rockets") become visible (Fig. 14.7). The lengths of these rockets are proportional to the antigen concentrations in the wells. Rocket electrophoresis can be used for the quantitative assay of many proteins, including immunoglobulins. The reverse modality with antigen incorporated in the agar can be used for the quantitation of specific antibodies.

G. Immunonephelometry

Under antibody excess conditions, mixing antigen and antibody results in the formation of soluble antigen-antibody complexes whose concentration can be determined by measuring light dispersion. A beam of light is passed through tubes containing mixtures of fixed amounts of antibody and variable concentrations of antigen, which form antigen-antibody complexes. The concentration of immune complexes in the test tube will determine how much light is scattered, which is measured at angles varying from near $0°$ to $90°$. Since antibody concentrations are kept constant, the light scattered is proportional to the concentration of antigen in the mixture. This principle is the basis for immunonephelometric assays, which by virtue of their sensitivity, speed, and expediency, have replaced radial immunodiffusion as the method of choice for the quantitation of immunoglobulins and other proteins that exist in concentrations greater than 1 mg/dl.

II. METHODS BASED ON AGGLUTINATION

When bacteria, antigen-coated particles, or cells in suspension are mixed with antibody directed to their surface determinants, the antigen-antibody reaction leads to the clumping (agglutination) of the cells or particles carrying the antigen. Quantitative analysis to determine the agglutinating antibody content of an antiserum involves dilution of the serum and determination an of end point, which is the last dilution at which agglutination can be observed. The reciprocal of this last agglutinating dilution is designated as antibody titer.

A. Agglutination of Whole Microorganisms

Agglutination of whole microorganisms or of products derived directly from microorganisms is used in the diagnosis of some infectious diseases, e.g., the Widal test for the diagnosis of typhoid fever and the Weil-Felix test for the diagnosis of typhus (based on the fact that certain stains of *Proteus* share antigens with several *Rickettsia* species).

B. Agglutination of Inert Particles Coated with Antigen or Antibody

Latex particles have been widely used as substrates on which antigen can be coated, and these particles are subsequently agglutinated in the presence of specific antibody. Conversely, specific antibodies can be easily adsorbed by latex particles and will agglutinate in the presence of the corresponding antigen.

1. Gamma-globulin-coated latex particles are used for the detection of anti-Ig factors (rhematoid factors) in the RA test (Fig. 14.8).
2. Latex particles coated with thyroglobulin are used in a thryoglobulin antibody test.
3. A wide variety of diagnostic tests for infectious diseases have been developed based on latex agglutination. In some cases the antigen is bound to latex and the test detects specific antibodies (e.g., tests for histoplasmosis, cryptococcosis, and trichinosis). More recently, tests for the rapid

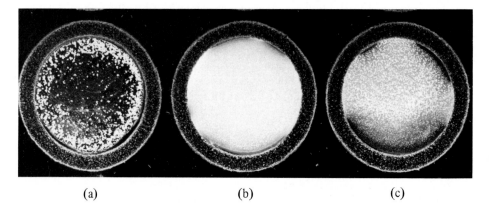

(a)   (b)   (c)

FIGURE 14.8 Detection of rheumatoid factor by the latex agglutination technique. A suspension of IgG-coated latex particles as mixed with a 1:20 dilution of three sera. Obvious clumping is seen in (a), corresponding to a strongly positive serum; no clumping is seen in (b), corresponding to a negative serum; very fine clumping is seen in (c), corresponding to a weakly positive serum.

diagnosis of bacterial and fungal meningitis have been developed by adsorbing the relevant specific antibodies to latex particles. The antibody-coated particles will agglutinate if mixed with CSF containing the relevant antigen. This procedure allows a rapid etiological diagnosis of meningitis, which is essential if proper therapy is to be initiated.

C. Hemagglutination

Hemagglutination tests are based on the agglutination of red blood cells, either by antibodies directed to native red cells or by antibodies directed against antigens artificially conjugated to the red cell.

1. Direct Hemagglutination

Direct hemagglutination is a method used to detect antibodies directed against antigenic determinants native to the RBCs. Determination of the ABO blood group is done by direct agglutination, as are the tests for isohemagglutinins (anti-A and anti-B antibodies) and for cold hemagglutinins (IgM antibodies that agglutinate RBCs at temperatures below that of the body), as illustrated in Figure 14.9. The Paul-Bunnell test, useful for the diagnosis of infectious mononucleosis, is a direct hemagglutination test that detects heterophile antibodies that induce the agglutination of horse erythrocytes.

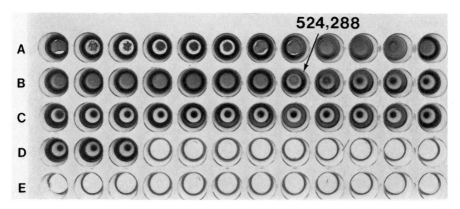

FIGURE 14.9 Detection of cold agglutinins by direct hemagglutination. The wells in the microtiter plate were first filled with serial dilutions of a patient's serum (rows A and B), serial dilutions of a control serum (row C) and saline (row D), and then with O+ red cells, incubated at 4°C and examined for agglutination. The normal control and saline control do not show agglutination, whereas the patient's serum shows a prozone followed by agglutination up to a dilution of 1:512,000.

2. Indirect Hemagglutination

Indirect hemagglutination detects antibodies that react with antigens present in the erythrocytes but that by themselves cannot induce direct agglutination, possibly by being bivalent IgG antibodies, which are not as efficient agglutinators of red cells as polymeric and polyvalent IgM antibodies. A second antibody directed to human immunoglobulins is used to induce agglutination. The best known example of indirect agglutination is the antiglobulin or Coombs' test, which is used in the diagnosis of autoimmune hemolytic anemia.

3. Passive Hemagglutination

Passive hemagglutination techniques use red blood cells as a substrate much as latex is used in tests involving inert particles. Antigen can be coated onto the red cells by a variety of methods, and the coated cells will agglutinate when exposed to specific antibody (Fig. 14.10). This system is very sensitive and has been used as basis for a variety of diagnostic procedures such as an antithyroid antibody test, the Rose Waaler test for anti-Ig factors present in the serum of patients with rheumatoid arthritis, and many tests to detect anti-infectious antibodies. Antigens can also be detected by this technique by determining whether a biological fluid suspected of containing them can reduce the agglutinating capacity of an antiserum (hemagglutination inhibition). In a first step, the antiserum and biological fluid are mixed. In a second step, red cells coated with antigen are added to dilutions of the mixture. The agglutinating titer of the antiserum is known, and if a fourfold or greater decrease in titer is observed, it

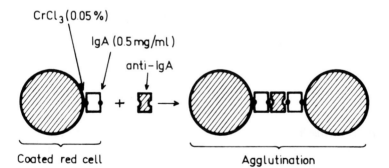

Coated red cell   Agglutination

FIGURE 14.10 Diagrammatic representation of a passive hemagglutination test to detect anti-IgA antibodies. Purified IgA was coated to chromium-chloride-treated RBC; the IgA coated red cells will be agglutinated by anti-IgA antibodies. (Original diagram of Dr. Jukka Koistinen, Finnish Red Cross, Helsinki, Finland.)

can be concluded that antigen was present in the tested biological fluid. Hemagglutination tests are difficult to standardize and reproduce and they are not too accurate (like all titration tests). Therefore, they have been progressively replaced by tests that are more sensitive, more accurate, and easier to reproduce, such as enzymoimmunoassays.

III. COMPLEMENT FIXATION

When antigen and antibodies of the IgM or IgG classes are mixed, complement is fixed to the antigen-antibody aggregate. If this occurs on the surface of a red blood cell, the complement cascade will be activated and hemolysis will occur. Complement fixation reactions have been widely used in a large number of tests designed to assist in the diagnosis of specific infections.

The method actually involves two antigen-antibody complement systems, a test system and an indicator system (Fig. 14.11). The indicator system consists of sheep red blood cells that have been coated with antibodies to RBC antigen; these are designated as sensitized red cells. In the test system, patient's serum, which has been heated to 56°C to inactivate the native complement and adsorbed with washed sheep RBC to eliminate Forssman-type cross-reactive antibodies, is mixed with purified antigen and with a dilution of fresh guinea pig serum as a controlled source of complement. The mixture is incubated for 30 minutes at 37°C to allow any antibody in the patient's serum to form complexes with antigen and fix complement. Sensitized red cells are then added to the mixture. If the red cells are lysed it indicates that there were no antigen-specific antibodies in the serum of the patient, so complement was not consumed in the test system and was available to be used by the anti-RBC antibodies, resulting in hemolysis. This reaction is considered negative. If the red cells are not lysed, it indicates that antibodies specific to the antigen were present in the test system and fixed complement, and that none was available to be activated by the indicator system. This reaction is considered positive.

Complement fixation has the advantage of being widely applicable to the detection of antibodies to almost any antigen. It is the basis of the Wasserman test for syphilis and can be used to detect antibodies to *Mycoplasma pneumoniae, Bordetella pertussis*, antibodies to many different viruses, and to fungi like *Cryptococcus, Histoplasma*, and *Coccidioides immitis*. But because of many technical difficulties in the test, the tendency is to replace it with newer methods.

IV. IMMUNOFLUORESCENCE

The primary reaction between antibody and cell or tissue-fixed antigens can be demonstrated by use of antibodies chemically combined with fluorescent dyes.

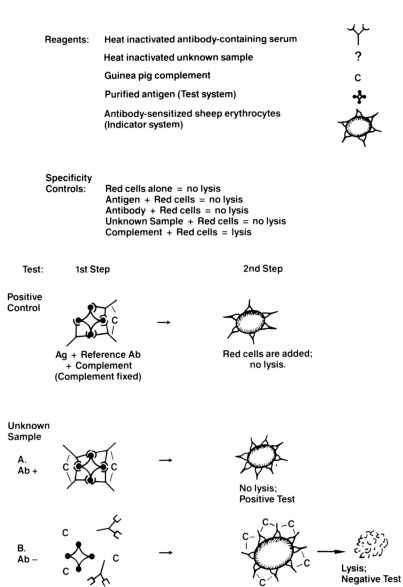

Reagents: Heat inactivated antibody-containing serum

              Heat inactivated unknown sample

              Guinea pig complement

              Purified antigen (Test system)

              Antibody-sensitized sheep erythrocytes
              (Indicator system)

Specificity
Controls: Red cells alone = no lysis
              Antigen + Red cells = no lysis
              Antibody + Red cells = no lysis
              Unknown Sample + Red cells = no lysis
              Complement + Red cells = lysis

Test: 1st Step   2nd Step

Positive
Control

             Ag + Reference Ab   Red cells are added;
             + Complement   no lysis.
             (Complement fixed)

Unknown
Sample

A.
Ab +

                                                   No lysis;
                                                   Positive Test

B.
Ab −

                                                   Lysis;
                                                   Negative Test

FIGURE 14.11   Diagrammatic representation of the general principles of complement fixation tests.

There are various methods that can be used to detect the presence of unknown antigen in cells or tissues and the presence of unknown antibodies in patient's serum (Fig. 14.12). In the *direct* method, antigen in a cell or tissue is visualized by direct labeling with fluorescent antibody, or tissue-deposited immune complexes can be revealed by reaction with a fluorescent anti-immunoglobulin antibody. In the *indirect* method, there are two steps, the first involving incubation of fixed antigen (e.g., in a cell or tissue) with unlabeled antibody to form an

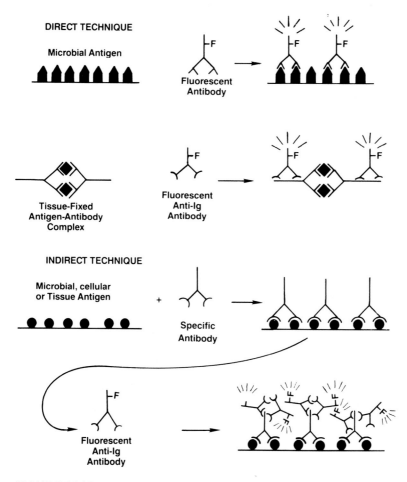

FIGURE 14.12 Diagrammatic representation of the general principles of direct and indirect immunofluorescence.

immune complex, and the second involving reacting the immune complex with labeled anti-immunoglobulin antibody so that it can then be visualized (Fig. 14.11). The indirect method has the advantage of using a single labeled anti-immunoglobulin antibody to detect many different specific antigen-antibody reactions occurring within a given species, such as the human.

Immunofluorescence has wide diagnostic applications. In microbiology it can be used to identify most bacterial species and also to detect specific anti-body bound to the microorganisms. An example is the use of an indirect fluorescence test for the diagnosis of syphilis. In a first step the patient's serum is incubated with killed *Treponema pallidum*; in the second step a fluorescent-labeled antihuman antibody is used to determine whether antibodies from the patient's serum become bound to the *Treponema*. Similar techniques have been used for some viral diseases using virus-infected cells as antigen-containing substrate. By using fluorescent labeled anti-IgM a greater degree of specificity and information concerning the nature of the infection (recent or past) can be obtained, because the presence of IgM antibodies is usually a hallmark of a very recent antigenic exposure.

Outside of microbiology, immunofluorescence has found many other applications, including the identification of lymphocyte subpopulations through the use of labeled monoclonal antibodies. The development of cytofluorographs, able to measure cell size and fluorescence intensity, the availability of a wide assay of monoclonal antibodies to different cell markers, and the possibility of double labeling some cells with two different antibodies labeled with two different fluorescent compounds (usually one green and one red) has resulted in great progress in the characterization of lymphocyte subsets in peripheral blood, as discussed in Chapter 16.

Immunofluorescence is also the technique of choice for the detection of autoantibodies such as antinuclear factor. Classically the suspect serum is incubated with an adequate tissue (rat kidney, HeLa cells), and indirect immunofluorescence is performed in a second step to detect antibodies fixed to the substrate. In a positive test the nuclei of the cells used as substrate will be fluorescent. Anti-dsDNA antibodies can also be detected by immunofluorescence using a flagellate (*Chritidia lucilliae*) that has a kinetoplast composed of pure dsDNA. Fixed organisms are incubated with patient's serum seen in the first step. Anti-dsDNA antibodies, if present, will bind to the kinetoplast and will be revealed with fluorescein-labeled anti-IgG antibody.

V. RADIOIMMUNOASSAY (RIA)

The classical radioimmunoassay methods were based on the principle of competitive binding. Unlabeled antigen competes with radiolabeled antigen for binding to antibody with the appropriate specificty. Upon addition of unlabeled

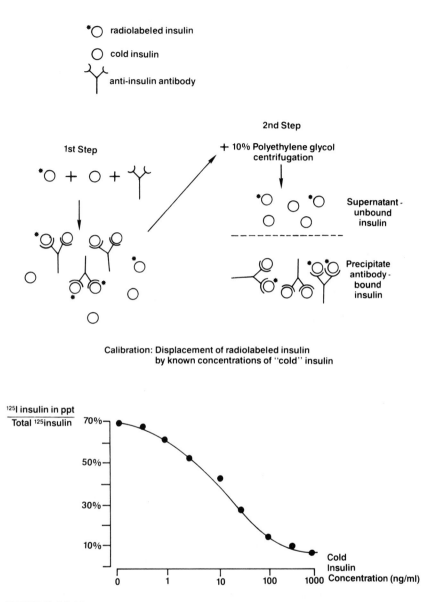

FIGURE 14.13 Diagrammatic representation of the general principles of competitive radioimmunoassays in fluid phase. In this type of technique (of which the quantitation of insulin levels is a good example) the free and antibody-bound antigens are separated either by physiochemical techniques, as shown in the diagram, or by using a second antibody (anti-immunoglobulin) to precipitate the antibody molecules that will carry with them any antigen they may have reacted with.

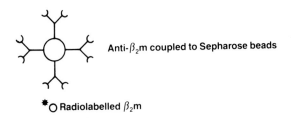

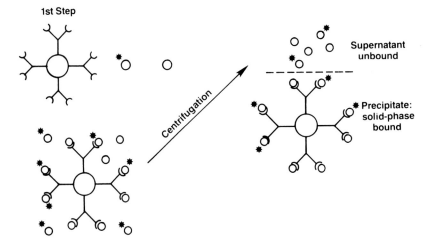

FIGURE 14.14   Diagrammatic representation of the general principles of competitive radioimmunoassays in solid phase. In this case (an assay for $\beta2$ microglobulin), because the antibody is bound to an insoluble matrix, the separation of free antigen from antibody-bound antigen is achieved by simple centrifugation. The calibration of the assay follows the simple principles shown in Figure 14.12.

antigen the amount of free (not bound to antibody) radiolabeled antigen is directly proportional to the quantity of unlabeled antigen added. A standard curve is constructed by plotting the percentage of antibody-bound radiolabeled antigen against known concentrations of a standardized unlabeled antigen (Fig. 14.13).

Any RIA requires a method of separating free and antibody-bound radiolabeled antigen so that the radiolabeled immune complexes can be quantitated. Solid-phase RIA is the easiest answer to this problem. The basic principle in solid-phase RIA is to attach the antibody to a test tube wall, or to an inert particle that can be centrifuged; the subsequent separation of free and bound antigen then becomes easier (Fig. 14.14). Solid phase RIA for the detection of specific antibodies has also been described. Most frequently, noncompetitive assays are used, in which the antigen is bound to solid phase and a radiolabeled antihuman immunoglobulin is used to quantitate specific antibody that becomes bound to the immobilized antigen.

Radioimmunoassays are extremely sensitive and have been used with extremely good results in the assay of many different hormones (insulin, aldosterone, human FSH, progesterone, testosterone, thyroxin, vasopressin, etc.), proteins (alpha-fetoprotein, carcinoembryonic antigen, IgE, hepatitis B surface antigen), vitamins (vitamin B12), drugs (digoxin, LSD, barbiturate derivates), enzymes (pepsin, trypsin), antibodies to DNA and to hepatitis B surface antigen (HBsAg), etc. Their main drawbacks lie in the cost of equipment and reagents, in the short shelf-life of radiolabeled compounds, and in the problems associated with the disposal of radiolabeled substances.

VI. ENZYMOIMMUNOASSAY

Enzymoimmunoassay (EIA, also known as ELISA for enzyme-linked immunosorbent assay), a technique introduced in the mid-1970s, has become perhaps the most widely used immunological assay method. Conceptually EIA is very close to solid-phase RIA; one of the components of the reaction (antigen if we want to assay antibodies; antibody if we want to assay antigens) is adsorbed onto a solid phase (e.g., polystyrene tubes, plastic microtiter plates, plastic or metal beads, plastic discs, etc.). The second step consists of an incubation with antigen or antibody-containing solutions, depending on the assay. Finally, an enzyme-labeled component (antigen or antibody) is added; its binding to the previous components is measured by adding an adequate substrate that, upon reaction with the enzyme (usually peroxidase or alkaline phosphatase), develops a color whose intensity can be measured by spectrophotometry. The method can be based on competitive binding, e.g., for the assay of IgG, anti-IgG is adsorbed to the solid phase and incubated with mixtures of enzyme-labeled and test IgG, or the assay can be noncompetitive, similar to indirect immunofluorescence. For example, to assay antibodies to tetanus toxoid, the toxoid is adsorbed to the solid phase, then incubated with test sera and calibrated sera; next, an enzyme labeled anti-Ig will react with the antibodies fixed to the toxoid; finally, a substrate is added that develops a color whose intensity is proportional to the amount of bound enzyme-conjugated antibody. Since the amount of enzyme-conjugated antibody bound to the plate is proportional to the amount of antitetanus toxoid bound in the first place, a correlation between known antibody concentration and color intensity can be established and used to calculate antibody concentrations in unknown samples.

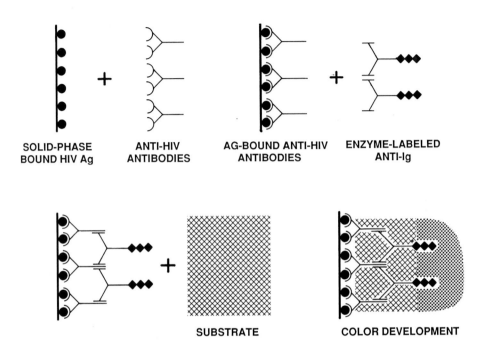

SOLID-PHASE   ANTI-HIV   AG-BOUND ANTI-HIV   ENZYME-LABELED
BOUND HIV Ag   ANTIBODIES   ANTIBODIES   ANTI-Ig

SUBSTRATE   COLOR DEVELOPMENT

FIGURE 14.15   Diagrammatic representation of an enzymoimmunoassay test for the diagnosis of HIV infection. The test uses solid-phase-bound HIV antigens; the patient's serum is incubated with the immobilized antigens, allowing the specific binding of anti-HIV antibodies; after washing unbound proteins, a second, enzyme-labeled antihuman immunoglobulin antibody is added to the reactants; this second antibody will bind to the patient's immunoglobulins that had reacted with the immobilized antigen in the first step; after washing unbound second antibody a substrate is added; the substrate is usually colorless, but in the presence of the enzyme bound to the second antibody it will develop a color. The development of color indicates positivity, and it allows quantitative measurements, because its intensity is directly proportional to the concentration of anti-HIV antibody added in the first incubation.

The sensitivity of enzymoimmunoassays allows the assay of nanogram amounts without great difficulty and can be further increased if the avidin-biotin peroxidase complex is used as indicator. The first step of the technique, antibody-substrate reaction, is identical to that of conventional assay, but the secondary antibody is labeled with biotin, and biotinilated peroxidase is used as indicator. Avidin, an egg-white protein with very high affinity for biotin, is added to the system and bridges the biotin molecules linked to the secondary antibody and to the enzyme (peroxidase). The amplifying character of this reaction results from the fact that the amount of peroxidase eventually bound to the secondary antibody is considerably in excess of what it would be if peroxidase were directly coupled to it.

Enzymoimmunoassays of one or another variety has progressively replaced RIA because of its comparable sensitivity, the longer shelf-life of enzyme-conjugated antibodies, and the lack of problems related to disposal of enzyme conjugates. Enzymoimmunoassays have been developed for a variety of antibacterial, viral, and parasite antigens (including the test for anti-HIV antibodies, illustrated in Fig. 14.15), as well as for antigen, hormone, and drug detections. In recent years, a variety of home tests based on EIA, particularly for pregnancy diagnosis, have been developed and successfully introduced. Usually the tests provide a dipstick with an absorbant pad to which monoclonal antibodies to hCG have been coupled. The dipstick is dipped into freshly collected urine; it will capture hCG proportionally to the concentration being excreted. After the tip of the dipstick is rinsed in running water, it is dipped in a solution containing alkaline-phosphatase-labelled anti-hCG monoclonal antibody, which will be bound to the dipstick in amounts proportional to those of captured hCG. After incubation the dipstick is washed and dipped into a solution containing (for example) bromochloroindolyl phosphate, a substrate that will react with alkaline phosphatase, becoming insoluble and turning indigo. The blue color is deposited on the pad where hCG was bound, indicating a positive result. A simplified ELISA home-assay for hCG has been introduced in which the urine is first mixed with enzyme-conjugated monoclonal anti-hCG, and the complexes formed between urinary hCG and the labelled antibody are then bound into a dipstick whose tip has a small absorbant pad with immobilized anti-hCG. After incubation and rinsing, the pad is immersed into a substrate solution that will react with the enzyme-labelled antibody and turn the pad deep blue (positive reaction). The convenience and simplicity of these tests has ensured their rapid diffusion, and it is expected that a variety of other tests based on similar principles will be introduced in the near future.

SELF-EVALUATION

Questions

Choose the one best answer.

14.1 A possible cause for false positivity in a complement fixation test could be
   A. The existence of antigen-antibody complexes in the unknown sample.
   B. Too much complement added.
   C. Inefficient complement inactivation in the unknown sample.

D. Old red cells.

E. Involuntary omission of antigen in the test.

14.2 The method of choice to quantitate serum immunoglobulins is

A. Direct immunofluorescence.

B. Double immunodiffusion.

C. Radioimmunoassay.

D. Radial immunodiffusion.

E. Immunonephelometry.

14.3 The antibodies detected in passive hemagglutination are

A. Directed against antigens of ABO system.

B. Directed against antigens of the Rh complex.

C. Incomplete red cell agglutinins.

D. Directed against antigens chemically coupled to red cells.

E. The result of passive immunization.

14.4 In a solid-phase enzymoimmunoassay for anti-tetanus toxoid antibody the intensity of color measured after adding the substrate in the final step is

A. Directly proportional to the concentration of antibody in the patient's serum.

B. Inversely proportional to the concentration of antibody in the patient's serum.

C. Directly proportional to the concentration of antigen in the solid phase.

D. Directly proportional to the concentration of enzyme-labelled antibody.

E. Inversely proportional to the concentration of substrate.

14.5 In a competitive radioimmunoassay,

A. Free antigen is preferentially precipitated with polyethylene glycol.

B. The calibration curve is established by measuring the displacement of labelled antigen by increasing concentrations of cold antigen.

C. The calibration curve is established by measuring the radioactivity corresponding to the binding of serial dilutions of antigen.

D. The antigen has to be coupled to a solid phase.

E. The antibody has to be coupled to a solid phase.

In questions 14.6-14.10, match the techniques with their application (each choice can be used once, more than once, or not at all): (A) radioimmunoassay; (B) direct immunofluorescence; (C) latex agglutination; (D) indirect hemagglutination; (E) immunonephelometry.

14.6 Quantitation of serum IgE levels.

14.7 Detection of antinuclear factors.

14.8   Detection of rheumatoid factor.

14.9   Detection of anti-red-cell antibodies in hemolytic anemia.

14.10   Characterization of lymphocyte subsets.

Answers

14.1 (A)   A positive CF test is the one in which complement is consumed and the red cells are not lysed. Excess of complement, endogenous or exogenous, would cause lysis (false negative). Omission of antigen would also result in nonconsumption of complement. Old red cells often lyse spontaneously or with minimal concentration of complement, also causing false negative results.

14.2 (E)   Immunonephelometry can be automated and is more sensitive and reproducible than radial immunodiffusion.

14.3 (D)

14.4 (A)   In ELISA assays the concentrations of immobilized antigen, enzyme-labelled second antibody, and substrate are kept constant; therefore the intensity of color developed when the reaction is completed is directly proportional to the concentration of antibody in the unknown sample (patient's serum) and in the samples with known antibody concentrations used to calibrate the assay.

14.5 (B)

14.6 (A)   IgE is usually present in concentrations below the sensitivity limits of immunonephelometry.

14.7 (B)

14.8   Detection of rheumatoid factor.

14.9 (D)

14.10 (B)

BIBLIOGRAPHY

Bogulaski, R. C., Maggio, E. T., and Nakamura, R. M. *Clinical Immunochemistry: Principles of Methods and Applications.* Little, Brown, Boston, 1984.
Collins, W. P. (Ed.). *Alternative Immunoassays.* John Wiley, New York, 1985. (Contains chapters about newer immunoassays.)
Collins, W. P. (Ed.). *Complementary Immunoassays.* John Wiley, New York, 1988. (Has two excellent reviews on in-office and in-home immunoassays.)

Grieco, M. H. and Meriney, D. K. *Immunodiagnosis for Clinicians*. Year Book Medical Publishers, Chicago, 1983. (A comprehensive review of the most widely used immunodiagnostic procedures, with emphasis on interpretation.)

Kaplan, L. A. and Pesce, A. J. *Non-Isotopic Alternatives to Radioimmunoassay*. Marcel Dekker, New York, 1981. (Includes several good chapters on enzymo-immunoassays.)

Langone, J. J. and VanVunakis, H. (Eds.). *Methods in Enzymology—Immuno-chemical Techniques*, Part A (Vol. 70), Part B (Vol. 73), Part C (Vol. 74), and Part D (Vol. 84). Academic Press, New York.

Nakamura, R. M., Dito, W. R., and Tucker, E. S., III (Eds.). *Immunoassays in the Clinical Laboratory*. Alan R. Liss, New York, 1979.

Ritchie, R. F. (Ed.). *Automated Immunoanalysis*, Parts 1 and 2. Marcel Dekker, New York, 1978.

15

Diagnostic Evaluation of Humoral Immunity

GABRIEL VIRELLA

One of the most frequent problems faced by clinical immunologists is the investigation of a possible immunodeficiency. The attention of the physician is often aroused by a patient who presents a history of repeated pyogenic infections that subside after adequate antibiotic therapy but recur a short time after antibiotics are withdrawn. This general picture may be presented by a patient of any age. In general, patients with primary immunodeficiencies develop symptoms at an early age, while patients over thirty are more likely to be suffering from a secondary immunodeficiency. In most cases, it is wise to investigate both humoral and cell-mediated immunity, since both might be compromised. It also must be stressed that frequently this is a frustrating investigation that fails to show any definite abnormalities. Three reasons account for this: the predisposition to contract repeated infections may result from local factors affecting nonspecific defense mechanisms; defects in granulocyte or macrophage function also can be responsible for a clinical picture of immunodeficiency and are difficult to investigate; finally, our methodologies are not yet refined enough for the study of the more subtle abnormalities of the immune system, such as those involving immunoregulatory circuits.

In the investigation of a humoral immunodeficiency it is usual to start with the simplest procedures and to proceed to more sensitive and complex tests as needed. The same sequence will be followed in this chapter.

I. IMMUNOGLOBULIN QUANTITATION

A. Assay of Serum Immunoglobulins

This is the most frequently performed screening test for humoral immunity. Usually it is sufficient to assay the three major immunoglobulin classes (IgG, IgA, and IgM), because there is no proof that deficiencies of IgD or IgE might have any pathological consequences.

The finding of significantly low levels of all immunoglobulins is considered as evidence of a deficient humoral immunity. However, in interpreting immunoglobulin levels in children it is very important to remember that normal values vary with age, as shown in Table 15.1.

Immunoglobulin quantitation is a fundamental element in the classification of immunodeficiencies (Table 15.2). If all immunoglobulin classes are depressed, we term the condition generalized hypogammaglobulinemia. If the depression is very severe, and the combined levels of all three immunoglobulins are below 200 mg/dl, we use the terms severe hypogammaglobulinemia or agammaglobulinemia. When only one or two immunoglobulin classes are depressed, we designate the condition as dysgammaglobulinemia.

Generalized hypogammaglobulinemia is often found in association with secondary immunodeficiencies, such as those of patients with plasma cell dyscrasias, the nephrotic syndrome, intestinal malabsorption, or long-term immunosuppression.

Agammaglobulinemia is usually seen in cases of primary immunodeficiency. Only in very rare cases will an agammaglobulinemic individual be asymptomatic.

Table 15.1 Normal Values for Human Immunoglobulins (mg/dl)

	IgG	IgA	IgM
Newborn	636-1606	0	6-25
1-2 mo	250-900	1-53	20-87
4-6 mo	196-558	4-73	27-100
10-12 mo	294-1069	16-84	41-150
1-2 yr	345-1210	14-106	43-173
3-4 yr	440-1135	21-159	47-200
5-18 yr	630-1280	33-200	48-207
8-10 yr	608-1572	45-236	52-242
>10 yr	639-1349	70-312	57-352

As determined by immunonephelometry in the Department of Laboratory Medicine, Medical University of South Carolina.

Table 15.2   Ig Levels in Immune Deficiency (mg/dl)

Patient	IgG	IgA	IgM	Interpretation
A	850	2.8	128	IgA deficiency
B	1990	39.4	145	IgA deficiency
C	131	28.2	Traces	Severe hypogamma-globulinemia
D	690	16.0	264	IgA deficiency
E	154	60.0	840	Hyper-IgM syn-drome

Among *dysgammaglobulinemias*, the most frequent by far is IgA deficiency, which is also the most frequent form of human immune deficiency. It needs to be stressed that at least 50% of IgA-deficient individuals are clinically asymptomatic. Those with recurrent infections often have associated IgG subclass deficiencies.

The frequency of IgA deficiency varies according to the sensitivity of the methodology used; when methods of very high sensitivity are used for the quantitation of IgA, fewer individuals are shown to be IgA deficient. However, for practical purposes, one should consider as IgA deficient those cases where IgA is unmeasurable by routine methods for immunoglobulin quantitation, such as radial immunodiffusion or immunonephelometry, with the understanding that only a small proportion of such cases will have an absolute lack of IgA. Based on this assumption, the frequency of IgA deficiency varies between 1:500 and 1:800 individuals.

One other relative frequent form of dysgammaglobulinemia is characterized by a combined deficiency of IgG and IgA, with elevated IgM (*hyper-IgM syndrome*). In some cases there is combined immunodeficiency with hyperactive suppressor cells associated with this type of dysgammaglobulinemia.

Deficiencies in the levels of IgG subclasses have also been reported. Total IgG concentration may be normal to slightly depressed, and one or two of the minor subclasses may be deficient. Particular attention has been given to IgG2 subclass deficiency, which may be associated to infections with bacteria with polysaccharide capsules. Coexisting IgG2 and IgA deficiency is also being detected with previously unsuspected frequency, and individuals with this combined deficiency are often symptomatic, suffering mostly from bacterial infections.

B. Assay of Secretory IgA and Secretory Component

Secretory IgA antibodies are the best characterized defense mechanism of the mucosal surfaces. Other defense mechanisms, however, must exist, because the absence of secretory IgA does not necessarily imply an inordinate predisposition toward mucosal infection. Large numbers of patients without secretory IgA live symptom-free. In many people IgM seems to take the place of IgA. In others, nonspecific mechanisms of defense, transudation of IgG antibodies, and, perhaps, cell-mediated immune mechanisms are sufficient to provide resistance against infection. Precipitating antibodies to milk and other food proteins, as well as autoantibodies, are frequently detected in IgA-deficient cases, the former reflecting abnormal absorption of antigenic proteins, the latter pointing to the coexistence of immunoregulatory defects.

In any case, in patients with serum IgA deficiency, or with repeated episodes of mucosal infection, the assay of secretory immunoglobulins may be indicated. In general, patients with serum IgA deficiency are deficient in secretory IgA and vice versa. However, there seems to be some degree of biological dissociation between the systemic and the secretory IgA system, and rare cases of secretory IgA deficiency in the presence of normal serum IgA levels have been reported, warranting the independent evaluation of both systems. With currently available methodologies, particularly immunonephelometry, it is possible to estimate with reasonable accuracy the level of immunoglobulins A, M, and G in secretions. Quantitation of IgA by radial immunodiffusion or immunonephelometry will not distinguish between secretory IgA molecules and exudated IgA molecules of systemic origin, because the antisera employed are specific for the alpha chain shared by both forms of IgA. Specific enzymoimmunoassay methods have been developed for the assay of secretory IgA, usually based on the recognition of secretory component, which is not associated with circulating IgA.

II. DETERMINATION OF ANTI-Ig IMMUNOGLOBULIN ANTIBODIES

In patients with immune deficiencies, particularly IgA deficiency, antibodies to human immunoglobulins are often detectable. The most common are anti-IgA antibodies, of variable specificities (anti-isotypic or anti-allotypic). The origin and role of such antibodies is controversial. Their presence in serum will result in rapid binding and elimination of exogenous or endogenous IgA, and in such a way that antibodies to IgA could contribute to perpetuate the IgA deficiency. A more significant consequence of the existence of such antibodies may be a severe reaction after whole blood transfusion or administration of plasma or gamma globulin preparations. Usually, severe reactions occur only when the antibody titers are greater than 1:80. In patients with known high titers of anti-IgA antibody undergoing elective surgery, an effort should be made to procure blood from a compatible IgA-deficient donor. If that is not possible, packed and extensively washed red cells (to wash out all plasma proteins) may be used. Packed but not washed red cells are unsafe; these preparations contain at least 20% plasma.

III. DETERMINATION OF COMMON ANTIBODIES

Another way to look at humoral immunity is to quantitate antibodies that are found in most normal individuals. Among such we usually include isohemagglutinins, anti-streptolysin O, and antibodies to common viruses (mumps, measles, polio).

In patients with severe immunodeficiency, these antibodies are often absent, and each absence confirms and reinforces the results of immunoglobulin quantitation. However, their determination may not provide useful information in cases where the deficiency is more subtle and is also mainly indicative of past immunoreactivity; such determination often fails to give any clue toward a secondary immunodeficiency of recent onset, in which the first function to be lost is the ability to mount a primary immune response.

IV. QUANTITATION OF ANTIBODIES AFTER ANTIGENIC CHALLENGE

The quantitation of antibodies after antigenic challenge is the ideal approach for the investigation of the humoral immune response, because it determines specifically the ability of the patient to sustain a functional antibody response after adequate challenge. This type of investigation can be carried out (1) to determine whether the individual is able to develop primary and secondary immune responses, or (2) to determine the ability of the individual to synthesize antibodies to a specific microorganism.

The first approach is part of the general investigation of a possible immunodeficiency. The individual is challenged with antigens chosen by the following criteria: lack of risk for the patient; availability of techniques for the measurement of the corresponding antibodies; adequacy of the antigen for the purpose in mind.

For evaluation of primary immune responsiveness one needs to use an antigen to which the individual has never been exposed. This is not an easy thing to do. In immunodeficient children, in whom good records of previous immunizations and infections are available, any component or killed vaccine (*never live attenuated*) to which there has been no previous exposure can be used. Proteins extracted from lower animals, such as keyhole limpet hemocyanin, can also be used. However, it is very difficult to exclude the possibility of having been exposed to a cross-reactive immunogen in the past, leading to detectable titers of natural antibodies prior to immunization. The best approach devised so far is

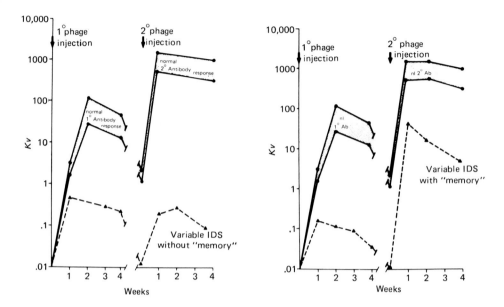

FIGURE 15.1   Primary and secondary response to bacteriophage ϕX174 in a patient with a variable immunodeficiency syndrome. The shaded area between the solid lines indicates the range for normal responses. The patient's response is the interrupted line. The patient studied on the left panel showed a definite but diminished antibody response; the secondary response was not greater than the primary, so that no memory/amplification occurred. The immunoglobulin class of antibody in both primary and secondary responses was entirely IgM. The patients studied on the right panel showed greater response to secondary immunization than to primary (memory/amplification), although both were diminished in comparison to the normal range. The immunoglobulin class of the seconary response was entirely IgM. (Reproduced with permission from Wedgewood, R. J., Ochs, H. D., and Davis, S. D. *Birth Defects Orig. Art. Ser.* *11*:331-338, 1975.)

the immunization with bacteriophage ϕX174. With this immunization we can follow not only the antibody levels through very sensitive techniques (Fig. 15.1) but also the initial phases of the immune response, determining whether there is an effective immune elimination of the bacteriophage (Fig. 15.2). Phage immunization has been carried out by several groups in different countries, and it has been proven to be a harmless procedure. At this point the main problems preventing the widespread use of this approach is the need for development of phage inactivation assays for the measurement of the antiphage antibody

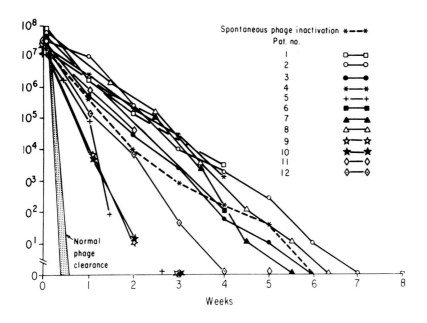

FIGURE 15.2 Antigen clearance using bacteriophage φX174 in 12 patients with infantile X-linked agammaglobulinemia. The normal response, the disappearance of phage circulating in the blood, is shown on the shaded area; phage is not found after 4 days. The sequential assays on each of the patients are indicated by the solid lines. The discontinuous line shows the spontaneous inactivation (or decay) of phage at 37°C in vitro. The rate of clearance in patients is markedly prolonged and is about the same rate as spontaneous inactivation. Immune antigen clearance is not demonstrable. (Reproduced with permission from Wedgewood, R. J., Ochs, H. D., and Davis, S. D. *Birth Defects Orig. Art. Ser. 11*:331-338, 1975.)

response, which is beyond the scope of possibilities for many clinical diagnostic laboratories.

The evaluation of the secondary immune response does not raise so many problems, but it is less informative, because the capacity to initiate a primary immune response seems to be the first (and sometimes the only) function affected by immunosuppressive agents or in diseases associated with immunodepression. If a primary immunization with bacteriophage has been previously carried out, the secondary immune response can be easily studied by rechallenging the patient (Fig. 15.3). Most frequently, diphtheria and tetanus toxoids are used. These are protein, noninfective vaccines, and the immune response

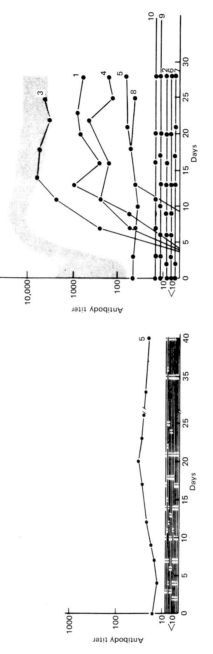

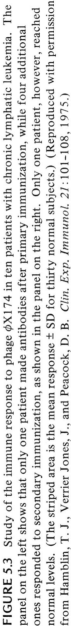

FIGURE 5.3 Study of the immune response to phage ϕX174 in ten patients with chronic lymphatic leukemia. The panel on the left shows that only one patient made antibodies after primary immunization, while four additional ones responded to secondary immunization, as shown in the panel on the right. Only one patient, however, reached normal levels. (The striped area is the mean response ± SD for thirty normal subjects.) (Reproduced with permission from Hamblin, T. J., Verrier Jones, J., and Peacock, D. B. *Clin. Exp. Immunol. 21*:101–108, 1975.)

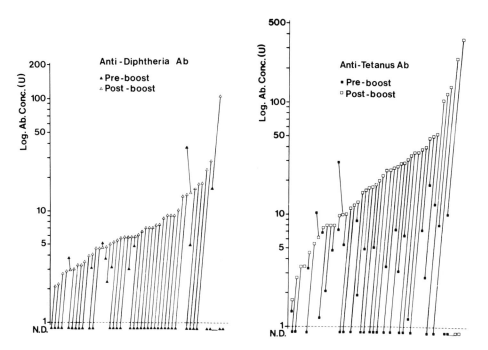

FIGURE 15.4   Pre- and postboost antibody titers to diphtheria and tetanus toxoid determined in 46 healthy children between 16 and 33 months of age. (Reproduced with permission from Virella, G., Fudenberg, H. H., Kyong, C. U., Pandey, J. P., and Galbraith, R. M., Z. *Immunitätsforsch.* 155:80-86, 1978.)

can be quantitated by a variety of techniques, such as enzymoimmunoassay.
Killed polio vaccine (Salk-type) can also be used. Given the lack of information
concerning normal values for these antibodies, and that the abnormality
searched for is the lack of an active response rather than a low level of antibody,
the approach used is to collect blood for a baseline study prior to a booster with
the corresponding antigen and to repeat the collection 10 to 14 days later.
Following this protocol we could detect active responses in all but two of a
group of children randomly selected from the population of a rural county of
South Carolina (Fig. 15.4). The existence of normal nonresponders needs to be
considered when evaluating a patient suspected of having an immunodeficiency.

   The second approach is the quantitation of antibodies to a specific microorganism. This approach is to be preferred in cases where a patient presents with
repeated infections by one microorganism or by a group of closely related microorganisms. In such cases, all investigations might be inconclusive except for the
measurement of antibodies to the infecting microorganism(s), which might reveal

an antigen-selective immunodeficiency. This approach requires, as a first step, the careful identification of the microorganism(s) involved; unfortunately, sufficiently specific and sensitive techniques for the assay of antibodies against many different microorganisms are not available. Whenever possible, however, this type of investigation should be performed, because it is the most direct approach to the diagnosis of a possible humoral immunodeficiency.

V. ADDITIONAL INVESTIGATIONS

The finding of an immunoglobulin deficiency or of the inability to mount a humoral immune response does not give many clues to the pathogenesis of the defect. Basically, a depressed or absent humoral response can correspond to either a primary or a secondary immunodeficiency. Primary humoral immunodeficiencies may result from a variety of defects, such as the absence or lack of differentiation of B cells, defects in intracellular synthesis or assembly of intracellular immunoglobulins, hyperactivity of suppressor cells, antibodies to T helper cells, etc. Secondary immunodeficiencies might result from a diversity of causes: protein losses in the urine or in the gut, malabsorption, malnutrition, immunosuppressive therapy, malignancies, viral infections (AIDS, measles), etc. The careful clinical investigation of conditions potentially associated with secondary immunodeficiency is an essential phase in the evaluation of these patients.

In primary immunodeficiencies, several investigations can be performed in order to clarify the nature of the immunodeficiency.

B-cell number in peripheral blood. This is usually investigated by determining the percentage of peripheral blood lymphocytes with surface immunoglobulins, or with specific B lymphocyte markers. The proportion of lymphocytes is identifiable as B cells in the peripheral blood by such techniques is between 4 and 10%.

Differentiation in B cells in vivo. The best approach is to look for germinal centers and immunoglobulin-producing cells in a lymph node biopsy from an area draining the site where an antigenic challenge has been carried out a week earlier (for example, with diphtheria or tetanus toxoids). The main drawback is the need for surgical excision of a lymph node.

Investigation of B-cell function in vitro. The easiest way is to separate peripheral blood lymphocytes (PBL) and to study their response to pokeweed mitogen (a T-dependent B-cell mitogen), *S. aureus*, or a T-independent B-cell activator such as *Salmonella paratyphi B* to determine whether the patient's B cells are able to differentiate into antibody-producing cells (Fig. 15.5).

In vitro testing of helper and suppressor functions. To determine whether the immunodeficiency is secondary to a defect in the immunoregulatory circuits, peripheral lymphocytes from the patient (before and after separation of

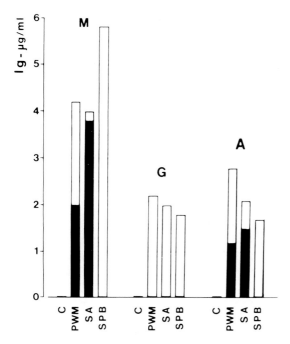

FIGURE 15.5   Study of the differential stimulation of PBL isolated from a patient and a normal control with common variable immunodeficiency with pokeweed mitogen, *S. aureus* (SA), and *Salmonella paratyphi B* (SPB). The levels of immunoglobulin M, G, and A quantitated on 7-day culture supernatants are shown by open bars for the control and closed bars for the patient. The patient's PBL responded with IgM and IgA production to stimulation with pokeweed mitogen and *S. aureus* but failed to respond to *Salmonella paratyphi B*. The induction of immunoglobulin secretion in vitro by *S. aureus* is believed to be T-dependent (in contrast to its mitogenic properties, believed to be T-independent), so these results appear to show that in this case, the stimulation of B cells without T help (believed to be a property of SPB) is not possible, and even when stimulation is achieved, IgG is not produced, which points to a genetic defect in the switch mechanism.

monocytes) are cocultured with lymphocytes from a normal individual, and the response to pokeweed mitogen is compared with that obtained with cultures of lymphocytes from normal controls. A reduction in the stimulation indexes in such mixed cultures, below that observed in a control coculture of lymphocytes from normal donors, will indicate suppressor activity by the patient's peripheral lymphocytes. An increased response in comparison to the

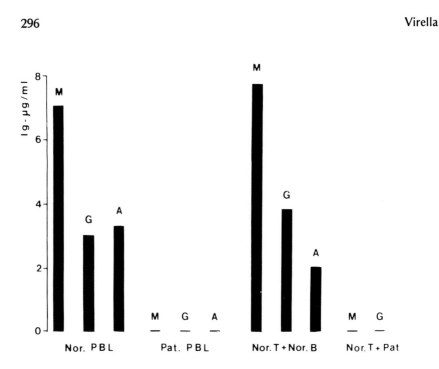

FIGURE 15.6 Coculture experiment designed to evaluate a possible immuno-regulatory defect in a patient with common variable immunodeficiency. Unfractionated patient's PBL failed to respond to pokeweed mitogen (PWM), while both unfractionated PBL and 1:1 mixture of T and B cells separated from the normal control responded to PWM stimulation by producing detectable amounts of IgM, IgG, and IgA (measured on 7-day culture supernatants). A coculture of patient's B cells and normal T cells (1:1) failed to produce immunoglobulins, suggesting that the patient's B cells are either unable to synthesize or unable to secrete immunoglobulins in a normal fashion.

the patient's control culture would indicate a deficiency in the patient's helper cells. A better characterization of the cellular defects involved will require purification of cell populations (monocytes, B lymphocytes, and T lymphocytes) from the patient and a normal control, and their coculture. In the example shown in Figure 15.6, coculture of a patient's B cells and T cells isolated from a normal donor failed to reconstitute the ability of the patient's B cells to produce and secrete immunoglobulins, which pointed to an intrinsic B-cell defect. If the patient's T cells have excessive suppressive activity or defective helper activity, the response of a mixture of normal B cells and patient's T cells will be deficient. A lack of helper T cells can be assumed if the patient's B cells recover their ability to produce immunoglobulins when mixed with normal T cells. Excessive suppressor activity is suggested if a mixture of patient's T cells plus nor-

Table 15.3 Sequence of Testing for a Patient with Suspected Humoral Immunity Deficiency

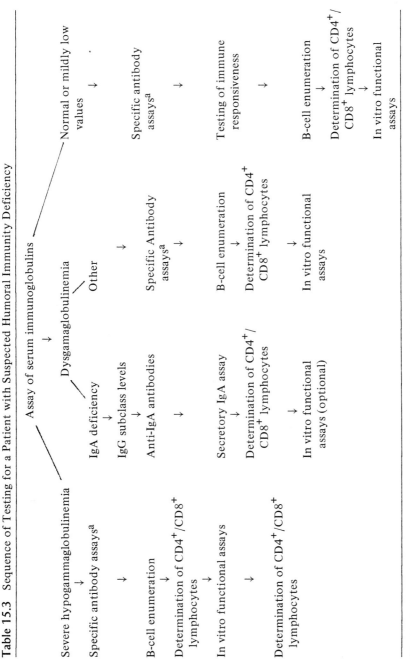

Assay of serum immunoglobulins →

Severe hypogammaglobulinemia / Dysgamaglobulinemia / Normal or mildly low values

Severe hypogammaglobulinemia
Specific antibody assays[a] →
B-cell enumeration →
Determination of CD4+/CD8+ lymphocytes →
In vitro functional assays →

Dysgamaglobulinemia
IgA deficiency / Other
IgG subclass levels →
Anti-IgA antibodies →
Secretory IgA assay →
Determination of CD4+/CD8+ lymphocytes →
In vitro functional assays (optional) →
Determination of CD4+/CD8+ lymphocytes

Other
Specific Antibody assays[a] →
B-cell enumeration →
Determination of CD4+ CD8+ lymphocytes →
In vitro functional assays →

Normal or mildly low values
Specific antibody assays[a] →
Testing of immune responsiveness →
B-cell enumeration →
Determination of CD4+/ CD8+ lymphocytes →
In vitro functional assays

[a]Antibody to agent or agents proven to cause infections to the patient being investigated.

mal T and B cells results in depressed B cell response. Finally, if B cell function is suppressed by unfractionated mononuclear cells (T cells and monocytes) but not by purified T cells, this suggests suppression by monocytes.

In the last few years, a great deal of interest and effort has been centered on the characterization and enumeration of T-cell subpopulations through monoclonal antibodies. This approach is considerably simpler and faster than functional testing, but the correlation between cell markers and function is not perfect. For example, there is data suggesting the existence of a suppressor/inducer subpopulation of $CD4^+$ cells, which are classically considered as helper. Also, $CD4^+$ cytotoxic T cells have been characterized both in mice and in humans. However, in situations such as AIDS, the degree of $CD4^+$ cell depletion correlates well with the degree of immunosuppression, as reflected by the increased incidence of opportunistic infections.

VI. PATIENT EVALUATION

Patients being evaluated for a possible humoral immunodeficiency should be tested following a logical sequence such as shown in Table 15.3. It should be noted that although the in vitro functional assays are essential from the investigative point of view, the rewards are likely to be clear-cut only in patients with severe hypogammaglobulinemia, and their cost and complicated nature often preclude their execution.

SELF-EVALUATION

Questions

Choose the one best answer for each of the following questions.

15.1 An IgA deficient patient is scheduled for surgery and in the preoperatory work-up found to be A, Rh positive and to have anti-IgA antibodies at a titer of 160. You should alert the blood bank for the possible need of
A. Packed A, Rh positive red cells.
B. Frozen plasma with normal IgA levels.
C. Fresh A, Rh positive blood.
D. A, Rh positive blood from an IgA deficient donor.
E. AB, Rh positive blood.

15.2 The easiest method of evaluating the ability of a patient to mount a secondary immune response is the
A. Titration of isohemagglutinins.
B. Quantitation of serum immunoglobulin levels (G, A and G).
C. Phage immunization.

    D. Determination of antibody titers to poliovirus before and after the administration of oral polio vaccine.

    E. Determination of antibody titers to tetanus toxoid before and after the administration of a booster injection.

15.3 A 21 year old female is seen as an outpatient with a history of repeated chronic pyogenic infections caused by *Streptococcus pneumoniae*. Preliminary investigations show that the patient's blood groups is O, but the blood has no detectable isoagglutinins; her immunoglobulin levels are strongly depressed, but her peripheral blood contains 4% surface Ig^+ cells. You would ask for all of the following texts except the

    A. Quellung test.

    B. Helper and suppressor T cell counts.

    C. Functional studies of the patient's T and B cells.

    D. Response to active immunization with multivalent pneumococcal vaccine.

    E. Quantitation of secretory immunoglobulins.

15.4 A four-year-old boy has had recurrent pneumonia since 3 months of age. Bacterial examinations have been repeatedly positive for *Haemophilus influenzae*. Immunological levels are IgG: 400 mg/dl; IgA: 40 mg/dl; IgM: 50 mg/dl. The most useful information will be given by the

    A. Tritration of isohemagglutinins.

    B. Assay of secretory IgA.

    C. Assay of antibodies to tetanus and diphtheria toxoids prior to and one week after a DPT booster.

    D. Study of the primary immune response to a bacteriophage.

    E. Determination of antibody titers to *Haemophilus influenzae* capsular polysaccharide.

15.5 Consider the following data from a coculture experiment in which B-cell activity was evaluated by quantitating immunoglobulins in culture supernatants harvested 7 days after pokeweed mitogen (PWM) stimulation using PBL from a patient with common variable immune deficiency and from a normal control.

	IgG[a]	IgA[a]	IgM[a]
Patient's unfractionated PBL	0	0	0
Control's unfractionated PBL	4	2	9
Patient's T + patient's B cells (1:1)	0	0	0
Control's T + control's B cells (1:1)	3	1.5	9
Patient's T + control's B cells (1:1)	0	p	0
Patient's T + control's unfractionated PBL (1:1)	0	0	0
Control's T + patient's B cells (1:1)	2	3	5

[a]Values in µg/ml of culture containing 1×10^6 PBL/ml.

These results indicate that the patient's humoral immune deficiency is due
to
A. Excess of suppressor T cells.
B. Lack of B-cell differentiation.
C. Lack of helper T cells.
D. Excess of suppressor monocytes.
E. Abnormal biosynthesis of immunoglobulins in the patient's B cells.

15.6   In a 4-year-old child with a history of repeated pyogenic infections caused
       by bacteria with polysaccharide-rich capsules, deficiency(ies) to be investi-
       gated is/are
       A. IgA deficiency.
       B. IgG1 deficiency.
       C. IgG2 deficiency.
       D. IgA and IgG2 deficiency.
       E. IgG and IgA2 deficiency.

15.7   In a normal 4-month-old child, you expect to see
       A. IgM as the quantitatively preponderant serum immunoglobulin.
       B. A concentration of IgG close to that of an adult, because of the per-
          sistence in circulation of maternally transferred IgG.
       C. A total immunoglobulin concentration (IgG + IgA + IgM) below 200
          mg/dl.
       D. Undetectable IgA.
       E. Lower levels of all immunoglobulin classes relative to normal adult
          levels.

15.8   All of the following are adequate antigens for use in evaluating the humor-
       al immune response of a suspected immune deficiency except
       A. Diphtheria and/or tetanus toxoids.
       B. Bacteriophage ϕX174.
       C. Measles vaccine.
       D. *S. typhi* vaccine.
       E. Keyhole limpet hemocyanin (KLH).

15.9   The diagnosis of IgA deficiency is based on
       A. Undetectable IgA by conventional assay techniques.
       B. Frequent episodes of mucosal infection and/or intestinal malabsorp-
          tion.
       C. Detectable autoantibodies and antifood precipitins.
       D. The simultaneous findings A, B, and C.
       E. The absence of IgA associated with either B or C.

15.10   The earliest functional evidence of secondary (or acquired) immuno-
deficiency in most individuals is
A. A depression of serum immunoglobulin levels.
B. A loss of immunological memory.
C. Lack of capacity to initiate a primary immune response.
D. An antigen-specific immune deficiency.
E. A depression in the peripheral lymphocyte count.

Answers

15.1 (D)   In the presence of anti-IgA antibody titers exceeding 80, the possibility that IgA-containing blood products may cause a serious transfusion reaction needs to be considered. Ideally, IgA-deficient A,
Rh positive blood should be used. If this is not possible, extensively
washed and packed A, Rh+ cells should be used (packed but not
washed red cells contain at least 20% plasma).

15.2 (E)   Toxoids are fully adequate for this purpose; attenuated vaccines, on
the contrary, should always be avoided.

15.3 (E)   The Quellung test would give an indication of the ability of the patient to respond to *S. pneumoniae*. Aactive immunization with *S.
pneumoniae* would further characterize whether the patient is able
to respond adequately to the infectious agent that causes clinical
problems. In most cases of adult-onset agammaglobulinemia the
number of B cells is normal but their function is not, often because
of immunoregulatory defects. Secretory IgA is likely to be low, and
its assay will not contribute any significant information in this type
of patient.

15.4 (E)   When a patient suffers from repeated infectious bouts caused by one
given microorganism, the most informative studies of humoral immunity are those measuring the response to the infecting agent.

15.5 (A)   The patient's T cells suppressed normal B cells, and normal T cells
helped the patient's B cells to produce normal amounts of immunoglobulins.

15.6 (D)   Combined IgA and IgG deficiency is frequently associated to increased frequency of infections with encapsulated pyogenic bacteria.

15.7 (E)

15.8 (C)   Live, attenuated vaccines should *never* be used in immunodeficient
patients unless the risks are outweighed by potential benefits, which
is not the case when an investigation of immune responsiveness is being carried out.

15.9 (A)   Most cases of IgA deficiency are asymptomatic.

15.10(C)

BIBLIOGRAPHY

Asherson, G. L. and Webster, A. D. B. *Diagnosis and Treatment of Immunode-ficiency Diseases.* Blackwell, Oxford, 1980.

IUIS/WHO Working Group. Use and abuse of laboratory tests in clinical immu-nology: Critical considerations of eight widely used diagnostic procedures. *Clin. Immunol. Immunopathol. 24*:122, 1982. (A critical perspective of the use and abuse of immunoglobulin quantitation, among other tests.)

Rose, N. R. and Friedman, H. *Manual of Clinical Immunology,* 2nd Ed. American Society for Microbiology, Washington, D.C., 1980. (Includes the section "Tests for humoral components of the immunological response.")

Rosen, F. S. Defects in cell-mediated immunity. *Clin. Immunol. Immuno-pathol. 41*:1, 1986.

WHO Scientific Group on Immunodeficiency. Primary immunodeficiency Diseases. *Clin. Immunol. Immunopathol. 28*:450, 1983.

16

Diagnostic Evaluation of Cell-Mediated Immunity

GABRIEL VIRELLA, CHRISTIAN C. PATRICK and JEAN-MICHEL GOUST

Cell-mediated immunity (CMI), as discussed in earlier chapters, is the result of a complex network of interrelated cellular reactions often resulting in the production and release of soluble factors that appear to mediate the cooperation between different cell populations and the expression of a variety of functions. Thus it is understandable that the tests used to evaluate CMI in humans are difficult to standardize and evaluate. However, a variety of tests, some in vivo, some in vitro, have been shown to correlate with different aspects or functions believed to depend primarily on the stimulation and activation of T lymphocytes.

I. IN VIVO TESTING OF DELAYED-TYPE HYPERSENSITIVITY

Skin testing and induction of contact sensitivity are the two classical approaches to measure delayed-type hypersensitivity (DTH) in vivo. The first approach is based on eliciting a secondary response to an antigen to which the patient was previously sensitized. The second approach will measure the ability of the tested individual to become sensitized to a substance to which he was not previously exposed.

A. Skin Testing

Skin testing was first described by Koch in 1891 and eventually led to the
definition of the DTH reactions. In simple terms, a small amount of soluble
antigen is injected intradermally on the extensor surface of the forearm, and the
area of the skin receiving the injection is observed for the appearance of erythema and induration. The antigens used are usually microbial in origin (e.g.,
purified protein derivative or PPD of tuberculin, mumps, candidin, coccidioidin,
histoplasmin, tetanus toxoid). Measurements of erythema and induration are
taken at 24 and 48 hours. A positive skin test is usually considered to be associated with an area of induration greater than 10 mm in diameter. If no reaction
is observed, the test may be repeated with a higher concentration of antigen. If
a patient has no reaction after being tested with a battery of antigens, it is assumed that a state of *anergy* exists. Anergy can be caused by immunological
deficiencies or infections (such as measles or chronic disseminated tuberculosis),
but it can also be the result of errors in the technique of skin testing.

Because the capacity to demonstrate DTH reactivity may persist for long
periods of time, a positive skin test may indicate either a past or a present illness. A word of caution is needed because immediate hypersensitivity reactions
do occasionally occur to the skin test antigens, and these reactions must not be
construed as DTH reactions. The distinction is made by the lack of induration
and by the greater speed that characterize immediate hypersensitivity, which
will appear and disappear usually in less than 18 hours. Although these tests
have the theoretical advantage of testing the function of the T-cell system in
vivo, they meet with a variety of problems due to the difficulty in obtaining
consistency among different sources and batches of antigens and reproducibility
in the technique of inoculation among different investigators. Also, the diagnostic meaning (as far as implying a cell-mediated immunodeficiency) of negative tests has to be carefully weighed. Negative results after challenge with antigens to which there is no record of previous exposure can always be questioned,
while a negative result with an antigen extracted from a microbial agent that has
been documented as causing disease in the patient has a much stronger diagnostic significance.

B. Contact Sensitivity

Contact sensitivity involves the application of a low-molecular-weight chemical
compound (e.g., dinitrochlorobenzene or DNCB) to intact skin. It is believed
that the chemical will bind covalently to skin proteins and elicit a delayed hypersensitivity reaction. After the initial application, a period of 7 to 10 days is
needed for contact sensitivity to develop, whereupon a challenge dose may be
given. Induration does not usually occur, as it does with skin testing, but instead a flare response is noted. Lack of reaction means inability to initiate a
cell-mediated immune response. This type of testing has been avoided in recent
years because of the carcinogenic properties of DNCB and related substances.

C. Patch Test

In the investigation of contact hypersensitivity (states of hypersensitivity acquired by skin contact with substances such as nickel, dyes, etc.) it is often necessary to determine the identity of the sensitizing substance. This can be accomplished by the patch test, in which several potential antigens are applied in a dilute, nonirritating form to the patient's back and covered with an occlusive dressing. Forty-eight hours later the dressing is removed, and if a reaction consisting of erythema, edema, and vesiculation is seen at the point of application of one of the atigens, that antigen is identified as the cause of the hypersensitivity reaction.

II. IN VITRO TESTING OF CELL-MEDIATED IMMUNE REACTIONS

Most in vitro lymphocyte testing requires a more or less purified population of lymphocytes. A truly purified population of lymphocytes is not usually obtained, but a highly enriched population of mononuclear cells depleted of erythrocytes and PMN leukocytes is used. This population is separated by the use of density gradient centrifugation, usually in Ficoll-Hypaque. This separation medium has a specific gravity of 1.077, which lies in between the density of human erythrocytes (1.092) and the density of human lymphocytes (1.070). By carefully centrifuging blood in Ficoll-Hypaque, a gradient is formed: erythrocytes and PMN leukocytes sink to the bottom of the tube, a thin layer containing lymphocytes and monocytes is formed, and a platelet-rich plasma layer develops on top. Approximately 80% of the cells recovered in the lymphocyte-rich layer are lymphocytes, and 20% are monocytes. Of the lymphocytes, approximately 80% are T-cell, 4-10% are B-cells, and the remaining are non-T, non-B lymphocytes.

III. ENUMERATION OF T CELLS

A. Erythrocyte Rosetting (E-Rosetting)

T cells have been shown to have certain membrane markers that are not found on other cell populations. The rosetting of sheep red blood cells (SRBC) by T cells is the membrane marker historically used to enumerate the total T-cell population. This pocedure is termed erythrocyte rosetting (E-rosetting). The test is performed by incubating "purified" peripheral blood lymphocytes in a balanced salt solution with serum and diluted SRBC. After a short incubation at $37°C$, the cells are pelleted by centrifugation and placed in the refrigerator ($4°C$) overnight. The cells are then gently suspended and counted. Lymphocytes with 3 or more SRBCs attached are considered T cells (Fig. 16.1). Peri-

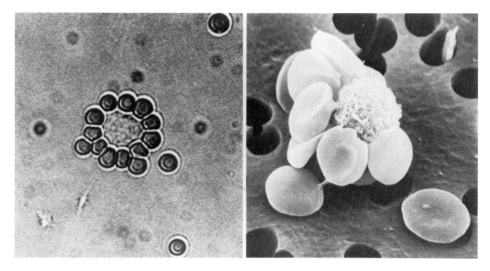

FIGURE 16.1   Human T-cell rosettes, as seen by conventional microscopy (left)
and scanning electron microscopy (right). (Reproduced with permission from
Immunology, R. D. Guthmann (Ed.). Upjohn, Kalamazoo, Michigan, 1981.)

pheral blood lymphocytes are 70-85% T cells by E-rosetting. In patients with
severe deficiencies of cell-mediated immunity, the E-rosette count is severely
depressed. In many situations, however, moderate depressions of the number
of E-rosette-forming cells can be present with or without clear symptoms of
immune deficiency. Rosette formation has been abandoned as a test for the
enumeration of T cells, but it is still frequently used as one of the steps in some
protocols for T-cell purification.

B.   Antibody-Defined Cell Populations

The first successful attempts to define T-cell subpopulations based on antigenic
differences were made using sera obtained from patients with systemic lupus
erythematosus of juvenile rheumatoid arthritis. However, those antisera presented problems of multispecificity and were not easily available; it was through
the development of murine hybridomas producing monoclonal antibodies to different T-cell markers that the serological definition of T-cell subpopulations
become available to all interested researchers. The development of monoclonal
antibodies to T cells pioneered by Reinherz and Schlossman at Harvard, has led
to a better understanding of T-cell ontogeny and cellular interactions. Total T
cells and a variety of T-cell subsets can be identified and enumerated by immu-

TABLE 16.1 Human T-Cell Markers Identified by Monoclonal Antibodies

Marker	Distribution	Biological significance
CD2 (T11)	All T cells	Cell-to-cell interaction through LFA-3
CD3 (T3)	All T cells	T-cell-receptor-associated
CD4 (T4)	Helper T cells	Interaction with MHC II
CD5 (T1)	All T cells	–
CD8 (T8)	Cytotoxic/suppressor T cells	Interaction with MHC I
CD25 (TAC)	Activated T and B cells	IL2 receptor
CD29	Helper/inducer T cells	–
CD45R	Suppressor/inducer T cells	–

CD = cluster of differentiation
LFA = leukocyte function antigen

nofluorescence procedure in which fluorescent-labeled monoclonal antibodies are used to detect the different T-cell antigens (Table 16.1).

The enumeration of lymphocytes carrying a specific marker recognized by a corresponding monoclonal antibody can be done manually by immunofluorescence microscopy or, in a more automated and reliable fashion, using flow cytometry. The principle of flow cytometry, illustrated in Figure 16.2 is relatively simple. Lymphocytes at high dilution flow into a cell as a unicellular stream and are analyzed through light-scattering and fluorescence. Light-scattering measurements allow sizing of the cells, and fluorescent measurements allow one to determine the number of cells expressing markers recognized by specific fluorescent-labeled monoclonal antibodies. By means of computer-assisted analysis, cell populations of homogeneous size can be segregated, allowing one to exclude from the final counts of fluorescent cells cross-reactive cell types that may express identical markers but be of a totally different nature. By using monoclonal antibodies labeled with diferent fluorochromes that emit fluorescent light at different wavelengths, it is possible to analyze cells for the simultaneous expression of two or three different markers. The study of T-cell subsets has found its main clinical application in the characterization of T-cell development abnormalities (such as in primary immune deficiencies), acquired abnormalities in the distribution of T-cell subpopulations (such as in AIDS), and aberrant representation of T-cell subpopulations (as in certain autoimmune diseases and leukemias).

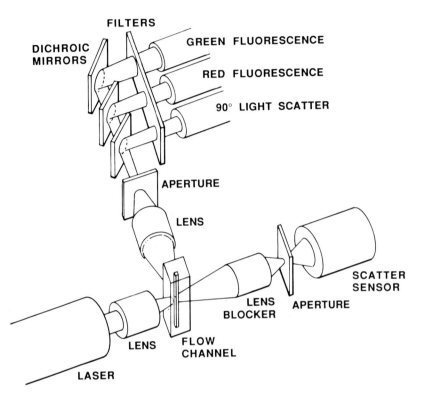

FIGURE 16.3   Diagrammatic representation of the principle of flow cytometry. A cells suspension is premixed with one or two different monoclonal antibodies to cell surface markers, and as it flows on an optic channel several parameters are analyzed: light scattered (forward and at a 90° angle) and emission of fluorescent light at two wavelengths. The light scattering data is processed by a microcomputer and used to discriminate different cell populations according to size. The ability to analyze fluorescence at two wavelengths enables the simultaneous analysis with two antibodies, providing each one is labeled with a different fluorochrome emitting fluorescence at a different wavelength. The simultaneous consideration of fluorescence data and size data enables the discrimination of cell populations by size and presence or absence of markers.

C.   Terminal Deoxynucleotidyl Transferase (TdT) Assay

TdT is a nuclear enzyme present in immature blood cells. It catalyses the polymerization of deoxynucleotide triphosphates in the absence of a template. Its presence, usually detected by immunofluorescence, is characteristic of immature T and B lymphocytes and of the undifferentiated lymphocytes in leukemias and lymphomas. Its interest, thereby, is mostly related to the investigation of lymphocyte ontogeny and to the classification of lymphocytic malignancies.

IV. ENUMERATION OF B CELLS

A. Assay for Surface Immunoglobulins

B cells have immunoglobulin (Ig) molecules attached to their membranes. Direct immunofluorescence can detect these Ig molecules using antihuman Ig or alternatively antihuman light chain antisera. Briefly, "purified" lymphocytes are incubated with fluorescein-labeled antibodies—aggregate-free or, preferably, $F(ab')_2$ fragments—for 20 to 30 min at $4°C$. The cells are then washed and counted using a fluorescence microscope. Normal B cells constitute 4-10% of the total circulating lymphocyte population. Lower counts are associated with humoral immune deficiencies, and elevated counts with B-cell malignancies.

B. Assay for Fc Receptors

B cells are predominant lymphocyte populating bearing immunoglobulin Fc receptors. Fc receptors, however, are also expressed by approximately 65% of granulocytes, as well as by platelets, monocytes/macrophages, and T cells. The presence of Fc receptors can be investigated by different assays. A rosetting assay, using non-rosette-forming red cells (human, for example) exposed to anti-D antibody of the IgG class, can be used to determine the number of EA rosettes, based on the binding of red cells through Fc receptors. Alternatively, fluorescein-labeled heat-aggregated gamma globulin can be used, knowing that it will be bound by any cell Fc receptors on the membrane, which will subsequently exhibit membrane fluorescence. Given the wide distribution of the Fc receptor, these assays do not yield an accurate B-cell count and will include monocytes and even some T cells.

C. Serological Identification of B Cells

Monoclonal antibodies specific for B-cell antigens have been raised and successfully introduced for diagnostic use. Circulating, mature B cells express CD19 (B4) and CD20 (B1), as well as Ia (MHC class II). For enumeration of B cells, antibodies to CD19 and CD20 are preferred, since MHC II is also expressed by monocytes in the peripheral blood. It should be noticed that CD19, CD20, and MHC II are not expressed by plasma cells; these cells express specific antigens, such as PCA-1.

V. ASSAYS FOR T-CELL ACTIVATION

T-cell activation can be induced either by specific antigens or by nonspecific substances. These nonspecific substances are termed mitogens and are mainly plant glycoproteins (lectins). A T cell, upon encountering a mitogen or its specific antigen, will express the IL2 receptor and undergo blastogenic transformation, becoming a lymphoblast. This transformation process with subsequent cell divisions involves, in order of occurrence, protein, RNA, and DNA synthesis. The expression of IL2 receptor can be measured by flow cytometry, using fluorescent-labeled anti-CD25 (TAC) antibodies. Blastogenic transformation can be evaluated by observing large lymphocytes under the light microscope, but the most common assay measures the incorporation of tritiated thymidine (^{3}HTdr) into the DNA of dividing lymphocytes. This latter technique is preferred to visual observation because of its quantitative nature and its independence from subjective factors.

A. Mitogenic Stimulation

Table 16.2 lists five commonly used lymphocyte mitogens. Three of these are plant lectins (PHA, ConA, PWM). Of these lectins, PWM stimulates both B cells and T cells, while PHA and ConA stimulate T cells only. The two other mitogens, (*S. Aureus*) protein A and SPB, are of bacterial origin; the mitogenic effect of protein A is virtually restricted to B lymphocytes, while SPB leads B cells to differentiate into immunoglobulin-secreting cells with minimal cell division.

The response to mitogens is usually carried out using peripheral blood lymphocytes separated by centrifugation in Ficoll-Hypaque gradients. The concentration of lymphocytes is usually adjusted to 1×10^6 lymphocytes/ml, and

TABLE 16.2 Lymphocyte Mitogens

Mitogen	T cell	B cell
Phytohemagglutinin (PHA)	+	−
Concanavalin A (ConA)	+	−
Pokeweed mitogen (PWM)	+	+[a]
Protein A (*Staphylococcus aureus* membrane component)	±[b]	+
Salmonella paratyphi B (SPB)	±	+

[a]PWM is mainly a T-cell mitogen, inducing also B-cell proliferation and differentiation through the release of soluble factors by T cells.

[b]T-cell cooperation is not required to induce B-cell division, but it is required for the functional activation of B cells into Ig-secreting cells.

the mitogen is then added in varying concentrations. The mixture is incubated for 72 h at $37°C$ with 5% CO_2, and ^3H Tdr is added for the last 6 to 8 h of incubation. The cells are pelleted and washed, and then the amount of radioactivity incorporated by the dividing cells is determined with a scintillation counter. A stimulation index can be calculated by dividing the counts per minute (CPM) in control lymphocytes without mitogen into the CPM corresponding to stimulated lymphocytes. By varying the amount of mitogen added, a dose-response curve can be generated.

Although the study of the mitogenic response is relatively simple to perform, the assays have a variety of problems, such as poor reproducibility and individual variations among normals. Perhaps the biggest pitfall is that the lymphocyte pool separated by centrifugation in Ficoll-Hypaque contains T cells, B cells, and monocytes in varying concentrations. Nevertheless, the finding of a very low uptake of ^3H-Tdr after stimulation with a T-cell mitogen suggests a deficiency of T-cell function.

B. Antigen-Specific Stimulation

This assay is analogous to the mitogen assay except for the replacement of the mitogen by a specific antigen and a longer incubation time, because only approximately 0.1% of lymphocytes will respond to a specific antigen. Incubation times are usually 5 to 7 days. The antigens used should be ones to which the patient has been exposed. These include purified protein derivative (PPD), *Candida albicans* antigens, tetanus toxoid, etc. Although this approach is, in principle, more physiological and functionally more relevant than the stimulation with mitogens, the technical difficulties that surround it have prevented its routine use in the evaluation of T-cell function.

C. Assays for Lymphokine Release

The lymphokines are soluble factors released by lymphocytes; they mediate a variety of actions, some amplifying and some regulating the immune response. Classically, the two lymphokines most commonly assayed to evaluate CMI were the migration inhibitory factor (MIF) and the leukocyte inhibitory factor (LIF). Their mechanism of action is to inhibit cell migration; MIF inhibits macrophages and LIF inhibits neutrophils (PMNs). Experimentally, the effects of MIF release can be easily demonstrated if capillary tubes filled with peritoneal cells from sensitized and control guinea pigs are placed so that the tips are surrounded by an adequate medium containing antigen (or not, as control); the area of cell migration around the tip of the capillary tubes is measured (Fig. 16.3). The release of MIF by human lymphocytes is usually assayed by observing the action exerted by supernatants from sensitized lymphocytes exposed to the sensitizing antigen upon the migration of guinea pig peritoneal macro-

NO ANTIGEN   WITH PPD

NORMAL
CELLS

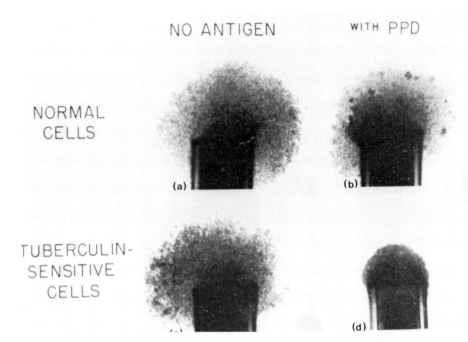

(a)   (b)

TUBERCULIN-
SENSITIVE
CELLS

(d)

FIGURE 16.3   Test for the release of MIF from guinea pig peritoneal cells.
Cells were obtained from a control guinea pig and a tuberculin-sensitive guinea
pig; the cells were packed into capillary tubes, and then the tip of each capillary
tube was dipped into a diffusion chamber filled with buffer or with a dilution
of PPD in the same buffer. As can be seen migration was inhibited only when
the cells were exposed to PPD. (Reproduced with permission from David, J. R.,
Al-Askari, S., Lawrence, H. S., and Thomas, L. Delayed hypersensitivity in
vitro. I. The specificity of inhibition of cell migration by antigens. *J. Immunol.*
93:264, 1964.)

phages from a capillary tube. Briefly, a two-stage procedure is used for the
MIF assay. Patient and control lymphocytes are separately mixed with an antigen and incubated. Afterwards, a cell-free supernatant is obtained by centrifugation from each mixture and placed into a chamber containing capillary tubes
packed with guinea pig peritoneal macrophages. If MIF has been released by
sensitized lymphocytes contacting their specific antigen, the macrophages
will not migrate out of the tube; but if no MIF is produced, the macrophages
will migrate out of the open end of the tube. The migration of cells from the
capillary tube is measured by the use of a planimeter. An alternative procedure
is to place the cells and supernatant in a well that is cut into an agarose medium;

the migration of macrophages around the well is measured in a manner similar to that of radial immunodiffusion. With either of these procedures, a migration index is obtained by dividing the average areas of migration with and without the antigen and multiplying by 100.

The release of LIF is tested in a similar manner using human neutrophils as the target cell population. LIF can be assayed in a one-stage or a two-stage procedure. In the first, patient or control leukocytes are incubated with either nonspecific mitogens or defined antigens and neutrophils, either in a capillary tube or in a well in a highly purified agarose gel around which the PMN in the mixture will diffuse to a greater or lesser degree, depending on the release of LIF (Fig. 16.4). The measurement of lymphokine release is one of the best approaches to the in vitro assay of the functional capabilities of the T-cell population, and as noted before it can be used to test the general reactivity of lymphocytes to mitogens or the specific response to a given antigen.

Recently, enzymoimmunoassays for IL2 have been introduced that are rapidly replacing the MIF and LIF assays because of their simplicity and their quantitative nature. Usually mononuclear cells are incubated with several concentrations of mitogenic substances for 24 h, and IL2 concentrations in the supernatants are measured. The addition of anti-IL2 receptor antibodies preventing IL2 uptake by activated T cells has been proposed as a way to increase the accuracy of the assay. Assays for other interleukins are likely to be developed in the near future. Low or absent release of IL2 has been observed in a variety of immunodeficient states, particularly in AIDS patients. Increased serum IL2 levels have been reported in multiple sclerosis, rheumatoid arthritis, and patients undergoing graft rejection, which probably reflects T-cell hyperactivity in those patients. Rejection of a renal allograft is also associated to increased urinary levels of IL2.

The availability of ELISA assays for the IL2 receptor (CD25) has also allowed the demonstration of elevated levels of soluble receptors (shed by activated T cells) in various biological fluids. In general, the results of assays for IL2 receptor show parallelism with the results of assays for IL2. Both assays are likely to become widely used in the monitoring of graft rejection, of autoimmune diseases, and of patients receiving immunosuppressive treatment.

D. Assays for Cytotoxic Effector Cells

Cytotoxicity assays are designed to allow the quantitation of cytotoxic effector cells. These include cytotoxic T lymphocytes, natural killer cells, and killer cells mediating antibody-dependent cell cytotoxicity (ADCC) reaction. These cells vary in their lytic rates and their recyclable capacity, so that these assays do not reflect an equipotential of lytic rate to cell-type number.

Two methods are generally used to assay cytotoxic effect. The first and oldest technique is by cell counting. Dead target cells are differentiation from

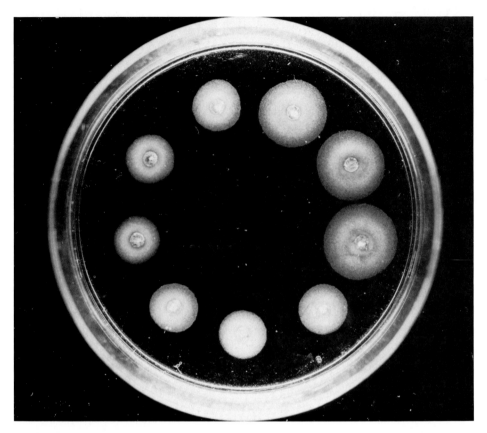

FIGURE 16.4   Assay of LIF release by diffusion in agarose. Mixtures of leukocytes from a PPD-sensitive individual with different dilutions of PPD were used
to fill wells carved in the agarose. After adequate incubation one can see different areas of leukocyte migration around the wells, directly proportional to antigen concentrations. (Courtesy of Dr. M. Arala-Chaves, Faculdade das Ciencias
Medicas, Porto, Portugal.)

live target cells by the uptake of vital dyes such as trypan blue. This technique,
however, is mostly used for the study of antibody-mediated cytotoxicity. The
technique most frequently used for measurement of cell-mediated cytotoxicity
is based on the measurement of the release of an isotope (^{51}Cr) from previously
labeled target cells.

The functional interest of cytotoxicity assays is evident. In the case of T
cells, these assays measure the functional adequacy of one of the major effector

T-cell subpopulations. Obviously, an abnormal result in a cytotoxicity assay does not necessarily mean that the cytotoxic population is abnormal; it could also reflect, for example, a defect in the helper-T-cell population. As for NK and K cells, their definition is basically dependent on cytotoxicity assays. K cells appear important in their collaboration with the humoral system in the destruction of microbial targets, although there has been not a single case reported of clinical immunodeficiency due to a deficiency of this population. NK cells have been postulated to play a crucial role in antitumor defense and perhaps in autoimmune diseases. A deficiency of this population has been reported to be characteristic of patients with symptomatic AIDS.

E. Mixed Lymphocyte Reaction (MLR)

One of the best ways to study the function of the T-lymphocyte system in vitro is the mixed lymphocyte reaction (MLR), which can be performed with a variety of protocols. For example, a two-way MLR is used to select a donor for a bone marrow graft. Lymphocytes from potential donors are mixed separately with lymphocytes from the patient, and after 4 to 5 days of incubation the incorporation of ^{3}H-Tdr is measured in the last 18 hours of culture. The donor-patient combination that results in a negligible ^{3}H-Tdr is considered the most suitable for grafting (Fig. 16.5).

The basis of the MLR is the recognition of antigenic differences mostly related to the expression of class II antigens on the membrane of mononuclear cells. For many years the MLR was used to type the so-called D-locus specificities, which were the first class II HLA specificities described. This was usually accomplished in a one-way MLR reaction, in which the mononuclear cells from a donor of known D-locus specificity were mitomycin-treated and became the stimulator cells (particularly the B-cell and monocyte populations that express the D antigens), while the mononuclear cells of the untyped individual, untreated and unfractionated, become the responder cells. A response in this system, as measured by ^{3}H-Tdr incorporation, was considered as indicating lack of identity of the D locus. With the progress of serological typing, three class II loci have been defined, and the MLR is currently used to define subgroups among individuals whose lymphocytes appear identical serologically, as detailed in Chapter 2.

The one-way MLR can also be used to evaluate T-cell function, by using B cells of genetically unrelated individuals as stimulators. As an endpoint, one can use ^{3}H-Tdr incorporation, or the generation of cytotoxic T cells. For this last assay, after a 5-day culture of inactivated stimulator cells and responder T cells, the stimulated T cells are mixed with viable target lymphocytes obtained from the same individual that provided the cells used as stimulators. If cytotoxic T cells are generated, the viable cells added in the second step will become their

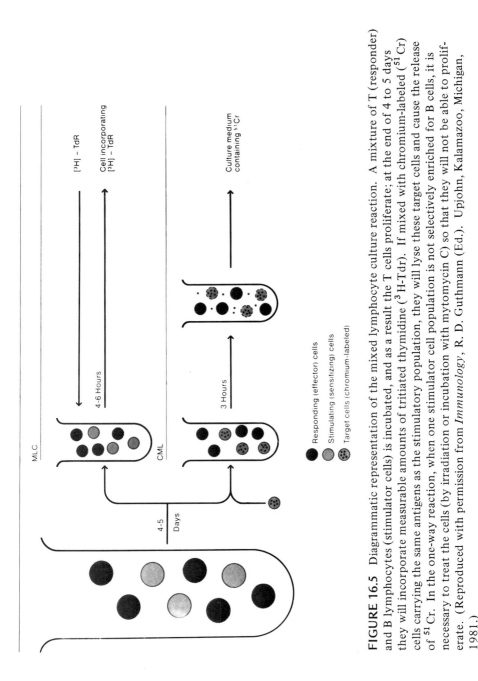

FIGURE 16.5 Diagrammatic representation of the mixed lymphocyte culture reaction. A mixture of T (responder) and B lymphocytes (stimulator cells) is incubated, and as a result the T cells proliferate; at the end of 4 to 5 days they will incorporate measurable amounts of tritiated thymidine (^{3}H-Tdr). If mixed with chromium-labeled (^{51}Cr) cells carrying the same antigens as the stimulatory population, they will lyse these target cells and cause the release of ^{51}Cr. In the one-way reaction, when one stimulator cell population is not selectively enriched for B cells, it is necessary to treat the cells (by irradiation or incubation with mytomycin C) so that they will not be able to proliferate. (Reproduced with permission from *Immunology*, R. D. Guthmann (Ed.). Upjohn, Kalamazoo, Michigan, 1981.)

targets and will be killed in a few hours, their death being measured, for example, by ^{51}Cr release (Fig. 16.5).

VI. EVALUATION OF A PATIENT WITH A SUSPECTED CELL-MEDIATED IMMUNITY DEFECT

A defect in cell-mediated immunity is suggested by an abnormal frequency of infections with agents known to be more efficiently controlled by CMI mechanisms than by circulating antibodies. These include viruses, particularly those that propagate from cell to cell, such as the viruses of the herpes family, intracellular bacteria, such as *Mycobacterium tuberculosis*, parasites such as *Pneumocystis carinii* and toxoplasma, and fungi, particularly Candida species.

A significant decrease in T cells will always be reflected by lymphopenia in the peripheral blood, because T cells represent 75-80% of the peripheral blood lymphocyte population; hence, a simple leukocyte count with differential helps in detecting a T-cell deficiency. If the deficiency is only functional, it may be unapparent or may be suggested by abnormal lymphocyte morphology.

The next step in the evaluation of a patient is usually the performance of skin tests using a battery of common antigens, as previously described. Usually, over 95% of a normal population will react to at least three out of five common antigens.

The enumeration of T cells and their subpopulations usually follows. This area is in constant evolution because of the development of new monoclonal antibodies. There is always some uncertainty about the perfect correlation between the cell markers that allow the enumeration of T cells and their subpopulations and the functional capabilities of the cells carrying these markers. It is clear that a marked decrease of $CD4^+$ (helper) T cells is generally associated with clinical immunodeficiency, but examples of dissociation between cell markers and function have been reported. Therefore, moderate deviations from normality in the distribution of T-cell subpopulations may not be paralleled by the expected functional abnormalities.

The evaluation of T cell function by in vitro assays should be the hallmark of the investigation of T-cell deficiencies, because many believe the in vitro tests to be more reproducible than skin tests. The easier in vitro assays are the studies of the response to T-cell mitogens (PHA, ConA), but these studies have an inherent lack of physiologic correspondence. Assays measuring the generation of cytotoxic T cells or the release of lymphokines, such as IL2, MIF, and LIF, tend to be considered the best available choices.

Finally, the functional evaluation of defective helper function or excessive suppressor function are the most difficult to perform, because they involve the separation of T and B lymphocytes from a patient and a normal and their mixture in different combinations to study the effect of normal cells on patient cells and vice versa.

TABLE 16.3   Sequence of Tests for a Patient with Suspected CMI Deficiency

Total lymphocyte count

Skin tests

Enumeration of T cells and T-cell subsets

Response to mitogens

Release of lymphokines (IL2, LIF, MIF)

MLR (with cytotoxicity assay, if necessary)

Functional studies of suppressor and helper activities

A sequence of laboratory studies in a patient with suspected CMI deficiencies is given in Table 16.3.

SELF-EVALUATION

Questions

Choose the one best answer:

16.1   All of the following tests can be used to evaluate cell-mediated immunity except
A. Quantitating IL2 release after mitogenic stimulation.
B. Determination of the CD4 (T4)/CD8 (T8) ratio.
C. Enumeration of CD3 (T3)$^+$ cells.
D. Enumeration of CD2 (T11)$^+$ cells.
E. Mitogenic response to $S.$ $aureus$ protein A.

16.2   A patient with chronic pulmonary tuberculosis is found to have negative skin tests to coccidioidin, candidin, and tetanus toxoid. On the basis of this observation you can state that the patient
A. Has a generalized cellular immune deficiency.
B. Is in a state of anergy associated with chronic tuberculosis.
C. Is unable to respond to polysaccharides.
D. Needs to be vaccinated against tetanus.
E. None of the above.

16.3   The test that gives the best indication of the ability of T cells to differentiate functionally after stimulation is the test for
A. Number of CD29$^+$ cells.
B. Number of CD25 (IL2 receptor)$^+$ cells.
C. ^{3}H Tdr incorporation after PHA stimulation.
D. ^{3}H Tdr incorporation after PWM stimulation.
E. Release of IL2 after mitogenic stimulation.

16.4 In vitro assays for cell-mediated immunity will not involve
   A. Measurement of the levels of IL2 in serum.
   B. Blastogenesis and DNA synthesis by peripheral lymphocytes measured by uptake of ^{3}H Tdr.
   C. Release of histamine after in vitro incubation with an antigen.
   D. Mixed lymphocyte reaction.
   E. Cytotoxicity to target cells bearing specific antigen on the surface by direct contact with cytotoxic T lymphocytes.

16.5 The mitogenic response of human T lymphocytes is best elicited with
   A. Pokeweed mitogen (PWM).
   B. *Staphylococcus aureus* (Cowan I).
   C. Phytohemagglutinin (PHA).
   D. *Salmonella paratyphi B* (SPB).
   E. Lipopolysaccharide (LPS).

16.6 Which of the following statements concerning mixed lymphocyte culture (MLC) is not correct?
   A. It is of great value in assessing the suitability of donor bone marrow for transplantation into an immune-deificient recipient.
   B. In man, it is currently used to define class II MHC subgroups.
   C. The responder cells are T lymphocytes.
   D. When positive, it is an indicator that reacting cells have been previously sensitized to some of the antigens present on the stimulator cells.
   E. Purified B cells can be used as the stimulator population.

16.7 A delayed hypersensitivity reaction to a given antigen is defined by
   A. Onset not earlier than 24 h after challenge.
   B. An area of induration of at least 10 mm in diameter at 24-48 h after challenge.
   C. An erythematous area of at least 10 mm in diameter at 24-48 h after challenge.
   D. A and B.
   E. A, B, and C.

16.8 Peripheral blood B lymphocytes
   A. Represent 20% of the total lymphocyte population.
   B. Have Fc receptors but lack C3b receptors.
   C. Are best defined by the EA-rosette assay.
   D. Show an intense proliferative response after PHA stimulation.
   E. Can be induced to proliferate and differentiate into immunoglobulin-secreting cells when unfractionated mononuclear cells are incubated with PWM.

16.9 The cell marker likely to be significantly depressed 6 days after stimula-
      tion of a normal lymphocyte culture with pokeweed mitogen (PWM) is
      A. PCA-1.
      B. CD19 (B4).
      C. CD25 (IL2 receptor).
      D. CD4 (T4).
      E. CD2 (T11).

16.10 When the MLC is followed by a cytotoxicity assay the target cells are
       A. Syngeneic with the stimulating cells.
       B. Syngeneic with the responding cells.
       C. Labeled with ^{125}I.
       D. Virally infected.
       E. Lysed by complement.

Answers

16.1 (E) The mitogenic response to *S. aureus* protein A is a B-cell property.

16.2 (E) The negative reaction to candidin, coccidioidin, and tetanus toxoid
           may reflect generalized immunodeficiency or a state of anergy, but it
           could also reflect lack of sensitization of a perfectly immunocompe-
           tent individual. Also, anergy is more common in patients with dis-
           seminated (miliary) tuberculosis. For the same reason, it is not pos-
           sible to claim that this patient does not respond to polysaccharides
           (and tetanus toxoid is a protein). Finally, protection against tetanus
           toxoid is antibody mediated, and a negative skin test has no mean-
           ing for the degree of protection.

16.3 (E) CD29 defines the population of helper/inducer cells but is not infor-
           mative about the functional activity of the cells expressing the
           marker. The expression of CD25 (IL2 receptor) is typical of activ-
           ated T cells. The mitogenic responses to PHA and PWM only give
           an indication about the general ability of T cells (as well as of B cells,
           when PWM is used) to proliferate. IL2 release is probably the major
           determinant of the initial expansion of T cells during an immune re-
           sponse, and therefore it can be considered the best way to assess the
           ability of T cells to differentiate functionally after stimulation.

16.4 (C) Histamine release is not directly or indirectly related to T lympho-
           cyte activation.

16.5 (C) All other mitogens listed stimulate preferentially the proliferation or
           activation of B lymphocytes.

16.6   (D) The need for a long incubation period in the MLC arises because the responding T cells are sensitized in vitro during that period.

16.7   (D)

16.8   (E)

16.9   (B) The proportion of cell expressing T-cell markers (CD4, CD2) will increase after PWM stimulation, because T cells will proliferate in response to this mitogen. Similarly, the proportion of cells expressing IL2 receptor (CD25) will be increased, reflecting the state of activation of the proliferating cells. On the other hand, the proliferation and differentiation of B cells into antibody-producing cells caused by PWM will be associated with the loss of B-cell markers (CD19, CD20) and increased expression of plasma cell markers (PCA-1).

16.10 (A) The responding cells proliferated and differentiated after specific antigenic stimulation by D-locus antigens on the stimulator cells.

BIBLIOGRAPHY

Klaus, G. G. B. *Lymphocytes: A Practical Approach.* IRL Press, Oxford/Washington, D.C., 1987.

Mishell, B. B. and Shiigi, S. M. (Eds.). *Selected Methods in Cellular Immunology.* W. H. Freeman, San Francisco, 1980.

Rose, N. R., Friedman, H. and Fahey, J. L. *Manual of Clinical Laboratory Immunology,* 3rd Ed. American Society for Microbiology, 1986. (Includes the section "Cellular Components.")

Stites, D. P. Clinical laboratory methods of detection of cellular immune function. In *Basic and Clinical Immunology,* 6th Ed. D. P. Stites, J. D. Stobo, and J. V. Wells (Eds.). Appleton and Lange, 1987, p. 285.

WHO Scientific Group on Immunodeficiency. Primary immunodeficiency diseases. *Clin. Immunol. Immunopathol. 28*:450, 1983. (Contains a good outline of the diagnostic approach to CMI deficiencies.)

17

Diagnostic Evaluation of Phagocytic Function

GABRIEL VIRELLA

As pointed out in earlier chapters, the failure or success of an immune response directed against an infectious agent depends greatly on the cooperation between the immune system and nonimmune antimicrobial systems. This is particularly true in the case of the humoral immune response, because the antimicrobial effects of antibodies depend entirely on their ability to trigger the complement system and/or to induce phagocytosis.

Most mammals, including man, have developed two well-defined systems of phagocytic cells: the polymorphonuclear leukocyte system and the monocyte/macrophage system. Both types of cells can engulf microorganisms and cause their intracellular death through a variety of enzymatic systems, but the two-cell systems differ considerably in their biological characteristics. For example, the PMN leukocyte is basically a wandering cell, able to recognize foreign matter by a wide variety of immunological and nonimmunological mechanisms. The monocyte/macrophage system plays other very important roles in collaboration with the immune system, particularly in the areas of immunoregulation and in the final effector stages of cell-mediated immune responses. A comparison of the main biological characteristics of the two phagocytic cell systems is shown in Table 17.1.

TABLE 17.1 Comparison of the Characteristics of PMN Leukocytes and Monocytes/Macrophages

Characteristic	PMN leukocytes	Monocyte/macrophage
Numbers in peripheral blood	$3\text{-}6 \times 10^3/\text{mm}^3$	$285\text{-}500/\text{mm}^3$
Resident forms in tissues	−	+ (macrophage)
Nonimmunological phagocytosis	+ +	+
Fc and C3b receptors	+ +	+ +
Enzymatic granules	+ +	+ +
Bactericidal enzymes	+ +	+ +
Ability to generate superoxide and H_2O_2	+ +	+ +
Synthesis and release of leukotrienes	+ (B4)	+ + (B4, C4, D4)
Synthesis and release of prostaglandins	−	+ +
Release of PAF	+ +	+
Release of interleukins	−	+ + (IL1, IL6)
Response to nonimmunologic factors	+	−
Response to C5a/C3a	+	−
Response to lymphokines	+	+ + (IFNγ)
Antigen processing	−	+ +
Expression of HLA class II antigens	−	+ +
Phagocytosis-independent enzyme release	+ +	−

I. PHYSIOLOGY OF THE PMN LEUKOCYTE

As stated earlier, PMN leukocytes are constantly circulating around the vascular network. The first step in the mobilization of these cells is believed to be the recognition of a chemotactic stimulus, which in most cases will be of bacterial origin. It can also be released as a consequence of tissue necrosis or as a result of complement activation. Among bacterial products, formyl-methionyl peptides, such as f-methionine-leucine-phenylalanine (f-met-leu-phe), are extremely potent chemotactic agents. Tissue damage may result in the activation of the plasmin system, which in turn initiate complement activation with generation of C5a, another extremely potent chemotactic agent. Many microorganisms can probably generate C5a by activation of the complement system through the alternative pathway. After an inflammatory process has been established, proteases released by activated PMN and macrophages can also split C5, and the same cells may release leukotriene B4, another potent chemotactic factor, attracting more PMN leukocytes to the site.

After receiving a chemotactic stimulus, the PMN leukocyte migrates to the extravascular compartment. This migration usually involves two stages: first, the PMN leukocytes express "adherence" molecules, become "sticky," and adhere to endothelial cells; then, through a process of diapedesis, they squeeze through the endothelial cell junctions into the extravascular compartment. This initial sequence of events appears to be initiated by changes in membrane potential, loss of membrane associated Ca^{2+}, and intracellular accumulation of Ca^{2+}. The cell membrane, which is smooth in the resting cell, becomes "ruffled," and the cell adhesiveness is markedly increased. This increased adhesiveness is associated with increased expression of adherence molecules, namely the CR3 (Mac-1) molecule and the LFA (leukocyte function antigen)-1 molecule. Both CR3 and LFA-1 are expressed by neutrophils and monocytes/macrophages, and their expression mediates a variety of cell-to-cell interactions such as those that lead to neutrophil aggregation and most importantly, those that mediate adhesion of neutrophils to endothelial cells. Soon thereafter, the locomotor apparatus of the neutrophils, which involves a contractile actin-myosin system stabilized by polymerized microtubules, is activated. An intact CR3 protein seems essential for the proper modulation of microtubule assembly, which will not take place in CR3-deficient patients.

At the area of infection, PMN leukocytes recognize the infectious agents, which are ingested and digested intracellularly. Several recognition systems appear to be involved, the best defined of which is the reaction with the Fc fragment of opsonizing antibodies. Surface binding of microorganisms to PMN through C3b receptors has been well established; this further enhances phagocytic uptake. Nonimmune recognition systems leading to phagocytosis appear responsible for the ingestion of polysaccharide-rich microbial components such as zymosan and particulate matter such as latex beads. Sugar receptors have been identified and probably mediate the phagocytosis of zymosan and of fungi with polysaccharide-rich capsules. The engulfment of latex particles can be mediated by Fc receptors, if latex is first incubated with serum or IgG, which is passively adsorbed to the particles. Plain, unopsonized latex particles can also be ingested by neutrophils; it has been suggested that the hydrophobic nature of the beads is responsible for their engulfment.

Ingestion is achieved through formation of pesudopods that surround the particle or bacterium; the pseudopods eventually fuse at the distal pole to form a phagosome. The cytoplasmic granules of the neutrophil (lysosomes) then fuse with the phagosomes, and their contents empty inside the phagosomes. This degranulation process is very rapid and delivers a variety of antimicrobial substances to the phagosome. The azurophilic or *primary granules* contain, among other substances, myeloperoxidase, lysozyme, acid hydrolases (such as β-glucuronidase), cationic proteins, and neutral proteases (including collagenase, elastase, and cathepsin C2). The *secondary granules* or lysosomes contain lysozyme and lactoferrin. From the antibacterial point of view, lysozyme, lactoferrin, and cationic proteins appear most important. Lysozyme is able to split the β-1,4 linkage between the N-acetylmuramic acid peptide N-acetylglucosamine on the bacterial peptidoglycan. However, the importance of this enzyme as a primary killing mechanism has been questioned, because of the relative inaccessibility of the peptidoglycan layer in many microorganisms, which may be surrounded by capsules (gram-positive bacteria) or by the outer membrane (gram-negative bacteria). Lactoferrin has antimicrobial activity by chelating iron and preventing its use by bacteria that need it as an essential nutrient. Cationic proteins can bind to negatively charged cell surfaces (such as the bacterial outer membrane) and interfere with growth.

From the bactericidal point of view, however, the activation of the superoxide generating system appears considerably more significant. This system is activated not only by opsonization but as a consequence of the recognition,

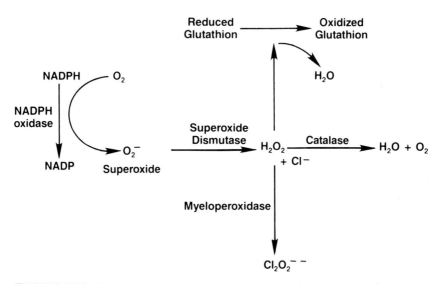

FIGURE 17.1 Diagrammatic representation of the major pathways of oxidative metabolism in phagocytic cells.

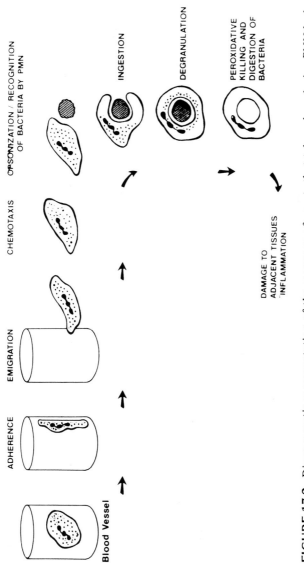

FIGURE 17.2 Diagrammatic representation of the sequence of events that takes place during PMN leukocyte phagocytosis. (Reproduced with permission from Wolach, B., Baehner, R. L., and Boxer, L. A. *Israel J. Med. Sci. 18:*897, 1982.)

through membrane receptors, of a variety of PMN-activating stimuli, ranging from f-met-leu-phe to C5a.

In simplified terms, a key enzyme (NADPH oxidase) is activated and reduces oxygen to form superoxide. This compound is quickly converted to H_2O_2 by superoxide dismutase, and H_2O_2 is detoxified by catalase and by the oxidation of reduced glutathione, which requires activation of the hexose monophosphate shunt (see Fig. 17.1). Both superoxide and H_2O_2 are extremely toxic, and their generation appears essential for intracellular killing of bacteria. Through myeloperoxidase, H_2O_2 can be peroxidated and led to form hypochlorite and other halide ion derivatives, which are potent bactericidal agents.

The sequence of the different stages involved in neutrophil function is diagrammatically summarized in Figure 17.2.

II. PHYSIOLOGY OF THE MONOCYTE/MACROPHAGE

Although th PMN leukocyte and the monocyte/macrophage share many common characteristics, such as the presence of Fc and C3b receptors on their membranes, their ability to engulf bacteria and particles, and their metabolic and enzymatic killing mechanisms, there are important differences between the two types of cells.

One important distinguishing feature is the ability of the monocyte/macrophage series of cells to participate in immunoregulatory mechanisms such as antigen processing and interleukin secretion, characteristics not shared by the PMN leukocyte. Also, the monocyte/macrophage cell series appears to be more sensitive to chemotactic factors released by T cells (such as MCF) and other leukocytes (such as LTB4) than to complement-derived chemotactic stimuli (such as C5a). It should be pointed out that these two types of phagocytic cells have different preferences in phagocytosis. The PMN leukocyte is avid to engulf inert particles such as latex but has very little ability to engulf antibody-coated homologous erythrocytes; the reverse is true for the monocyte/macrophage.

The circulating monocytes and the tissue-fixed (resident) macrophages are usually resting cells that can be activated in vitro by several types of stimuli, including microorganisms (bacteria, viruses, or protozoa) or their products (*C. parvum* or *Mycobacterium* products), T-lymphocyte mediators, or nonspecific substances such as the carcinogen phorbol myristic acetate, glycogen, or thioglycolate.

The stimulation of monocytes/macrophages by the above-mentioned microbes and substances results in morphological and functional changes. Morphologically the activated macrophage is larger, and its cytoplasm tends to spread and attach to surfaces. This reaction appears to be mediated by a cleavage product of factor B of the alternative complement pathway, which is synthesized by the macrophage themselves. The composition of the plasma membrane is changed, and the rates of pinocytosis and engulfment are increased (phagocytosis through C3b receptors is seen only after activation). Intracellularly there is a marked increase in enzymatic contents, particularly of plasminogen activator, collagenase, and elastase, and the oxidative metabolism (leading to generation of superoxide and H_2O_2) is greatly enhanced.

The intracellular killing mechanisms of the macrophage appear similar to those of the PMN leukocyte, and most of the killing-related metabolic pathways are probably similar, in contrast to other functions and metabolic pathways, which differ considerably (see Table 17.1).

III. LABORATORY EVALUATION OF PHAGOCYTIC FUNCTION

The evaluation of phagocytic function is usually centered on the study of polymorphonuclear leukocytes, which are considerably easier to purify than monocytes or macrophages. Phagocytosis by PMN can be depressed as a result of neutropenia or as a result of a functional defect. Functional defects affecting every stage of the phagocytic response have been reported and have to be evaluated by different tests.

A. Polymorphonuclear Leukocyte Count

The PMN leukocyte count is the simplest and one of the most important tests, because phagocytic defects due to neutropenia are by far more common than the primary, congenital, defects of phagocytic function.

It is believed that as a general rule a neutrophil count below $1000/mm^3$ represents an increased risk of infection, and when neutrophil counts are lower than $200/mm^3$ the patient will invariably be infected.

B. Adherence

The first stage of PMN leukocyte activation is an increased adherence of the cell, which is related to its margination in the vessels. The aggregation of PMN can be measured in aggregometers, and C5a desarg (a nonchemotactic derivative of C5a generated by exposing freshly drawn serum to a substance such as zymosan, which activates the alternative pathway of complement) is the most frequently used chemotactic stimulus. Other tests measure the adherence to nylon wool fibers or other artificial substrates. With the availability of monoclonal antibodies directed to the different components of CD11, which include CR3 and LFA-1, it has become possible to define patients with hereditary defects of these adherence molecules.

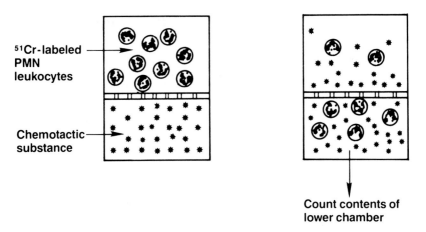

⁵¹Cr-labeled
PMN
leukocytes

Chemotactic
substance

Count contents of
lower chamber

FIGURE 17.3   Schematic representation of the principle of chemotaxis assays using the Boyden chamber and ⁵¹Cr-labeled PMN leukocytes.

C. Chemotaxis and Migration

The migration of phagocytes in response to chemotactic stimuli is usually studied using the Boyden chamber. The basic principle of all versions of the Boyden chamber is to have two compartments separated by a membrane whose pores are too tight to allow PMN leukocytes to diffuse passively from one chamber to the other but large enough to allow the active movement of these cells from the upper chamber, where they are placed, to the lower chamber. The movement of the cells is stimulated by adding to the lower chamber a chemotactic factor such as C5a or the tetrapeptide f-met-leu-phe. The results are usually obtained either by counting the number of cells that reach the bottom side of the membrane or by the indirect determination of the number of cells reaching the bottom chamber using ⁵¹Cr-labeled PMN (as illustrated in Figure 17.3).

In vivo, the capacity to recruit PMN into an area of inflammation can be measured by the Rebuck's skin window technique. A superficial abrasion of the skin is covered with a glass cover slip, which thus forms a small diffusion chamber ("skin window"). Inflammatory cells reaching it will adhere to the glass and can be stained and counted.

D. Ingestion

Ingestion tests are relatively simple to perform and reproduce. They are usually based on incubating PMN with opsonized particles and, after an adequate incubation, determining either the number of ingested particles or a phagocytic index obtained by applying the following formula:

$$\text{Phagocytic index} = \frac{\text{No. of cells with ingested particles}}{\text{Total No. of cells}} \times 100$$

Several types of particles have been used, including latex, zymosan (fragments of fungal capsular polysaccharidic material), killed *C. albicans*, and IgG-coated beads (immunobeads). All these particles will activate complement by either one of the pathways and become coated with C3, although opsonization with complement is not the major determinant of phagocytosis. The easiest particles to visualize once ingested are fluorescent latex beads; their use considerably simplifies the assay (Fig. 17.4).

E. Degranulation

When the contents of cytoplasmic granules are released into a phagosome, there is always some leakage of their contents into the extracellular fluid. The tests to study degranulation involve ingestion of particulate matter, as mentioned above, but in this case the supernatants are analyzed for their contents of substances released by the PMN granules such as myeloperoxidase, lysozyme, β-glucuronidase, and lactoferrin.

F. Oxidative Burst

The biological significance of the generation of superoxide and $H_2 O_2$ has been discussed in earlier sections of this chapter. Four basic assays can be used to measure the oxidative burst.

1. Chemiluminescence

The chemiluminescence assay is based on the superoxide ion's instability, so that its dissociation can be measured either directly or indirectly after addition of luminol activated during superoxide dissociation. This is perhaps the most sensitive and directly quantitative assay for the oxidative burst, but it has a major drawback in that it requires special instrumentation.

2. Reduction of Cytochrome C

The reduction of cytochrome C can be used to measure superoxide release, because this pigment, when reduced by superoxide, will change its light absorbance properties. The change in color of cytochrome C can be measured with a conventional spectrophotometer. The main drawbacks of the assay are its relatively low sensitivity and difficulties in reproducibility.

3. Nitroblue Tetrazolium Reduction

Oxidized NBT, colorless to pale yellow in solution, is transformed by reduction into blue formazan. There are several technical variations of the test, the sim-

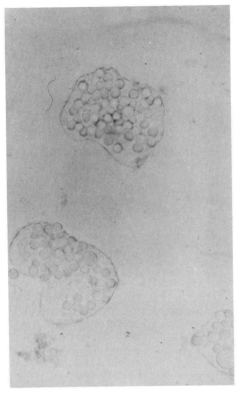

FIGURE 17.4 Use of fluorescent latex beads for evaluation of phagocytosis. The panel on the left reproduces a photograph of microscopic field showing the phagocytic cells that have ingested latex beads under visible light. The panel on the right shows the same field under UV light.

plest consisting of incubating PMN simultaneously with some particles (zymosan, immunobeads) and soluble, unreduced NBT. The particles and NBT are ingested, the oxidative burst causes the reduction of NBT, and the results of the test are determined by counting the number of PMN with blue-stained cytoplasms. This microscopic assay has been criticized as misleading and nonspecific, and modifications have been proposed. Some authors prefer tube tests in which the PMN are simultaneously exposed to opsonized latex particles and NBT; the change of color of the supernatant, from pale yellow to gray or purple (as a result of the spillage of oxidizing products during phagocytosis), is measured. A variant of this assay in which the reduction of NBT is followed by kinetic colormetry appears sensitive, specific, and reproducible. Others prefer to extract intracellular NBT with pyrimidine and measure its absorbance at 515 nm (which

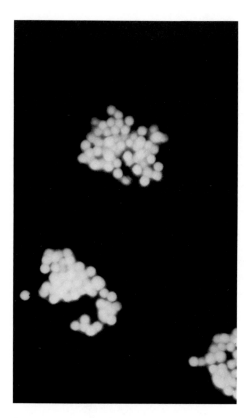

FIGURE 17.4 (continued)

corresponds to the absorbance peak of reduced NBT). This last NBT test is extremely sensitive and accurate, but it is the most difficult to perform.

4. Flow Cytometry

The most recently developed methods for the measurement of the superoxide burst are based on the oxidation of $2',7'$-dichlorofluorescin diacetate (nonfluorescent), which results in the formation of $2',7'$-dichlorofluorescein (highly fluorescent). The superoxide burst is induced with phorbol myristate acetate (or any other soluble PMN activator), and the numbers of fluorescent cells, and the fluorescence intensity of activated and nonactivated PMN suspensions from patients and suitable controls, can be determined by flow cytometry. In patients with chronic granulomatous disease, both the mean fluorescence intensity and the numbers of fluorescent cells after stimulation are considerably lower than those determined in normal, healthy volunteers.

G. Killing

The main function of the PMN is to kill ingested microorganisms. This ability can be tested using a variety of bacteria and fungi that are mixed with PMN in the presence of normal human serum (a source of opsonins); after a time, the cells are harvested and lysed, and the number of intracytoplasmic viable bacteria is determined. The assays are difficult and cumbersome, and they require close support from a microbiology laboratory. For this reason they have been less frequently used than the indirect killing assays based on detection of the oxidative burst of the PMN, mentioned in the previous section. Alternative and simpler approaches to the evaluation of intracellular killing by the differential uptake of dyes (such as acridine orange) between live and dead bacteria have been proposed but not yet sufficiently evaluated.

IV. DISEASES OF PHAGOCYTIC FUNCTION

Phagocytic function can be negatively affected by a variety of factors, some of a quantitative nature, some of a qualitative nature. Figure 17.5 diagrammatically

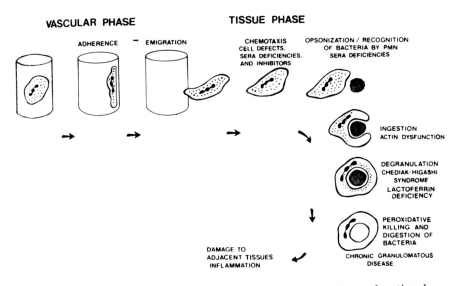

FIGURE 17.5 Diagrammatic representation of the major primary functional derangements of neutrophils that have been characterized in man. (Reproduced with permission from Wolach, B., Baehner, R. L., and Boxer, L. A. *Israel J. Med. Sci. 18*:897, 1982.)

TABLE 17.2   Causes of Neutropenia

Congenital

Secondary (acquired)
   Depressed bone marrow granulocytosis
     Drug-induced
     Tumor invasion
     Nutritional Deficiency
     Unknown cause (idiopathic)
   Peripheral destruction of neutrophils
     Autoimmune (Felty's symdrome)[a]
     Drug-induced

[a]An association of rheumatoid arthritis, splenomegaly and neutropenia.

illustrates the aspects of PMN function that can be affected in different pathological situations.

A. Neutropenia

A depression of the total number of neutrophils is the most frequent cause of infection due to defective phagocytic function. Although there are congenital forms of neutropenia of variable severity, most frequently neutropenia is secondary to a variety of causes (see Table 17.2).

B. Disorders of Adherence

A rare congenital disease, inherited as an autosomic recessive trait, has been recently described; it is characterized by the lack of CR3, LFA-2 and related proteins. The first sign of disease in many instances is a delayed separation of the umbilical cord, and during childhood these individuals suffer from repeated pyogenic infections and, with less frequency, from fungal infections.

C. Disorders of Chemotaxis

Those disorders can be secondary to the lack of generation of chemotactic factors (e.g., complement deficiencies) or to cellular deficiencies. Neutrophil adherence can also be affected by many drugs such as corticosteroids, salicylates, alcohol, and colchicine.

D. Job's Syndrome (Hyper-IgE Syndrome)

This syndrome is characterized by dermatitis, very high levels of serum IgE, and recurrent staphylococcal infections of the lungs and cutaneous abscesses. Other types of pyogenic infections, particularly of the upper airways, and chronic candidiasis can also be present. A defect of monocyte chemotaxis has been reported in most patients, but its severity is quite variable, and many doubt that it is, indeed, the primary defect. An alternative hypothesis to explain the syndrome is the generation of inhibitor(s) of chemotaxis by mononuclear cells. The high levels of IgE correspond, at least in part, to the production of IgE anti-*S. aureus* antibodies; in contrast, IgA antibodies to *S. aureus* are abnormally low, and other indices of humoral immune function (responses to toxoid boosters and to in vitro stimulation with PWM) are similarly depressed.

E. Disorders of Phagocyte Killing

1. Chronic Granulomatous Disease

This rare disease, affecting about one in one million persons, is characterized by recurrent life-threatening pyogenic infections. Both types of phagocytic cells (PMN leukocytes and monocytes) are affected by a defect in the oxidative metabolism. The nature of this defect is heterogeneous, but it results in a deficient activation of NADPH oxidase, the enzyme responsible for the generation of superoxide. As a consequence, superoxide and H_2O_2 generation are impaired, and intracellular killing is defective. The killing defect, however, affects mostly the elimination of catalase positive organisms such as *S. aureus, Aspergillus* sp., *Chromobacterium violaceum, Pseudomonas cepacia*, and *Nocardia* sp. Catalase-negative, peroxidase-generating microorganisms such as *Streptococcus pneumoniae* are not usually involved in these patients' infections. This is because catalase negative organisms, when ingested, continue to generate H_2O_2 that they cannot break down. The H_2O_2 generated by the bacteria progressively accumulates in the phagosome, eventually reaching bactericidal levels.

Clinically, the most frequent infection site is the lungs followed by the lymph nodes and the skin and soft tissues. It should be noted that in over 50% of febrile episodes suffered by these patients no microorganism is recovered from any suspected site of infection.

The infections are characterized by microabscess and granuloma formation; lymphadenopathy with suppuration and draining of the lymph nodes is one of the first manifestations of the disease. Hepatosplenomegaly, osteomyelitis, and hypergammaglobulinemia are frequent. Diagnosis is usually based on one of the variations of the NBT test, which, if abnormal, should be confirmed by a killing test.

Therapy is usually limited to the use of antimicrobials, based on sensitivity studies if bacteria have been recovered from infection sites. Prophylactic use of trimethoprim-sulfamethoxazole has been recommended and has met with success in some trials.

2. Chediak-Higashi Syndrome

This rare disease is due to abnormalities in the cytoplasmic granules so that the killing of certain microorganisms is impaired. It is believed that the primary defect may be in the regulation of membrane activation. The PMN leukocytes are able to ingest microorganisms, but the cytoplasmic granules tend to coalesce into giant secondary lysosomes, with reduced enzymatic contents, that are inconsistently delivered to the phagosome. As a consequence, intracellular killing is slow and ineffecient.

Clinically the symdrome is characterized by mucocutaneous albinism, recurrent neutropenia, and unexplained fever and peripheral neuropathy. Later the patients may develop hepatosplenomegaly and lymphadenopathy, and this is associated with recurrent bacterial and viral infection, fever, and prostration. At that stage, the prognosis is very poor.

The diagnosis is usually confirmed by the morphological features (giant lysosomes) and abnormal results in microbial killing tests. Therapy is usually symptomatic with antibiotics, but recent evidence suggests that ascorbic acid administration results in functional and clinical improvement in some patients. This improvement may be related to an effect of ascorbic acid on membrane fluidity, which is abnormally high in the patient's PMN leukocytes and is normalized by ascorbic acid. Whether as a result of changes in membrane fluidity or not, ascorbic acid administration is associated with increased bactericidal activity.

SELF-EVALUATION

Questions

Choose the one best answer.

17.1 Among the listed clinical situations associated with depressed phagocytic function, the one you expect to be most frequent is
A. Chronic granulomatous disease.
B. Job's disease.
C. Chediak-Higashi syndrome.
D. Drug-induced neutropenia.
E. CR3-LFA1 deficiency.

17.2 The killing defect in chronic granulomatous disease is related to a deficiency of
A. Lactoferrin.
B. Myeloperoxidase.
C. Lysozyme.
D. Secondary granule formation.
E. Activation of NDPH oxidase.

17.3 Among the microorganisms that cause recurrent infections in patients with chronic granulomatous disease, one expects to find all of those listed below except
A. *Staphylococcus aureus.*
B. *Streptococcus pneumoniae.*
C. *Staphylococcus epidermidis.*
D. *Pseudomonas cepacia.*
E. *Aspergillus fumigatus.*

17.4 Prophylactic therapy in the Chediak-Higashi syndrome may involve
A. Monthly injections of penicillin-benzatin.
B. Daily administration of trimethoprim-sulfamethoxazole.
C. Daily administration of ascorbic acid.
D. Splenectomy.
E. None of the above.

17.5 Phagocytosis of zymosan through a C3b receptor requires the presence of
A. Antizymosan antibodies.
B. EDTA.
C. Ca^{2+}.
D. Fresh normal human serum.
E. All of the above.

17.6 The NBT test is considered as an indirect measurement of killing capacity because
A. The reduction of NBT reflects the adequacy of the oxidative metabolic pathways.
B. NBT is oxidized in the presence of lactoperoxidase, and this enzyme is the major killing mechanism in PMN leukocytes.
C. This test reflects the ability to form phagolysosomes.
D. It does require the measurement of viability of intracellular bacteria previously incubated with PMN leukocytes and NBT.
E. None of the above.

In questions 17.7-17.10, for each numbered work or phase, select the one lettered heading that is most closely related to it. The same heading may be used once, more than once, or not at all: (A) Boyden chambers; (B) Rebuck skin window; (C) Latex particles; (D) Chemiluminescence; (E) NBT reduction test.

17.7   Used in measurement in vitro of chemotaxis.

17.8   Used to measure the generation of superoxide.

17.9   Used to assess ingestion.

17.10   Used to screen patients with suspected chronic granulomatous disease.

Answers

17.1 (D)   Primary phagocytic disorders are extremely rare disorders.

17.2 (E)   NDPH oxidase is responsible for the conversion of O_2 into superoxide, which is the initial event that triggers the generation of
H_2O_2 and halide ion derivatives involved in bactericidal activity.

17.3 (B)   Catalase negative organisms such as *S. pneumoniae* are not usually
involved as pathogens in chronic granulomatous disease.

17.4 (C)   Ascorbic acid appears to stabilize the fluidity of cell membranes,
and this appears to correct (at least in some cases) the phagocytic
defect associated with Chediak-Higashi syndrome.

17.5 (D)   Zymosan will activate the alternative pathway, and C3b will become adsorbed to the surface of the zymosan particles. This reaction does not require specific antibody, does require fresh serum
as complement source, and requires Mg^{2+} but not Ca^{2+}. If EDTA
is added to the culture, phagocytosis will be prevented, because
this reagent chelates both CA^{2+} and Mg^{2+}.

17.6 (A)   NBT is colorless to pale yellow, and it turns purple after reduction;
hence, the reduction of NBT is considered an indirect verification
of the adequacy of the oxidative metabolism in a phagocytic cell.

17.7 (A)

17.8 (D)

17.9 (C)

17.10 (E)   Usually, a variant of the NBT test is used for the initial screening of
chronic granulomatous disease. If available, chemiluminescence
and flow cytometry tests can be used either to screen or to confirm
a positive screening test result.

BIBLIOGRAPHY

Gallin, J. I., Brescher, E. S., Seligmann, B. E., Nath, J., Gaither, T., and Katz,
P. Recent advances in chronic granulomatous disease. *Ann. Intern. Med. 99*:
657, 1983.
Hanan, N. F., Douglas, S. D., and Campbell, D. E. Clinical evaluation of defects
in neutrophil oxydative metabolism. *Clin. Immunol. News. 9*:37, 1988.
Malech, H. L. and Gallin, J. I. Neutrophils in human diseases. *New England J.
Med. 317*:687, 1987.

Root, R. K. Host defenses against infection: Importance of phagocytic mechanisms from the study of genetic disorders of leukocyte function. *Bull. N. Y. Acad. Med. 58*:669, 1982.

Twomey, J. J. Disorders of macrophages. In *The Pathophysiology of Human Immunologic Disorders*, J. J. Twomey (Ed.). Urban & Schwarzenberg, Baltimore, 1982.

Wolach, B., Baehner, R. L., and Boxer, L. A. Review: Clinical and laboratory approach to the management of neutrophil dysfunction. *Israel J. Med. Sci. 18*:897, 1982.

III
Clinical Immunology

18

Hypersensitivity Reactions

GABRIEL VIRELLA

The immune response is basically a mechanism used by vertebrates to eliminate whatever is not recognized as self. The most obvious application of this mechanism is the eradication of infectious agents that succeed in penetrating the natural barriers. However, the immune response can be the cause of tissue damage either as an undesirable effect of an immune response directed against an exogenous antigen or as a consequence of an autoimmune reaction.

I. HYPERSENSITIVITY AND ALLERGY

If a harmful reaction to a given antigen occurs because of an abnormal state of reactivity, this is termed *hypersensitivity*. Hypersensitivity states can result in pathologic reactions when a given individual encounters an antigen to which he is hypersensitive. Such reactions can be distinguished by the time elapsed between the exposure to the antigen and the appearance of clinical symptoms and are categorized as immediate and delayed reactions. Immediate hypersensitivity reactions are those that are primarily involved in the field of allergy.

II. GELL AND COOMBS' CLASSIFICATION OF HYPERSENSITIVITY REACTIONS

Two British immunologists, Phillip Gell and Robin Coombs, proposed a classification of hypersensitivity states into four types that, despite its lack of per-

341

TABLE 18.1   General Characteristics of the Four Types of Hypersensitivity
Reactions as Defined by Gell and Coombs

Type	Manifestation	Lag between exposure and symptoms	Mechanism
I	Immediate hypersensitivity reactions	Minutes	IgE and possibly IgG4
II	Cytotoxic reactions	Variable	IgG and IgM
III	Antigen-antibody complexes	6 h[a]	IgG mainly
IV	Delayed hypersensitivity	12-14 hr	Sensitized lympho-cytes

[a]For the Arthus reaction

fect correspondence with many clinical situations, is still widely used (see Table 18.1).

The reactions of types I, II, and III are basically mediated by antibodies with or without participation of the complement system; type IV reactions are cell mediated. It must be emphasized that in many pathological processes one sees a combination of mechanisms belonging to several types of hypersensitivity reactions; but in spite of its obvious artificiality, the division of hypersensitivity states into four broad types aids considerably in the understanding of the pathogenesis of clinical conditions associated with hypersensitivity.

III.   IMMEDIATE HYPERSENSITIVITY (TYPE I HYPERSENSITIVITY REACTIONS, ALLERGIC STATES)

The most dramatic demonstration of a state of immediate hypersensitivity can be easily obtained by injecting an antigen such as egg albumin into a guinea pig previously sensitized against the same protein. Guinea pigs tend to produce large amounts of homocytotropic antibodies, and the challenge of a sensitized animal is followed by a massive release of vasoactive amines from cells to which the antibody has bound. This reaction is very rapid (it is observed within a few minutes after the challenge) and results in the death of the animal in anaphylactic shock. The speed of the reaction has led to the adoption of the term immediate hypersensitivity.

A wide variety of hypersensitivity states can be classified as immediate hypersensitivity reactions. Some have a predominantly cutaneous expression; others are of a systemic nature. The latter are often designated as *anaphylactic reactions*, of which anaphylactic shock is the most severe form. Both types of reactions share common pathways in their pathogenesis, because the primary event is the predominant synthesis of specific IgE antibodies by the allergic individual; these IgE antibodies bind with high avidity to the membranes of basophils and mast cells. When exposed to the sensitizing antigen, the reaction with cell-bound IgE triggers the release of histamine, through degranulation, and the synthesis of leukotrienes C4, D4, and E4 (this mixture constitutes what was formerly known as slow reacting substance of anaphylaxis or SRS-A). These substances are potent constrictors of smooth muscle and vasodilators.

The expression of generalized anaphylaxis is species specific. The guinea pig usually has bronchoconstriction and bronchial edema as the predominant expression, leading to death in acute asphyxiation. Generalized vasodilation and acute hypotension can also occur but are not predominant features. In the rabbit, on the contrary, the most affected organ is the heart, and the animals die of right heart failure. In man, bronchial asthma in its most severe forms closely resembles the reaction of the guinea pig. Systemic anaphylactic reactions in humans usually present with itching, erythema, vomiting, abdominal cramps, diarrhea, respiratory distress, and in severe cases, laryngeal edema and vascular collapse leading to shock that may be irreversible.

Most frequently, human type I hypersensitivity has a localized expression, such as the bronchoconstriction and bronchial edema that characterize bronchial asthma, the mucosal edema in hay fever, and the skin rash and subcutaneous edema that defines urticaria (hives). The factor(s) involved in determining what target organs are affected in different types of immediate hypersensitivity reactions are not well defined, but the route of exposure to the challenging antigen seems an important factor. Systemic anaphylaxis is usually associated with antigens that are directly introduced into the systemic circulation, such as in the case of hypersensitivity to insect venoms or to systemically administered drugs; allergic (extrinsic) asthma and hay fever are usually associated with inhaled antigens; for less clear reasons urticaria is seen as a frequent manifestation of food allergy.

A. Passive Transfer of Anaphylactic Reactions

One of the earliest observations that suggested the crucial role of antibodies in type I hypersensitivity was the transfer of sensitization by injection of serum from a sensitized individual to a nonallergic recipient. This can be observed both in animals and in man. For example, if serum from a guinea pig sensitized seven to ten days earlier with a single injection of egg albumin in adjuvant is transferred to a nonimmunized animal that is challenged 48 h later with egg albumin, this passively sensitized animal will develop acute symptoms and may die in anaphylactic shock,

This passive transfer of hypersensitivity can take less dramatic aspects if the reaction takes place in the skin. In these experiments, nonsensitized animals are injected intradermally with the serum from a sensitized individual. After 24 72 h (to allow for homocytotropic antibodies to diffuse and bind to mast cell membranes) the antigen in question is injected intravenously mixed with Evans blue dye. When the antigen reaches the area of the skin where antibodies were injected and are now bound to basophils, a localized type I reaction will take place, characterized by a small area of vascular hyperpermeability that results in edema and redness. When the reaction is performed with Evans blue the affected area will have a blue discoloration due to the transudation of the dye and will be easier to read. This reaction is known as passive cutaneous anaphylaxis (PCA).

A reaction with a similar principle, practiced initially in human subjects, is the Prausnitz-Kustner (PK) reaction. This reaction results from injecting serum from an allergic patient intradermally into a nonallergic recipient and after 24 to 48 h challenging the area of the skin where the serum was injected with the antigen that is suspected of causing the symptoms in the patient. A positive reaction consists of a wheal and flare appearing a few minutes after injection of the antigen. The rationale for this reaction was to avoid the risk of inducing a severe (potentially fatal) reaction if the antigen were injected directly into the skin of the allergic individual, but it has a considerable risk of transmitting hepatitis and other infections. The reaction was also performed in lower primates, which were injected intravenously with the serum of an allergic individual and challenged later with intradermal injections of a battery of antigens that could be implicated as the cause of the allergic reaction. With more controlled conditions for direct skin testing of allergic individuals and the introduction of in vitro procedures for the screening of specific IgE antibodies (also designated as reagins), the PK reaction is mentioned only for its general interest as historic development that helped our understanding of the immediate hypersensitivity reaction.

B. Atopy

In medicine the term atopy is used to designate the tendency of some individuals to become sensitized to a variety of *allergens* (antigens involved in allergic reactions) including pollens, spores, animal danders, house dust, and foods. These individuals, when skin tested, are positive to several allergens, and successful therapy must take this multiple reactivity into account. A genetic background for atopy is suggested by the familial prevalence of this condition.

IV. CYTOTOXIC REACTIONS (TYPE II HYPERSENSITIVITY)

Type II hypersensitivity involves, in its most common forms, complement-fixing antibodies (IgM or IgG) directed against cellular or tissue antigens.

A. Autoimmune Hemolytic Anemia

Autoimmune hemolytic anemia can be considered as a prototype cytotoxic reaction. The patients with this condition synthesize antibodies directed to their own red cells, mostly of the IgG class. Those antibodies bind to the patient's red cells and can cause hemolysis by two main mechanisms. If complement is activated up to C9, the red cells can be directly hemolysed (intravascular hemolysis). If complement activation stops at C3, the red cells become coated with antibody and C3b but are not hemolysed. Their destruction will be carried out by phagocytic cells that will recognize the Fc fragment of anti-red-cell antibodies and the C3b component and proceed to ingest the red cells that will be lysed intracellularly. This sequestration and destruction of red cells takes place mostly in the spleen and liver, and when there is a marked predominance of splenic sequestration, splenectomy can be of therapeutic benefit, leading to a longer half-life of the patient's red cells.

B. Goodpasture's Syndrome

Reactions due to antitissue antibodies have been traditionally classified as cytotoxic or type II reactions. The classical example is Goodpasture's syndrome, in which anti-basement-membrane antibodies bind to antigens of the glomerular and alevolar basement membranes. This results in the in situ formation of antigen-antibody complexes, and from then on this variety of type II reaction is really indistinguishable from the reactions mediated by the deposition of soluble immune complexes (type III). Essentially, complement will be activated by the in-situ-formed antigen-antibody complexes, and as a result C5a and C3a will be generated. These complement components have a variety of important properties: they are chemotactic for PMN leukocytes, and C5a can increase vascular permeability directly or indirectly (by including the degranulation of basophils and mast cells); this increase of vascular permeability favors the exsudation and tissue accumulation of PMN leukocytes. Once in the tissues the PMN will recognize the Fc region of tissue-bound antibodies, as well as any C3b bound to the corresponding immune complexes, and it will release their enzymatic contents, which include proteases and collagenase. These enzymes will cause tissue damage (i.e., destruction of the basement membrane), which is the end of the reaction triggered by the binding of antibody to the basement membrane or to any other structure. Using fluorescein-conjugated antisera, the deposition of immunoglobulins and complement in patients with Goodpasture's syndrome appears, as a rule, as a linear, very regular pattern, following the glomerular or alveolar basement membranes. Elution studies have resulted in the production of immunoglobulin-rich preparations that when injected into primates can induce a disease similar to Goodpasture's syndrome in humans. The pathogenic role of antiglomerular basement-membrane antibodies is also sug-

gested by the recurrence of the disease in patients who receive kidney transplants.

C. Nephrotoxic (Masugi) Nephritis

In several animal species it has been demonstrated, following the seminal work
of Masugi, that the injection of heterologous anti-basement-membrane antibodies into a healthy animal results in the induction of a nephritis due to the
binding of the antibodies to the basement membrane, particularly at the glomerular level.

This experimental model has been extremely useful in demonstrating the
pathogenic importance of complement activation and of neutrophil accumulation. If, instead of complete antibodies, one injects Fab or $F(ab')_2$ fragments
which do not activate complement, no accumulation of PMN leukocytes in the
kidney is seen. Similar results are observed if the animal is rendered C3 deficient by injection of cobra venom factor. If the infiltration of PMN leukocytes
is prevented, either as a consequence of the manipulations described above or as
a result of having induced neutropenia in the experimental animals, tissue damage will be minimal or nonexistent.

V. HYPERSENSITIVITY REACTIONS SECONDARY TO THE
DEPOSITION OF SOLUBLE IMMUNE COMPLEXES
(TYPE III HYPERSENSITIVITY)

In the course of acute or chronic infections, or as a consequence of the production of autoantibodies, soluble antigen-antibody complexes are likely to be
formed and remain in circulation until clearance by the phagocytic system. In
most cases this will be an inconsequential sequence of events, but in other cases
inflammatory reactions can be triggered by the deposition of those immune
complexes in tissues. A simplified sequence of events leading to immune-complex-induced inflammation is shown in Figure 18.1. It can be easily noticed
that once the immune complexes are deposited extravascularly the sequence
of events is virtually identical to that observed in cases of in situ immune reactions involving tissue antigens and the corresponding antibodies.

A. The Arthus Reaction

This reaction was first described at the turn of the century by Arthus, who observed that the intradermal injection of antigen into an animal previously sensitized in a local inflammatory reaction. This reaction is edematous in the early
stages, but later can become hemorrhagic and, eventually, necrotic. A human
equivalent of this reaction can be observed in some vaccinal reactions to booster
doses in individuals who have already reached high levels of immunity. Basic-

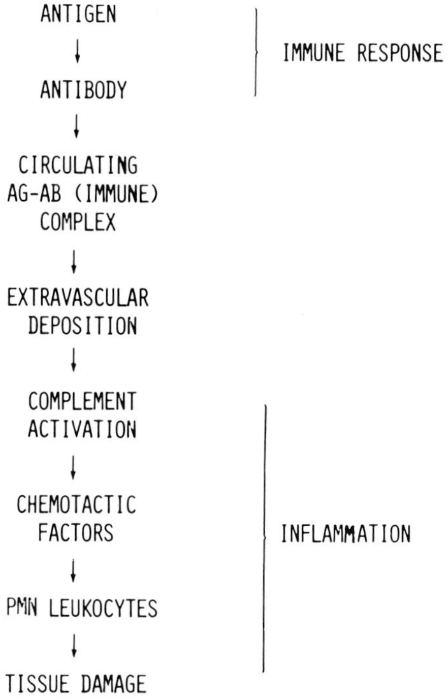

```
ANTIGEN
    ↓                    │ IMMUNE RESPONSE
ANTIBODY                 │
    ↓
CIRCULATING
AG-AB (IMMUNE)
  COMPLEX
    ↓
EXTRAVASCULAR
 DEPOSITION
    ↓
 COMPLEMENT              │
 ACTIVATION              │
    ↓                    │
CHEMOTACTIC              │
  FACTORS                │ INFLAMMATION
    ↓                    │
PMN LEUKOCYTES           │
    ↓                    │
TISSUE DAMAGE            │
```

FIGURE 18.1   Diagrammatic representation of the sequence of events triggered
by the deposition of soluble immune complexes that eventually results in tissue
damage.

ally, the reaction is due to the reaction fo complement-fixing IgG antibodies
(produced, as a rule, in hyperimmune states in most species) and tissue-localized
antigens. The lag time between antigen challenge and the reaction is usually 6 h,
which is a considerably slower onset than that of an immediate hypersensitivity
reaction but considerably faster than that of a delayed hypersensitivity reaction.
Although Arthus reactions are typically elicited in the skin, the same pathogenic
mechanisms can lead to organ lesions whenever the antigen, although intrinsically soluble, is unable to diffuse freely and remains retained in or around its
penetration point (e.g., the perialveolar spaces for inhaled antigens).

   The Arthus reaction, as induced in experimental animals, has been an extremely well studied model of immune-complex disease. Immunohistological
studies have shown that soon after antigen is injected in the skin IgG antibody
and C3 will form perivascular aggregates at the site of injection. The in situ
formation of immune complexes and consequent activation of the complement

system will trigger the sequence of events summarized in Figure 18.1. Again, if the animals are made neutropenic by administration of nitrogen mustard or of antineutrophil serum, the inflammatory reaction is prevented. The central role of the neutrophil in the pathogenesis of immune-complex-induced inflammation will be discussed in detail in a later chapter. At this point it should be noted that in spite of their pathogenic role, the neutrophils will actively engulf and eliminate the tissue-deposited IC, eliminating the initial trigger for the inflammatory reaction. As the IC are eliminated, the cellular infiltrate changes from having predominance of neutrophils and other granulocytes to having a predominance of mononuclear cells (macrophages), which is usually associated with the healing stage.

B. Serum Sickness

In the preantibiotic era the treatment of severe bacterial pneumonia and other infections with heterologous antisera was often tried in the hope that passive immunization would help the patient to survive. In many instances the pneumonia episode was successfully treated, but 7 to 10 days after the injection of heterologous antiserum the patient developed what was termed *serum sickness*, a combination of cutaneous rash (often purpuric), fever, arthralgias, mild acute glomerulonephritis, and carditis. Currently, serum sickness, as a complication of passive immunotherapy with heterologous antisera, is usually related to the injection of heterologous antisera to snake venoms, to the experimental use of mouse monoclonal antibodies in cancer immunotherapy, and to the administration of heterologous (monoclonal or polyclonal) antilymphocyte and antithymocyte sera in transplant patients. It can also be a side effect of some forms of drug therapy, particularly with penicillin and its congeners. The disease is extremely easy to reproduce in experimental animals through the injection of heterologous proteins. Basically two types of experimental serum sickness can be induced: acute, by one (or at the most two) immunizations with a large dose of protein; or chronic, by repeated daily injections of small doses of protein. The acute disease is reversible, while chronic serum sickness, which closely resembles human glomerulonephritis, is usually associated with irreversible damage.

In all types of serum sickness the initial event is the triggering of a humoral immune response, which explains the lag period of 7 to 10 days between the injection of heterologous protein (or drug) and the beginning of clinical symptoms. Evidently, this lag period will be shorter and the reaction more severe if there has been presensitization to the antigen in question. As soon as antibodies are secreted, they will combine with the antigens that then are still present in relatively large concentrations in the serum of the injected individual or experimental animal. Soluble immune complexes will be formed, and in the very early stages there will be great antigen excess, and the complexes will be small and nonpathogenic. With time, a situation of mild antigen excess, with formation of intermediate-sized immune complexes, will be reached, and those are potentially pathogenic, because they are not too large to cross the endothelial barrier (particularly if vascular permeability is increased) and are large enough to activate complement and induce inflammation. The deposition can take place in different organs, such as the myocardium (causing arthritis and myocardial inflammation), skin (causing erythematous rashes), joints (causing acute glomerulonephritis). Soluble immune complexes can also indirectly affect cells such as the neutrophils and platelets (as will be discussed in detail in later chapters), and purpuric rashes due to thrombocytopenia are frequently seen in serum sickness. As in the case of the Arthus reaction, the inflammatory changes associated with serum sickness do not take place or are very mild if complement or neutrophils are depleted.

VI.   DELAYED (TYPE IV) HYPERSENSITIVITY REACTIONS

In contrast to the other types of hypersensitivity reactions discussed earlier, type IV or delayed hypersensitivity is a manifestation of cell-mediated immunity. In other words, this type of hypersensitivity reaction is mediated by specifically sensitized T lymphocytes rather than by specific antibodies.

The prototype of a delayed hypersensitivity reaction is the tuberculin test, which consists of the intradermal injection of tuberculin or PPD followed by visual inspection of the injection site 24 and 46 h later. If the individual is hypersensitive, 24 h after the injection there will be a positive reaction characterized by an area of redness and induration with a diameter greater than 10 mm. Histologically the reaction is characterized by mononuclear cell infiltration, with perivascular cuffing. Macrophages can be seen infiltrating the dermis. If the reaction is severe, a central necrotic may develop. The cellular infiltration, which contrasts with the predominantly edematous reaction in type I hypersensitivity, is responsible for the induration that characterizes cell-mediated hypersensitivity reactions.

It is evident that in most immune responses both the humoral and the cellular arms of the immune system are activated. For example, when guinea pigs are immunized with egg albumin and adjuvant, not only do they become allergic, as discussed earlier, but also they develop cell-mediated hypersensitivity to the antigen. This duality can be demonstrated by passively transferring serum and lymphocytes from a sensitized animal to different unsensitized recipients of the same strain and challenging the passively immunized animals with egg albumin. The animals that received serum will develop an anaphylactic response immediately after challenge, while those that received lymphocytes will show only signals of a considerably less severe reaction after at least 24 h have elapsed from the time of challenge.

A. Contact Hypersensitivity

Very little is known about the pathogenesis of systemically induced delayed hypersensitivity, while extensive data is available concerning the induction of contact hypersensitivity. Experimental sensitization through the skin is relatively easy to induce by percutaneous application of low-molecular-weight substances such as picric acid or dinitrochlorobenzene (DNCB). The initial application leads to sensitization, and a second application will elicit a delayed hypersensitivity reaction in the area where the antigen is applied. Sensitization to those substances, which by themselves should not be antigenic, appears to involve their spontaneous coupling to an endogenous carrier protein, and this coupling will allow the small chemical compound to act as a hapten, while at the same time it will change the antigenicity of the protein that will act as a carrier. The haptenic group has to bind covalently to the carrier protein, and with simple chemicals, Cl, F, Br, and SO_3H groups are the most reactive. In the case of natural sensitization to drugs, chemicals or metals, it is believed that the haptenic substance diffuses into the dermis mostly through the sweat glands (hydrophobic substances appear to penetrate the skin more easily than hydrophilic substances); once in the dermis, the haptenic groups will react spontaneously with carrier proteins and trigger an immune reaction. The initial steps of sensitization appear to involve antigen processing and focusing of processed antigen on the membranes of Ia^+ cells, namely the Langerhans cells of the epidermis. These cells could actually carry out both functions (processing and presentation), because they share other properties with monocytes/macrophages besides the expression of Ia antigens, namely, the ability to secrete large amounts of interleukin 1. As a consequence of antigen-Ia recognition and of the nonspecific stimulatory signal that interleukin 1 represents, the sequence of events leading to clonal expansion of antigen-specific T lymphocytes is triggered. Later, when the sensitized individual is challenged with the same antigen, the recognition of this antigen by sensitized T cells will turn them into functionally active cells, releasing a variety of lymphokines, which are chemotactic for monocyte/macrophages, basophils, eosinophils, and neutrophils. In classical delayed hypersensitivity reactions, the cellular infiltrate is predominantly constituted by mononuclear cells (monocytes, macrophages, and lymphocytes). Those cells are probably kept in the area where the antigen has penetrated by lymphokines such as the migration inhibitory factor (MIF); local proliferation of lymphocytes under the influence of mitogenic factors is also likely to take place.

The tissue damage that takes place in this type of reaction is not likely to be due to the direct effects of cytotoxic T cells but rather to the effects of soluble agents released by the infiltrating cells. Proteases, collagenase, and cathepsins released by phagocytic cells and tumor necrosis factors α and β are likely to play important roles. Tumor necrosis factor α (TNFα, cachectin) is released predominantly by activated macrophages, while the structurally related tumor necrosis factor β (lymphotoxin) is released predominantly by activated T lymphocytes. Together with interleukin 1 (many of whose effects overlap with those of TNF), these factors appear to mediate many facets of inflammatory reactions. For example, TNFβ mediates the cytotoxicity that characterizes severe delayed hypersensitivity reactions, and together with TNFα it causes increased adhesiveness of endothelium for leukocytes, which is an important step leading to the formation of cellular infiltrates. TNFα and β are also known to activate neutrophils and macrophages (in the case of TNFα this represent an autocrine signal), and TNFα, like IL1, is a pyrogenic factor. Since TNFα activates the release of IL1 by endothelial cells and monocytes, it can cause fever both directly, at the hypothalamic level, and through the release of IL1. Prolonged release of TNFα, on the other hand, may have deleterious effects, because this factor contributes to the development of cachexia. The way in which TNFα causes cachexia has been recently elucidated: the factor inhibits lipoprotein lipase, and as a consequence there is an accumulation of triglyceride-rich particles in the serum and a lack of the breakdown of triglycerides into glycerol and free fatty acids. Thus the incorporation of triglycerides into the adipose tissue is inhibited, and this inhibition results in a negative metabolic balance: the cells continue to break down stored tryglycerides by other pathways to generate energy, and the used triglycerides are not replaced. Cachexia is often a preterminal development in patients with severe chronic infections or with disseminated neoplasia.

In some severe cases, a contact hypersensitivity reaction may take an exsudative, edematous, and highly inflammatory character. It seems likely that the release of proteases from monocytes and macrophages may trigger the complement-dependent inflammatory pathways by directly splitting C3 and C5; as noted before, increased vascular permeability is a constant feature of complement-dependent inflammatory processes.

B. Contact Hypersensitivity in Man

Contact hypersensitivity reactions can be observed with some frequency in man because of spontaneous sensitization to a variety of substances. Plant cathecols are apparently responsible for the hypersensitivity reactions in poison ivy and poison oak. A variety of chemicals can be implicated in hypersensitivity reactions to cosmetics and leather. Topically used drugs, particularly sulfonamides, often cause contact hypersensitivity. Metals, such as nickel, can be involved in reactions triggered by the use of bracelets, earrings, or thimbles. The diagnosis is usually based on a careful history of exposure to potential sensitizing agents and on the observation of the distribution of lesions, which can be informative about the source of sensitization. Patch tests using small pieces of filter paper, impregnated with suspected sensitizing agents, taped to the back of the patient can be used to pinpoint the exact nature of the sensitizing substance.

C. The Jones-Mote Reaction

Following challenge with an intradermal injection of a small dose of a protein to which an individual has been previously sensitized, a delayed reaction (with a lag of 24 h) somewhat different from a classical delayed hypersensitivity reaction can be seen. The reaction is more erythematous and less indurated, and the infiltrating cells are mostly lymphocytes and basophils, the last sometimes predominating. The reaction has also been described, for this reason, as *cutaneous basophil hypersensitivity*. Experimentally it has been demonstrated that like classic delayed hypersensitivity this reaction is triggered as a consequence of the antigenic stimulation of sensitized T lymphocytes.

D. Homograft Rejection

A striking clinical manifestation of a delayed hypersensitivity reaction is the rejection of a graft. In a classical chronic rejection, the graft recipient's immune system is first sensitized to tissue antigens of the donor. After clonal expansion, the T lymphocytes will reach the target organ, recognize the foreign antigen, and initiate a sequence of events that leads to inflammation and eventual necrosis of the organ. This topic will be discussed in detail in a later chapter.

E. Transfer of Delayed Hypersensitivity Reactions

Given the role played by T lymphocytes in delayed hypersensitivity reactions, it is not surprising that this type of hypersensitivity can only be transferred by isolating T lymphocytes from a sensitive animal and injecting them into either an immunosuppressed or a genetically identical animal.

In man, however, Sherwood Lawrence observed that delayed hypersensitivity reactions could also be transferred by means of dialysable extracts from the leukocytes of a sensitized individual. This was initially attributed to a putative "transfer factor." The classical experiments showed that if a leukocyte extract from a tuberculin-positive individual was injected into a tuberculin-negative volunteer, as early as 6 h after the injection the receipient would become tuberculin positive.

The lack of precise knowledge about the chemical nature of transfer factor, and the lack of standardized quantitative assays for transfer-factor activity in leukocyte extracts, have greatly hampered progress in the therapeutic use of leukocyte extracts, although there is considerable evidence suggesting that the administration of transfer factor can have beneficial effects in a wide variety of conditions, including chronic infections with agents usually eliminated by cell-mediated immune mechanisms, deficiencies of the T-lymphocyte system, and some neoplasias, particularly osteosarcoma.

Currently it is accepted that the dialysable leukocyte extracts (DLE) contain a variety of factors, some that transfer specific sensitivities, others that are apparently nonspecific. The term transfer factor is reserved for an antigen-specific factor that can be partially purified and whose chemical structure is still being investigated.

SELF-EVALUATION

Questions

Choose the one best answer.

18.1 Cutaneous hypersensitivity to nickel
   A. Is mediated by IgE antibodies.
   B. Results from the sensitization against a nickel-protein complex.
   C. Is characterized by marked basophilic infiltration.
   D. Can be effectively treated with antihistamines.
   E. Can be diagnosed by a PK reaction.

18.2 A delayed hypersensitivity reaction is not likely to be elicited in a skin test using
   A. Tuberculin.
   B. Tetanus toxoid.
   C. Mumps antigen.
   D. Diphtheria toxoid.
   E. Ragweed pollen.

18.3 The Arthus reaction is primarily associated with
   A. IgM antibodies.
   B. Mononuclear cell infiltrates.
   C. Complement activation by the classical pathway.
   D. Histamine release.
   E. IgE antibodies.

18.4 The skin biopsy of a patient having a delayed hypersensitivity reaction is characteristic because of
   A. Deposit of immunoglobulins and complement in the arterial wall.
   B. Neutrophil infiltrates around the arteries.
   C. Necrosis of the epidermis.

D. Mononuclear cell infiltrates surrounding small vessels.

E. Edema.

18.5 The immediate hypersensitivity reaction (type I)

A. Requires the synthesis of IgG antibodies.

B. Is characterized by the release of tumor necrosis factors α and β.

C. Takes about 24 h to become clinically evident.

D. Is exclusively observed in man.

E. Can persist for several hours because of the synthesis and release of leukotrienes C4, D4, and E4.

18.6 In type II (cytotoxic) hypersensitivity reactions,

A. Cytotoxic antibodies are directly responsible for cell lysis.

B. Complement activation is involved in at least two possible pathways leading to cell or tissue damage.

C. Cytotoxic T lymphocytes are involved in the later stages of the reaction.

D. Release of histamine plays an important role in the early stages.

E. K Cells are the main cells responsible for cell lysis.

18.7 The cells that appear to play the most significant role in the induction of tissue damage in human IC complex disease are

A. Erythrocytes.

B. PMN leukocytes.

C. Monocytes.

D. Platelets.

E. Lymphocytes.

The group of questions below consists of a set of lettered headings followed by a list of numbered words or phrases. For each numbered word or phrase select the one lettered heading that is most closely related to it. The same heading can be used once, more than once, or not at all: (A) Anaphylaxis; (B) Cytotoxic hypersensitivity; (C) Immune complex hypersensitivity; (D) Delayed hypersensitivity.

18.8 Shock following a penicillin injection.

18.9 Malaria-associated glomerulonephritis.

18.10 Chronic "drug" dermatitis in the upper eyelids of a 24-year-old woman.

Answers

18.1 (B)   The substances involved in contact dermatitis are often small molecules that apparently act as haptens after spontaneously reacting with an endogenous protein that will serve as a carrier.

18.2 (E)   Pollens are usually involved in type I hypersensitivity, and the skin tests with pollens elicit typical immediate hypersensitivity reactions.

18.3 (C)   The Arthus reaction involves primarily complement-fixing antibodies. The cellular infiltrate is mainly composed of PMN leukocytes.

18.4 (D)   In contrast to type II hypersensitivity, the cellular infiltrates in delayed hypersensitivity show usually a predominance of mononuclear cells.

18.5 (E)   The initial phase of the immediate hypersensitivity reaction is due to mast cell and basophil degranulation with release of stored histamine. In later stages, the reaction is sustained by the secretion of SRS-A, a mixture of leukotrienes C4, D4, and E4, which are synthesized after the cells have been stimulated by an allergen.

18.6 (B)   Complement activation is the key element and will lead either to direct cytolysis or to phagocytosis.

18.7 (B)

18.8 (A)

18.9 (C)   Many chronic infections can be associated with glomerulonephritis secondary to the deposition of immune complexes involving microbial antigens and the corresponding antibodies.

18.10 (D) Sensitization to cosmetics such as eye shadow is not uncommon, and it involves a type IV reaction, usually induced by formalin, which is added as a preservative.

BIBLIOGRAPHY

Altman, L. C. Basic immune mechansims in immediate hypersensitivity. *Med. Clin. N. Am. 65*:941, 1981.

Hokama, Y. and Nakamura, R. M. (Eds.). *Immunology and Immunopathology.* Little, Brown, Boston, 1982.

Lachmann, P. J. and Peters, D. K. (Eds.). *Clinical Aspects of Immunology*, 4th Ed. Blackwell Scientific, Oxford/Boston, 1982.

Lawrence, H. S. Transfer factor in cellular immunity. *Harvey Lect. 68*:239, 1974.

Old, L. J. Tumor necrosis factor. *Sci. Am.*, May 1988, p. 59.

Rudle, N. H. and Homer, R. The role of lymphotoxin in inflammation. *Progress in Allergy 40*:162, 1988.

Sell, S. *Immunology Immunopathology and Immunity*, 4th Ed. Elsevier, New York, 1987.

19

Immediate Hypersensitivity

JEAN-MICHEL GOUST

The main characteristic of immediate hypersensitivty reactions is the short time lag (seconds to minutes) between antigen exposure and the onset of clinical symptoms. This is because the initial symptoms of immediate hypersensitivity depend on the release of preformed mediators stored in cytoplasmic granules of basophils and mast cells; the release is triggered by the reaction of membrane-bound IgE with the corresponding antigen (also known as *allergen*, by being involved in allergic reactions).

Immediate hypersensitivity or allergic reactions can have a variety of clinical expressions, including systemic anaphylaxis, bronchial asthma, urticaria (hives), and vasomotor rhinitis (hay fever). Table 19.1 summarizes the morbidity and mortality data for the two most severe types of allergic reactions, systemic anaphylaxis and bronchial asthma.

I. THE MAJOR CLINICAL EXPRESSIONS OF TYPE I HYPERSENSITIVITY

A. Systemic Anaphylaxis

Systemic anaphylaxis is an acute IgE-mediated reaction usually affecting multiple organs. The time of onset of symptoms depends on the level of hypersensitivity and the amount, diffusibility, and site of exposure to the antigen. In a typical case, manifestations begin within 5 to 10 min after antigenic challenge. Reactions that appear more slowly tend to be less severe. Intervals longer than

357

TABLE 19.1 Morbidity and Mortality From Systemic Anaphylaxis and Bronchial Asthma in the United States

	Morbidity	Mortality
Systemic anaphylaxis		
Caused by antibiotics	10-40:100,000 injections	1:100,000 injections
Caused by insect bites	10:100,000 persons/yr	10-80/yr
Asthma	10 million persons (4-5% of U.S. population)	5-30 years of age: 0.5/100,000/yr >60 years of age: 10:100,000/yr

TABLE 19.2 Major Characteristics of Allergic and Nonallergic Bronchial Asthma

Symptoms	Dyspnea with prolonged expiratory phase; may be associated with courgh and sputum.	
Chest x-rays	Hyperlucency (reflecting impaired expiratory capacity), bronchial thickening	
	Allergic	*Nonallergic*
Blood	Eosinophilia	Normal eosinophil count
Sputum	Eosinophilia	No eosinophils
ESR	Normal	Raised (PAN)
Total IgE	Raised	Normal
Antigen-specific IgE	Raised	None
Pathology	Obstruction of airways due to smooth muscle constriction and mucosal edema Hypertrophy of mucous glands Eosinophil infiltration	
Frequency		
Children	80%[a]	20%
Adults	60%[a]	40%

[a]% of total number of bronchial asthma cases seen in each age range.

2 h leave the diagnosis of anaphylaxis open to question. Multiple organ systems are usually affected, including the skin (pruritus, urticaria, angioedema), respiratory tract (bronchospasm and laryngeal edema), and cardiovascular system (hypotension and cardiac arrhythmias). As a rule, most of the manifestations subside within 1 or 2 h. When death occurs, it is usually due to laryngeal edema, shock, or cardiac arrhythmias within the first 1 or 2 h.

B. Atopy

Atopy is defined a as a genetically determined state of hypersensitivity. Its most common clinical manifestations include asthma, hay fever, rhinitis, nasal polyposis, and atopic dermatitis. Of those, allergic bronchial asthma, by its potential severity and frequency, is the most important. Not all cases of asthma are of proven allergic etiology. The differential characteristics of allergic (extrinsic) and nonallergic (intrinsic) bronchial asthma are summarized in Table 19.2.

II. PATHOGENESIS OF IMMEDIATE HYPERSENSITIVITY

Immediate hypersensitivity reactions involve three main components, (1) the immune system, which produces reagins (IgE antibodies in man); (2) cells (basophils and mast cells) to which the reagins bind and which when reexposed to the antigen synthesize and release mediators; (3) smooth muscle, vascular endothelium, and mucous glands, which are the main targets for the mediators released by basophils and mast cells.

A. Immunoglobulin E Antibodies (Reagins)

The first demonstration that serum contains a factor capable of mediating specific allergic reactions was published in 1921 by Prausnitz and Kustner. The injection of serum from a fish-allergic person (Kustner) into Prausnitz's skin, and the subsequent exposure of Prausnitz to fish antigen injected in the same site, resulted in an allergic wheal and flare response. It was not until 1967 that the IgE class of immunoglobulin responsible for this reaction was isolated from the serum of ragweed-allergic individuals. But even in those individuals it was present at concentrations of several orders of magnitude lower than that of all the other classes of immunoglobulins, making it necessary to detect its presence by cumbersome and often unreliable bioassays. Several IgE myelomas were subsequently discovered, and this source of very large amounts of monoclonal IgE greatly facilitated further studies of IgE structure and the production of anti-IgE antibodies. The availability of anti-IgE antibodies, in turn, allowed the development of radioimmunoassays sufficiently sensitive to quantitate serum IgE levels accurately (Fig. 19.1).

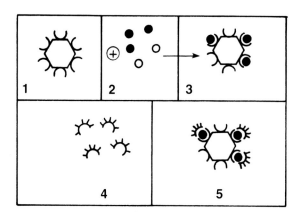

1. Anti-IgE coupled to paper disc
2. Serum IgE
3. Binding of Serum IgE to paper disc
4. Radiolabeled anti-IgE
5. Binding of the Radiolabel to disc-bound IgE

FIGURE 19.1   Diagrammatic representation of the general principles of the radioimmunosorbent test for IgE quantitation (PRIST = paper disc radio immunosorbent test).

An example of one of the available assays for serum IgE is the paper disc radioimmunosorbent test (PRIST), in which anti-IgE antibodies are covalently bound to small pieces of filter paper. The IgE present in the serum will attach to the solid-phase bound anti-IgE. ^{125}I-labeled anti-IgE antibodies are subsequently added and will bind to the paper-bound IgE. The radioactivity counted in the solid phase is directly related to the IgE level in the serum tested. The results are expressed in nanograms/ml (1 ng = 10^{-6} mg) or in International Units (1 IU = 2.5 ng/ml); 190 ng/ml is considered the upper limit for normal individuals. Allergic individuals often have elevated levels of IgE, but a significant number of asymptomatic individuals may also have elevated IgE levels (see Fig. 19.2). Therefore, a diagnosis of immediate hypersensitivity cannot be based on the determination of abnormally elevated IgE levels. From the diagnostic point of view the quantitation of antigen-specific IgE is considerably more relevant. The test used for this purpose is the radioallergosorbent test (RAST) (Fig. 19.3). In the RAST test the allergen itself (ragweed antigen, penicillin, β-lactoglobulin, etc.) is covalently bound to polydextran beads; serum is added, and the antigen-specific IgE, if present, will bind to the antigen on the bead. After washing off unbound immunoglobulins, radiolabeled anti-IgE is added. The amount of bead-bound radioactivity counted after

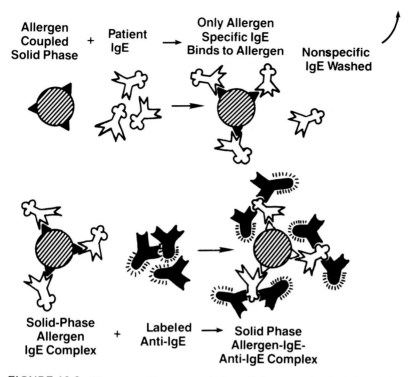

FIGURE 19.2 Diagrammatic representation of the general principles of the radioallergosorbent test (RAST) for quantitation of specific IgE antibodies.

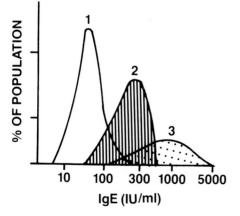

FIGURE 19.3 Distribution of IgE levels in a population of nonallergic individuals. Three subpopulations appear to exist: one constituted by low-responder individuals (1), one by high responder individuals (3), and a third population of individuals with intermediate levels of IgE (2).

washing off unbound labeled antibody is directly related to the concentration of antigen-specific IgE present in the serum. Although this assay is highly sensitive and accurate, it is expensive, and the range of antigens for which there are available tests is limited. Therefore, skin testing is preferred by many specialists for the diagnosis of IHS because it allows testing for a wider array of antigens and because the results obtained with the skin test appear to correlate better with clinical data. However, in highly sensitized individuals, there is always a risk of anaphylactic shock even after minimal challenge. Because of this risk, these tests should always be performed in a properly equipped clinical facility.

B.   The Immunoglobulin E Antibody Response

Parasitic infections stimulate very marked increases of IgE in virtually all mammals, including humans. IgE antibodies have a major role in the protection against parasites (particularly nematodes). Levels of circulating IgE considered normal in a developing country with endemic parasitism are two to three orders of magnitude higher than in the western world; in contrast, allergic disorders as we know them are practically unknown in developing countries.

IgE is predominantly synthesized in lymphoid tissues of the respiratory and gastrointestinal tract, through which the vast majority of allergens enters the body. Only the small minority of B lymphocytes with ϵ chains on their surfaces will become IgE-producing plasma cells.

1.   Genes Influencing IgE Production

The study of total IgE levels in normal nonallergic individuals (Fig. 19.2) shows a distribution into three groups: high, intermediate, and low producers. Family studies further suggest that the ability to produce high levels of IgE is a recessive trait, controlled by unknown genes independent of the HLA system. On the other hand, the tendency to develop allergic disorders in response to specific allergens is HLA-linked. For instance, the ability to produce antigen-specific IgE after exposure to the Ra5 antigen of ragweed is observed more often in HLA B7 DR2 individuals than in the general population. If the same HLA B7 individual is also genetically a high IgE producer, he will have a more severe allergic disorder than a low responder.

2.   T-B Cooperation in Antigen-Specific IgE Production

The influence of the MHC genes on the response to some allergens is probably because the IgE response is T-dependent. Using rats infected with helminths as experimental models (rats, like humans, exhibit a marked and persistent primary and secondary IgE response), it was found that the height and duration of the IgE-producing immune response are explained by a predominance of helper T cells over relatively low numbers of suppressor T cells. It has also been found that IL4 plays an important role in the final differentiation of IgE-producing B cells and could be overproduced in allergic individuals. Therefore, it is obvious that the genetic factors that control T cell activity are likely to have an effect on T cell responses.

A general rule also observed both in humans and in rats is that during the primary immune response to an allergen or a parasite most of the IgE synthesized appears to be non-antigen-specific (or, alternatively, is antibody of such a low affinity for the allergen that it cannot be detected by the RAST assay). This is probably the reason why allergic reactions very seldom develop after the first exposure to an allergen. This has clinical relevance for the evaluation of abnormal responses to a putative allergen. If the symptoms developed unquestionably after a first exposure, IgE is less likely to be responsible for the reaction. Allergen-specific IgE antibodies develop mostly after a second exposure (Fig. 19.4). Repeated exposures that further stimulate memory cells will increase the proportion of antigen-specific IgE, which in patients suffering from severe pollen allergies may constitute up to 50% of the total IgE.

As with helminth-infected rats, the production of allergen-specific IgE in humans persists long after the second exposure. This may result from a persistent

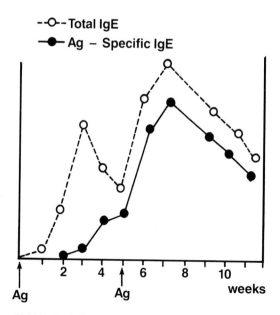

FIGURE 19.4 Longitudinal evolution of total IgE and antigen-specific IgE levels during an immune response to an allergen.

predominance of helper over suppressor T cells in allergic individuals. This seems to be due to a deficiency in IgE suppressor T cells, because when purified T cells from normal individuals are added to lymphocyte cultures from allergic individuals, a suppression of IgE production is observed. However, if we add T cells isolated from allergic individuals to cultures of lymphocytes from other allergic patients, no suppression of in vitro IgE synthesis is observed. Another argument for the importance of T-cell control over IgE synthesis is the observation that high IgE levels are found in conditions associated with depressed cell-mediated immunity such as the Wiskott-Aldrich and DiGeorge syndromes.

C. Interaction of Immunoglobulin E with Cell Surface Receptors

Basophils and mast cells contain characteristic metachromatic cytoplasmic granules, which contain preformed mediators such as histamine. They are also the only human cells that possess membrane receptors that specifically bind the Fc fragment of IgE with extremely high affinity. The Fc_ϵ receptor is closely associated with adenylate cyclase in the plasma membrane. The interaction between the receptor and IgE is consistent with a simple bimolecular forward reaction and a first-order reverse reaction:

$$\text{IgE} + \text{receptor} \underset{k^{-1}}{\overset{k^1}{\rightleftharpoons}} \text{IgE-receptor complex}$$

The affinity constant of the interaction, $KA = k^1/k^{-1}$, ranges from 10^8 to 10^{10} M/liter^{-1}. These very high affinity values are comparable to those of interactions between polypeptide hormones and their receptors, and they help to understand the persistence of sensitivity for up to several weeks after passive transfer of IgE antibodies into the skin of normal humans. IgE binds rapidly and very strongly to mast cells receptors, and it is released from the cells very slowly. However, conversely to what happens with polypeptide hormones, the cell behavior is not modified by IgE attachment. As long as the cell-bound IgE molecules are left alone, the mast cells and basophils carrying them are not activated. Receptor-bound IgE must be cross-linked in order for basophils and mast cells to release their intracellular mediators (Fig. 19.5). The physiological cross-linking agent is the allergen. In the laboratory, multivalent antigens or carrier-bound haptens can be used to activate basophils carrying the appropriate IgE antibodies. Univalent haptens, blocking each Fab fragment without cross-linking two molecules of IgE, do not cause degranulation and inhibit further reaction. Anti-IgE, its divalent $F(ab')_2$ fragment, and aggregated Fc_ϵ fragments are equally efficient in inducing the release of mediators. Biologically, IgE serves as an antigen receptor for mast cells and basophils. The receptor discriminates among antigens, binding exclusively those to which the patient has become sensitized. The IgE molecules are not produced by the mast

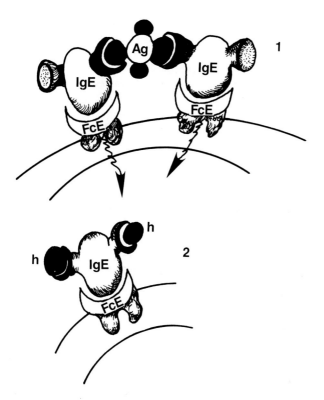

FIGURE 19.5 Diagrammatic depiction of the conditions required for stimulation of mediator release by mast cells and basophils. In panel 1 the reaction of membrane-bound IgE with a polyvalent antigen, leading to cross-linking of IgE molecules, is represented. This type of reaction leads to mediator release. In panel 2 the reaction of membrane-bound IgE with a monovalent hapten is illustrated. This reaction does not lead to mediator release.

cells and basophils, so there is no clonal restriction at the cell level. In other words, if the patient produces IgE antibodies to more than one allergen, IgE antibodies of different specificities may be bound by each basophil or mast cell.

Cross-linking of IgE is not the only signal leading to the liberation of mediators from basophils and mast cells; these cells also respond to C3a, C5a, basic lysosomal proteins, a histamine-releasing lymphokine, and kinins. It is apparent that there are multiple pathways for mast cell activation and that the participation of cell-bound IgE is not always needed.

D. Intracellular Events Triggered by the Reaction of an Antigen with Membrane Immunoglobulin E

The stimulation of mast cells and basophils does not lead to cell death. The cells release their preformed mediators but maintain their viability after the reaction has taken place. Thus the cells remain able to synthesize other substances, and this is the basis for the existence of two phases in most IHS reactions. Clinical observations were first to suggest that the allergic reactions had two phases: the early phase lasting from a few minutes to 6 hours and a later phase that starts shortly afterward but may persist up to 24 hours. In the case of asthma the early phase is characterized by shortness of breath and nonproductive cough. Around the sixth hour, the cough starts to produce sputum, signaling the onset of the late phase, during which the dyspnea may become more severe. In very severe cases, death may occur because of persistent peribronchial inflammation leading to severe airflow obstruction from mucous plugging. In the case of skin testing, the early phase resolves in 30 to 60 minutes, and the late phase generally peaks at 6 to 8 hours and is resolved at 24 hours. This clinical observation was substantiated by the finding that different mediators are responsible for the symptoms of each phase.

E. Early and Late Phases in Type I Hypersensitivity

1. Early Phase

Cross-linking of antigen-specific cell-bound IgE by the allergen triggers a very rapid sequence of events. The first change to be detected is the polymerization of microtubules, which is energy-dependent (inhibited by 2-deoxyglucose); it is enhanced by the addition of 3-5 GMP and inhibited by the addition of 3-5 AMP and colchicine. This polymerization of microtubules allows the transport of the intracytoplasmic granules to the cell membrane, to which they fuse. The fusion is followed by the release of histamine and other preformed mediators, such as chemotactic factors for eosinophils and neutrophils, into the surrounding medium. In vitro, this sequence of events takes 30 to 60 seconds. Histamine is the mediator responsible for most of the symptoms observed during the early phase of allergic reactions.

2. Late Phase

The mediators responsible for the late phase of the response are not detected until several hours after the release of histamine and other preformed mediators. Investigators had first identified, in the supernatants of IgE-coated mast cells challenged with the proper allergen, a substance they named the *slow reacting substance of anaphylaxis (SRS-A)*. It differs from histamine not only because it accumulates more slowly (reaching effective concentrations only 5

TABLE 19.3 Mediators of Immediate Hypersensitivity Produced by Mast Cells and Basophils

Mediators	Structure	Actions
Preformed		
Histamine	5-β-imidazolylethylamine (MW 111)	Smooth-muscle contraction; increased vascular permeability; many others.
Eosinophil chemotactic factors of anaphylaxis (ECF-A)	Acidic tetrapeptides (MW 360-390); others (MW 500-3000)	Chemotactic for eosinophils
Proteolytic enzymes	Trypsin and other enzymes in human mast cells; chymotrypsin in rat mast cells	Actions in vivo unknown, possible include C' activation
Heparin	Acidic proteoglycan (mw ≈ 750,000)	Anticoagulant C' inhibitor
Neutrophil chemotactic factor	Poorly characterized activity with MW > 750,000	Chemotactic for neutrophils
Other granuloproteins	Numerous poorly characterized peptides	In vivo significance not yet known
Newly formed (upon stimulation of mast cells or basophils)		
Slow-reacting substance of anaphylaxis (SRS-A)	Leukotrienes C4,D4,E4 (derived from arachidonic acid, MW 439-625)	Smooth-muscle contraction; increased vascular permeability
Prostaglandin D2	Cyclooxygenase product of arachidonic acid	Smooth-muscle contraction
Platelet activating factor (PAF)	Phospholipid (MW 300-500)	Platelet aggregation and release reaction
Leukotriene B4	Eicosotetraenoate product of arachidonic acid (MW 336)	Increased vascular permeability; chemotactic for eosinophils and neutrophils; neutrophil aggregation

6 hours after challenge) but also because in contrast with histamine, whose effects wane in a few minutes, the effects of SRS-A on the target cells last for several hours. The long latency period between cell stimulation and detection of SRS-A suggested that this substance was synthesized by mast cells after stimulation. It is now known that SRS-A is constituted by a mixture of three leukotrienes (LT) designated as LTC4, LTD4, and LTE4 and that the initial triggering of the cell stimulates the metabolic pathway leading to their synthesis. LTC4 and LTD4 are several times more potent than histamine in causing constriction of the peripheral airways, and they also induce mucous secretion in human bronchi. Another important mediator of late phase reaction is platelet activating factor (PAF), a phospholipid released by a variety of cells, whose effects range from inducing platelet aggregation and release of vasoactive amines to increased vascular permeability. The most important mediators of type I hypersensitivity are listed in Table 19.3. The extent of the clinical symptoms is directly related to the amount of mediators released and produced, which in turn is determined by the number of sensitized cells stimulated by the antigen. Both phases of the acute allergic response have built-in controls in normal individuals that terminate the acute event in a few hours. The control of IHS reactions is basically dependent on chemotactic factors for eosinophils, ECF-A, and leukotriene B4, and this explains the appearance of large numbers of eosinophils in the asthmatic's sputum at the late "humid" phase of the attack. The function of these cells appears to be the production and release of enzymes, such as histaminase, which degrade histamine, and phospholipase D, which degrades platelet activating factor. Oxygen products released by stimulated granulocytes, including eosinophils and perhaps neutrophils (which are also attracted by ECF-A and LTB4), cause the breakdown of SRS-A. Histamine itself can contribute to the downregulation of the reaction, by binding to a type II histamine receptor expressed on basophils and mast cells; the occupancy of this receptor leads to an intracellular increase in the level of cAMP, which inhibits further release of histamine (negative feedback).

III. THERAPY OF IMMEDIATE HYPERSENSITIVITY REACTIONS

Every event leading to the release of mediators and the corresponding steps in the activation sequence of target cells and tissues may be modified by one type of treatment or another. Environmental control, trying to prevent exposure to the allergen, is possible in monoallergies; however, it cannot be easily achieved by individuals with multiple allergies. Hyposensitization is one of the most popular approaches, also useful mostly in monoallergies. This therapy consists of injecting very small quantities of the sensitizing antigen, starting at the nanogram level, and increasing the dosage on a weekly basis. This induces (1) the production of IgG blocking antibodies and (2) an increase in the number of

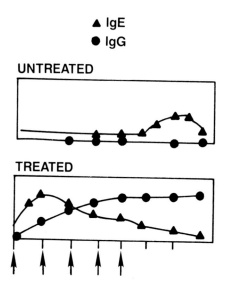

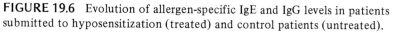

FIGURE 19.6   Evolution of allergen-specific IgE and IgG levels in patients submitted to hyposensitization (treated) and control patients (untreated).

antigen-specific suppressor cells, with a concomitant decline of serum IgE levels. Because both effects tend to be simultaneous, both appear to be correlated with a decrease of the allergic symptoms (Fig. 19.6). The circulating blocking antibodies of the IgG class have a protective effect, because they combine with the antigen before it reaches the cell-bound IgE. These blocking antibodies do not interfere with a RAST assay for IgE antibodies. A significant clinical improvement correlates better with an increase in blocking IgG than with a decrease in antigen-specific IgE. The beneficial effect of the competition between IgG and IgE antibodies is easy to understand in cases of insect venom anaphylaxis in which the allergen is injected directly in the circulation where it can be blocked by circulating IgG; however, it is more difficult to understand the protective mechanism involved in respiratory allergies, when the allergen has almost direct access to the sensitized cells without entering the systemic circulation. Hyposensitization is not always effective, but it has been claimed that it can be beneficial to up to 70% of patients with allergy to pollens.

A. Drug Therapy

Various drugs are used to treat or prevent immediate hypersensitivity reactions. Some inhibit or decrease mediator release by mast cells or basophils; others block the effect of mediators. The complex interactions of different drugs able

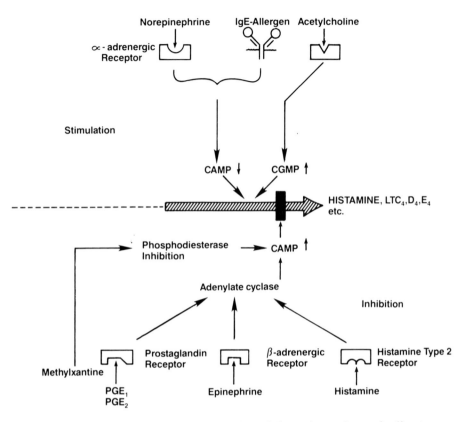

FIGURE 19.7 Diagrammatic representation of the major pathways leading to stimulation and inhibition of mediator release by basophils and mast cells. (Modifed from David, J. and Rocklin, R. E. Immediate hypersensitivity. In *Scientific American Medicine*, Sect. 6, Chap. 9, E. Rubinstein and D. D. Federman, (Eds.). Scientific American, Inc., New York, 1983.)

to influence mediator release are summarized in Figure 19.7. Among the antiallergic drugs able to inhibit mediator release the most important are the following.

1. Methylxanthines

Methylxanthines (e.g., theophylline) block phosphodiesterases, thus leading to a persistently high intracellular level of cAMP, which in turn inhibits histamine release.

2. β-Adrenergic Receptor Stimulators

β-Adrenergic receptor stimulators (epinephrine, isoproterenol, salbutamol) increase cAMP levels by stimulating membrane adenylcyclase directly. Their effect is rapid and of short duration. Epinephrine is the drug of choice for the treatment of severe allergic reactions such as systemic anaphylaxis or severe asthma. However, it can be abused by patients who expect fast relief, because the β-adrenergic receptors lose their sensitivity to a point where the symptoms become unresponsive unless the patients increase the dosage until the cardiac effects of the drug become dominant. Cholinergic agents have the opposite effects; hence their use must be avoided in asthmatic patients because they can aggravate the symptoms.

3. Disodium Cromoglycate

Disodium cromoglycate (cromolyn), not shown in the figure, is a very efficient prophylactic drug; its mechanism of action is related to a stabilization of the membrane of the mediator-containing granules.

The drugs competing at the target cell level are mostly *antihistaminics*, which compete with histamine in binding to the histamine type I receptor. They are widely consumed, but they are effective only if given prophylactically or very early after the beginning of symptoms. They are also more effective in the treatment of urticaria and vasomotor rhinitis than in the treatment of bronchial asthma, and they are totally ineffective in cases of systemic anaphylaxis.

Corticosteroids can be efficient both in acute situations, given intravenously, or as prophylactics in chronic situations, because they can prevent the development of the severe late phase reactions (in this modality, steroids are usually administered orally). Steroids are also indicated in patients in whom β-adrenergic stimulation is inefficient, as discussed above. Prolonged steroid therapy can lead to a variety of side effects, and there is always a risk of severe rebound when they are discontinued, if the allergen is still in the environment. The effects of corticosteroids in immediate hypersensitivity are probably anti-inflammatory, although when given for prolonged periods of time their weak immunosuppressive action may also be significant, by reducing the magnitude of the IgE response.

SELF-EVALUATION

Questions

Choose the one best answer.

19.1 The site of IgE molecules that bind with very high affinity to mast cell membrane receptors is located in the

A. Fab fragment.
B. CH_2 domain.
C. Variable H-chain region.
D. Hypervariable H-chain region.
E. Fc fragment.

19.2 At the mast cell level, theophylline is likely to induce
A. Activation of phosphodiesterases.
B. β-adrenergic stimulation.
C. Membrane stabilization.
D. Stimulation of adenylate cyclase.
E. Increased intracellular levels of cAMP.

19.3 During successful hyposensitization, IgE
A. Increases in serum.
B. Decreases in serum.
C. Is not significantly affected.
D. Is replaced by IgG at the cell membrane level.
E. Combines with the injected allergen and forms circulating immune complexes.

19.4 In a patient with suspected anaphylaxis, you should consider the immediate administration of
A. Epinephrine.
B. Sodium cromoglycate.
C. Methylxanthines.
D. Antihistaminics.
E. Cholinergic drugs.

19.5 Coupled to the solid phase in a RAST assay is
A. IgE.
B. Anti-IgE.
C. Antibodies to a given allergen.
D. A given allergen.
E. The patient's serum.

19.6 A patient with hay fever has a serum IgE level of 2000 ng/ml and a positive RAST test for ragweed. The antigen this patient would likely be positive for in his HLA phenotype is
A. HLA-B27.
B. HLA-B8.
C. HLA-B7.
D. HLA-DW3.
E. HLA-DW4.

19.7   The release of histamine from the mast cells of a ragweed-sensitized indi-
       vidual may be induced by
       A. Fab from an anti-IgE antibody.
       B. F(ab')$_2$ from an anti-IgE antibody.
       C. IgG antiragweed.
       D. A univalent fragment of ragweed.
       E. IgE antiragweed.

19.8   Eosinophils can be attracted to the area in which an immediate hyper-
       sensitivity reaction is taking place by
       A. ECF-A.
       B. LT B4.
       C. Both A and B.
       D. Neither A nor B.

19.9   Not involved in negative-feedback reactions in immediate hypersensitivity
       is
       A. Histamine.
       B. Phospholipase D.
       C. Histaminase.
       D. Prostaglandin D2.
       E. Leukotriene B4.

19.10 The isolated finding of a serum IgE level of 1000 ng/ml means that
       A. The individual is allergic.
       B. Atopy is likely to be the cause of the patient's symptoms.
       C. HLA-B7 is likely to be represented on the individual's phenotype.
       D. The individual is a high IgE producer.
       E. Hyposensitization is not likely to be effective.

Answers

19.1 (E)

19.2 (E) Methylxanthines, such as theophylline, inhibit the action of phospho-
      diesterase, and as a result the intracellular levels of cAMP increase.

19.3 (B) Hyposensitization appears to induce and increase the activity of
      antigen-specific suppressor cells that will lead to a decrease in serum
      IgE levels.

19.4 (A) Epinephrine, given intravenously, is the drug of choice for treatment
      of systemic anaphylaxis.

19.5 (D) The allergen is coupled to the solid phase; if IgE antibodies are present
      in the patient's serum, they will become bound to the antigen in the

solid phase, and their presence can be revealed with a radiolabeled anti-IgE antibody.

19.6 (C) HLA-B7 is frequently associated with a high response to the Ra5 antigen of ragweed.

19.7 (B) The release of histamine requires the cross-linking of membrane IgE, which can be induced by complete anti-IgE antibodies, bivalent $F(ab')_2$ fragments of anti-IgE antibodies. or multivalent antigen of the right specificity.

19.8 (C)

19.9 (D) Histamine, by reacting with type II histamine receptors in basophils and mast cells, will inhibit further histamine release; phospholipase D degrades PAF; histaminase degrades histamine; LT B4 is chemotactic for eosinophils, which release phospholipase D, histaminase, and other protective factors.

19.10 (D) Many nonallergic individuals may have IgE values above the upper limit of normalcy.

BIBLIOGRAPHY

Austen, K. F. Tissue mast cells in immediate hypersensitivity. In *The Biology of Immunologic Disease*, F. J. Dixon and D. W. Fisher (Eds.). Sinauer, Sunderland, Massachusetts, 1983, p. 223.

Bracquet, P., Touqui, L., Shen, T. Y., and Vargaftig, B. B. Perspectives in platelet-activating factor research. *Pharmacological Revs. 39*:97, 1987.

Godfrey, R. C. Respiratory disorders including atopy. In *Immunology in Medicine*, 2nd Ed., E. J. Holborow and W. G. Reeves (Eds.). Grune & Stratton, New York, 1983, p. 393.

Goetzl, E. J., Payan, D. G., and Goldman, D. W. Immunopathogenetic role of leukotrienes in human diseases. *J. Clin. Immunol. 4*:79, 1984.

Holgate, S. T. Mast cells and their mediators. In *Immunology in Medicine*, 2nd Ed., E. J. Holborow and W. G. Reeves (Eds.). Grune & Stratton, New York, 1983, p. 80.

Kay, A. B. Mediators and inflammatory cells in allergic disease. *Ann. Allergy 59*:35, 1987.

Lockey, R. F., and Bukantz, S. D. (Eds.). Primer on allergic and immunologic diseases, 2nd Ed. *J. Amer. Med. Assoc. 258*:2829, 1987. (Includes several chapers on hypersensitivity diseases.)

20

Immunohematology

GABRIEL VIRELLA and MARY ANN SPIVEY

I. INTRODUCTION: BLOOD GROUPS

A. The ABO System

The first human red-cell antigen system to be characterized was the ABO group system, which was discovered in 1900 by Karl Landsteiner when he studied the effects of mixing red cells and sera from different donors. This is, basically, a very simple system in which one, both, or neither of two immunogenic substances (A and B) are expressed in the cells, and antibodies are found in serum to the substance (or substances) not expressed, as shown in Table 20.1. A third substance (H), a nonimmunogenic precursor of the A and B antigens, is present in large quantities on the cells not carrying either A or B, but the typing of cells as group O is usually done by exclusion (a cell not reacting with anti-A or anti-B is considered to be of blood group O).

The anti-A and anti-B isoagglutinins, classical examples of natural antibodies, are synthesized as a consequence of cross-immunization with enterobacteriaceae, which have outer membrane oligosaccharides strikingly similar to those that define the A and B antigens. As an example, a group A newborn will not have IgM isoagglutinins in his serum, because he has had no opportunity to undergo cross-immunization. When his intestine is eventually colonized by the normal microbial flora, the infant will start to develop anti-B antibodies but will not produce anti-A antibodies because of his tolerance to his own blood group antigens (see Table 20.1).

375

TABLE 20.1 The ABO System

Red cell antigen	Serum isoagglutinins	Blood group
A	Anti-B	A
B	Anti-A	B
A and B	None	AB
None	Anti-A and anti-B	O

The inheritance of the ABO groups follows simple Mendelian rules, and for practical purposes we can consider only three allelic genes, A, B, and O (A can be subdivided into A_1 and A_2), of which any individual will carry two, one inherited from the mother and one from the father.

The ABO group of a given individual is determined by testing both cells and serum. The subject's red cells are mixed with serum containing known antibody (forward grouping), and his serum is tested against cells possessing known antigen (reverse grouping). For example, the cells of a group-A individual are agglutinated by anti-A serum but not by anti-B serum, and his serum agglutinates type B cells but not type A cells.

B. The Rh System

In 1939, Philip Levine discovered that the sera of most women who gave birth to infants with hemolytic disease contained a low-molecular-weight antibody that reacted with the red cells of the infant and with the red cells of 85% of Caucasians. In 1940, Landsteiner and Wiener injected blood from the monkey *Maccacus rhesus* into rabbits and guinea pigs and discovered that the resulting antibody agglutinated both rhesus monkeys' red cells and the red cells of about 85% of normal human donors. At that time, it was believed that the antigens responsible for hemolytic disease of the newborn were identical to those present on rhesus monkeys' red cells. The donors whose cells were agglutinated by the antibody to rhesus red cells were termed Rh positive, and those whose cells were not agglutinated were termed Rh negative. Later, Wiener and Peters found anti-Rh antibodies in the sera of individuals that had transfusion reactions following ABO group compatible transfusions. It is now known that the antibody obtained by Landsteiner and Wiener reacts with an antigen (LW) different from (but closely related to) the one that is recognized in human hemolytic disease. For historical reasons, however, the antigenic system responsible for hemolytic disease is still designated Rh.

With further investigation it became clear that the Rh system is antigenically heterogeneous. Fisher and Race proposed a theory and a nomenclature that are widely used and easy to understand. According to these authors, the Rh gene complex could be considered the result of the combination of three pairs of allelic genes: *Cc, Dd, Ee*. The possible combinations are *Dce, DCe, DcE, DCE, dce, dCe, dcE*, and *dCE*. According to Fisher and Race, the three gene loci of the system would be so closely linked that they would be inherited as a gene complex. Thus a *Dce/DcE* individual can only pass *Dce* or *DcE* to his offspring and no other combination. The antigen d has never been discovered, and the symbol *d* is used to denote the absence of *D*. All individuals lacking the *D* gene are termed Rh negative. The most frequent genotype of D-negative individuals is *cde/cde*. The lack of one of the postulated alleles seems to imply that the genetic basis of the Fisher-Race theory and nomenclature is not correct, but the use of this nomenclature has been retained, because it is easier to understand than any other.

The second most common nomenclature is that proposed by Wiener, who visualized multiple alleles at a single complex locus, each locus determining its particular agglutinogen comprising multiple factors, that were designated by bold-face type. The equivalents of the most common Rh factors in the Fisher-Race and Wiener nomenclature are shown in Table 20.2.

C. Kell, Duffy, and Kidd Systems

Aside from reactions due to ABO mismatch, which usually involve clerical error, the majority of transfusion reactions are due to sensitization against

TABLE 20.2 Comparison of the Fisher-Race and Wiener notations for the Rh System

Fisher-Race notation		Wiener notation		
Gene complex	Antigens	Genes	Agglutinogens	Factors
Dce	D,c,e	R^0	Rh_0	Rh_0,hr$'$,hr$''$
DCe	D,C,e	R^1	Rh_1	Rh_0,rh$'$,hr$''$
DcE	D,c,E	R^2	Rh_2	Rh_0,hr$'$,rh$''$
DCE	D,C,E	R^z	Rh_z	Rh_0,rh$'$,rh$''$
dce	d,c,e	r	rh	hr$'$,hr$''$
dCe	d,C,e	r'	rh$'$	rh$'$,hr$''$
cdE	d,c,E	r''	rh$''$	hr$'$,rh$''$
dCE	d,C,E	r^y	rh$_y$	rh$'$,rh$''$

antigens of the Rh, Kell, Duffy, and Kidd systems. Similarly, fetomaternal iso-immunization, which is most frequently observed within the Rh system, can also involve the Kell, Duffy, and Kidd Systems.

The Kell system is moderately polymorphic and it involves several antigens: Kell or K, Cellano or k, Kp^a, Kp^b, Js^a, Js^b, and others. The K antigen, present in about 9% of Caucasians, is relatively immunogenic though not as potent as D. The antibodies elicited are usually IgG.

The Duffy system has only two major antigens, Fy^a and Fy^b, the former being more immunogenic than the latter. All Caucasians carry at least one of the alleles coding for the antigens, but 60% of Blacks have neither Fy^a nor Fy^b antigens. The antibodies against these antigens are also usually of the IgG class.

The Kidd system, similar to the Duffy system, has two major antigens, Jk^a and Jk^b. The antibodies are usually IgG, but their detection may require anti-complement antibodies.

D. Laboratory Determination of Rh Phenotypes

The determination of Rh antigens is carried out using antisera able to recognize C, D, E, c, and e. Homozygosity and heterozygosity can be determined for C and E, because anti-C, anti-c, anti-E, and anti-e are available. Classically the antisera used for Rh typing have been obtained from sensitized humans, but monoclonal antibodies are currently being tested. With anti-D, homozygosity and heterozygosity are impossible to establish, because the d antigen has never been identified; so a positive result is recorded as D-positive and a negative as D-negative.

Rh phenotyping can be done in the laboratory using several different techniques. Because most anti-Rh antibodies are "incomplete" IgG antibodies unable to agglutinate saline-suspended red cells, considerable effort has been applied to the development of one-step techniques for Rh typing. There are basically two approaches: to modify the test conditions so that the cells become easier to agglutinate by IgG antibodies, or to use antibodies that are directly able to agglutinate red cells.

The first approach basically involves a reduction of the cell's negative zeta potential, or other measures that allow the red cells to approach each other more closely, so that they may be directly agglutinated by IgG antibodies. This involves preparation of the antiserum using a diluent containing high protein concentrations. Under these conditions an IgG anti-Rh antibody will agglutinate red cells positive for the antigen.

The second approach relies on the use of agglutinating anti-Rh antibodies either of the IgM class (which are difficult to obtain and require a relatively long incubation of the antisera and the cells) or IgG antibodies chemically modified by mild reduction of their interchain disulfide bonds to produce "unfolded" molecules capable of agglutinating red cells.

E. Direct and Indirect Antiglobulin (Coombs) Tests

In 1945, Coombs, Mourant, and Race described the use of antihuman globulin serum to detect red-cell-bound nonagglutinating antibodies. In 1957, Dacie showed that antihuman globulin serum also reacted with red-cell-bound human complement components.

There are two basic types of antiglobulin or Coombs tests. The direct antiglobulin test is performed to detect in vivo sensitization of red cells or, in other words, sensitization that has occurred in the patient (Fig. 20.1); the indirect antiglobulin test detects in vitro sensitization, which is sensitization that has been allowed to occur in the test tube under optimal conditions (Fig. 20.2). In the direct test, antihuman immunoglobulin G (and/or antihuman complement) is added to the patient's washed red cells, which are observed for agglutination (positive result). In the indirect test, a serum suspected of containing anti-red-cell antibodies is incubated with normal red blood cells; after washing unbound antibodies the red cells are tested with antihuman IgG (and/or anti-complement) antibodies as in the direct test.

The direct antiglobulin test is an aid in diagnosis and investigation of (1) hemolytic disease of the newborn, (2) autoimmune hemolytic anemia, (3) drug induced hemolytic anemia, and (4) hemolytic transfusion reactions. The indirect antiglobulin test is useful in (1) detecting and characterizing anti-red-cell antibodies using test cells of known antigenic composition (antibody screening), (2) crossmatching, and (3) phenotyping blood cells for antigens not demonstrable by other techniques.

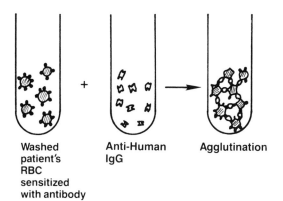

Washed patient's RBC sensitized with antibody   Anti-Human IgG   Agglutination

FIGURE 20.1 Diagrammatic representation of a direct Coombs test using anti-IgG antibodies.

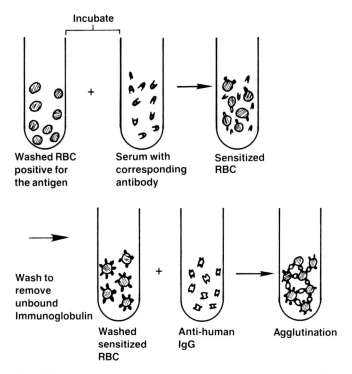

FIGURE 20.2 Diagrammatic representation of an indirect Coombs test.

II. BLOOD TRANSFUSION IMMUNOLOGY

A. Blood Testing

1. Compatibility Testing

Before a blood transfusion, a series of procedures needs to be done to establish the proper selection of blood for the patient. Basically, these procedures try to establish the compatibility between donor and recipient ABO and Rh systems (by typing both the donor and the blood to be transfused) and to rule out the existence of antibodies in the recipient's serum that could react with transfused red cells. A general antibody screening test is performed with red cells of known antigenic composition that are first incubated with the patient's serum to check for agglutination; if the direct agglutination test is negative an indirect Coombs test is performed. These two tests will determine whether the patient has anti-red-cell antibodies.

2. The Crossmatch

The most direct way to detect antibodies in the recipient's serum that could cause hemolysis of the transfused red cell is to test the patient's serum with the donor's cells (*major crossmatch*). The complete crossmatch also involves the same tests as the antibody screening test described above. Currently, an abbreviated version of the crosmatch is often performed in patients with a negative antibody screening test. This consists of immediately centrifuging a mixture of patient's serum and donor cells to detect agglutination; this primarily checks for ABO incompatibility. The *minor crossmatch*, which consists of testing the patient's cells with donor serum, is of little significance; any donor antibodies would be greatly diluted in the recipient's plasma and rarely cause clinical problems. Furthermore, donor blood found to contain antibodies can be safely transfused as packed red cells, containing very little plasma. This is a routine blood bank procedure, and no whole blood units containing clinically significant anti-red-cell antibodies are issued; such blood is, in all cases, issued as packed red cells and the plasma is discarded.

B. Blood Transfusion Reactions

Severe hemolytic blood transfusion reactions usually occur as a consequence of an ABO mismatch due to some clerical error; the result is the transfusion of the wrong blood (Table 20.3). Transfusion of blood incompatible for other blood groups to a patient previously sensitized during pregnancy or as a consequence of earlier transfusions can also cause a hemolytic reaction.

Not all transfusion reactions are hemolytic, and not all are due to immune phenomena. Table 20.4 presents a simplified classification of transfusion reactions.

C. Intravascular Hemolytic Reactions

The acute intravascular hemolytic reaction is triggered by the binding of complement-fixing antibodies to the red cells. By activating the complement system these antibodies cause red cell lysis; also, due to the massive release of soluble complement fragments (e.g., C3a and 5a) with anaphylatoxic properties, the patient may suffer generalized vasodilation, hypotension, and shock. Because of the interrelationships between the complement system and the clotting system, disseminated intravascular coagulation may occur during a severe transfusion reaction. As a consequence of the nephrotoxicity of hemoglobin released by the lysis of red cells, the patient may develop acute renal failure, usually due to acute tubular necrosis.

The most common initial symptom in a hemolytic transfusion reaction is fever, frequently associated with chills. Red or wine-colored urine (due to hemo-

TABLE 20.3 Summary of Fatal Transfusion Reactions[a]

Causes	No.
Clerical errors	
Wrong samples	7
Laboratory mix-up	9
Wrong patient	30
Wrong blood from warmer	1
Laboratory errors	
Mistyping	4
Undetermined antibody	4
Miscellaneous causes	
Blood "cooked" in warmer	1
Anaphylaxis	4
Multiple antibodies, urgent blood needed	5
Delayed reactions	3
Graft-vs.-host reaction	1
Respiratory distress syndrome	4
Gram-negative endotoxemia	2
DIC, undetermined type[b]	2
Total	77

[a]Reported to the Food and Drug Administration from April 3, 1976 to June 9, 1979.
[b]DIC indicates disseminated intravascular coagulation.
Source: Reproduced with permission from Myhre, B. A. *J. Amer. Med. Assoc. 244*:1333, 1980.

TABLE 20.4 Classification of Transfusion Reactions

Nonimmune
   Immune
      Red cell incompatibility
      Incompatibilities associated with platelets and leukocytes
      Incompatibilities due to antiallotypic antibodies (anti-Gm or anti-Am antibodies)

globinuria) may be the first symptom noticed by the patient. During surgery, the only symptom may be bleeding and/or hypotension. With progression of the reaction the patient may experience chest pains, dyspnea, hypotension, and shock. Generalized bleeding is the most serious manifestation of disseminated intravascular coagulation. Renal damage is indicated by back pain, oliguria, and in most severe cases, anuria.

Confirmation of intravascular hemolysis may involve one or several of the following tests in which the results obtained postreaction should, whenever possible, be compared with the results obtained in prereaction specimens.

1. Visual or photometric determination of free hemoglobin (pink) or bilirubin (yellow-brown) in serum.
2. Measurement of unconjugated bilirubin in serum of blood drawn 5 to 7 h after transfusion.
3. Determination of free hemoglobin and/or hemosiderin in urine
4. Measurement of serum haptoglobin (if no hemoglobin is detected in the serum by visual inspection)

D. Serologic Investigations in Transfusion Reactions

1. Serologic Investigations of Red-Cell Incompatibility

1. Repeat ABO and Rh determination on prereaction and postreaction samples and on the unit of transfused blood
2. Perform direct Coombs test on prereaction and postreaction samples
3. Crossmatch prereaction and postreaction samples with red blood cells from unit of transfused blood

2. Serologic Investigations of White-Cell and Platelet Incompatibilities

1. HLA typing of patient and donor
2. Investigation of cytotoxic antibodies (HLA-specific and non-HLA-specific). These antibodies may be responsible for severe febrile reactions.

3. Serologic Investigations of Anti-Immunoglobulin Antibodies

Investigate the presence of anti-IgA and anti-IgG antibodies. The anti-IgG and anti-IgA antibodies are often directed to allotypic markers of the Gm and Am system and are usually found in immunoglobulin-deficient patients that have been repeatedly transfused or received replacement therapy (gamma globulin or normal plasma) for relatively long periods of time. They may cause severe anaphylactic reactions.

III. HEMOLYTIC DISEASE OF THE NEWBORN (ERYTHROBLASTOSIS FETALIS)

Immunological destruction of fetal and/or newborn erythrocytes is likely to occur when IgG antibodies are present in the maternal circulation directed against the antigen(s) present in the fetal red blood cells (only IgG antibodies can cross the placenta and reach the fetal circulation).

Clinically, the two types of incompatibility most usually involved in hemolytic disease of the newborn are anti-D and anti-A or anti-B antibodies. Anti-A or anti-B antibodies are usually IgM, but in some circumstances IgG antibodies may develop. This can be secondary to immune stimulation (some vaccines contain blood-group substances or cross-reactive polysaccharides), or it may occur without apparent cause. IgG anti-A and/or anti-B antibodies are more frequently produced by group O mothers. One in five pregnancies are ABO incompatible, but the frequency of clinical symptoms is relatively low (1/150 of all infants develop jaundice), and the frequency of cases requiring therapy even lower (1/3000).

The frequency of clinically evident hemolytic disease of the newborn was estimated to be about 0.5% of total births, with a mortality rate close to 6% among affected newborns, prior to the introduction of immunoprophylaxis. Recent figures are considerably lower—0.15 to 0.3% incidence of clinically evident disease—and the perinatal mortality rate appears to be declining to about 4% of affected newborns. Clinically, Rh incompatibility has been associated with about 95% of the cases of hemolytic disease of the newborn requiring therapy; the majority of those cases were due to sensitization against the D antigen. With the introduction of immunoprophylaxis, the proportion of cases due to anti-D antibodies is decreasing, while the proportion of cases due to anti-c and anti-E antibodies, and to antibodies to antigens of other systems, is increasing.

The usual clinical features of this disease are anemia and jaundice present at birth or, more frequently, in the first 24 h of life. In severe cases, the infant may die in utero. Other severely affected children who survive until the third day develop signs of central nervous system damage attributed to the high unconjugated bilirubin concentrations (kernicterus). The peripheral blood shows reticulocytes and circulating erythroblasts.

A. Mechanisms of Sensitization

Although the exchange of red cells between mother and fetus is prevented by the placental barrier during pregnancy, about two-thirds of all women, after delivery (or miscarriage), have fetal red cells (or fetal hemoglobin) in their circulation. If the mother is Rh negative and the infant Rh positive, the mother may produce antibodies to the D antigen. Usually the first child is not affected, because the red cells that cross the placenta after the 28th week of gestation do so in small numbers and do not elicit a strong immune response. The immune response is usually initiated at term, when large amounts of fetal red cells reach maternal circulation. In subsequent pregnancies, even the small number of red cells crossing the placenta during pregnancy are enough to elicit a strong secondary response, with production of IgG antibodies that will cross the placenta, bind to the Rh positive cells, and cause their destruction in the spleen through Fc-mediated phagocytosis (and perhaps K-cell activity). IgG anti-D antibodies do not appear to activate the complement system, perhaps because the distribution of the D antigen on the red-cell surface is too sparse to allow the formation of IgG doublets with sufficient density of IgG molecules to induce complement activation. Complement, however, is not required for phagocytosis, which can be mediated by the Fc receptors in monocytes and macrophages.

B. Immunological Diagnosis

A positive direct Coombs (antiglobulin) test with cord RBC is invariably found in cases of Rh incompatibility, although 40% of the cases with positive reaction do not require treatment. In ABO incompatibility, the direct antiglobulin test is usually weakly positive and may be negative, and best results are obtained by eluting antibodies from the infant red cells and testing the eluate with adult A and B cells.

C. Prevention

The serological investigation of antibodies in pregnant women, particularly those who are Rh negative, is important in preventing serious hemolytic disease of the newborn. Amniocentesis is usually performed if a clinically significant antibody with an antiglobulin titer greater than 16 is present in the serum or if the woman has a history of a previously affected child. The amniotic fluid is examined for bile pigments at appropriate intervals, and the severity of the disease is assessed according to those levels. The amniotic fluid may also be used to assess fetal lung maturity by determining the ratio of lecithin to sphingomyelin.

If these test results so indicate, and if pregnancy is over 32 weeks, labor may be induced and, if necessary, the baby can be exchange-transfused after delivery. If pregnancy is less than 32 weeks or fetal lung maturity is inadequate, intrauterine transfusion may be performed by transfusing O, Rh negative red cells to the fetus.

An interesting observation concerning Rh hemolytic disease of the newborn is its rarity when mother and infant are incompatible in both Rh and ABO systems. In such cases, the ABO isoagglutinins in the maternal circulation appear to eliminate any fetal red cells before maternal sensitization occurs. This observation led to a very effective form of prevention for hemolytic disease of the newborn, achieved by the administration of anti-D IgG antibodies (Rh immune globulin) to Rh negative mothers. If this administration is carried out in the first 72 h after delivery of the first baby (before sensitization has had time to occur), the passively administered anti-D IgG prevents the emergence of maternal anti-D antibodies. The rate of success is 98 to 99%. Recently, antepartum administration of a full dose of Rh immune globulin at the 28th week of pregnancy has been recommended in addition to the postpartum administration. The rationale for this approach is to avoid sensitization due to prenatal spontaneous or posttraumatic bleeding. Prenatal anti-D prophylaxis is also indicated in any case in which an Rh negative pregnant woman is submitted to amniocentesis. If prophylaxis is initiated before the 28th week of pregnancy, it should be repeated 12 weeks later (or at 28 weeks gestation) and a third dose given after delivery if the infant is Rh positive, even if anti-D antibodies are detectable in maternal blood at the time of delivery.

The therapeutic anti-D antibody is prepared from the plasma of previously immunized mothers with persistently high titers, or from male donors immunized against Rh positive RBC. The recommended full dose is 300 μg IM, which can be increased if there is laboratory evidence of severe fetomaternal hemorrhage (by tests able to determine the number of fetal red cells in maternal peripheral blood, from which one can calculate the volume of fetomaternal hemorrhage). Smaller doses (50 μg) should be given after therapeutic or spontaneous abortion in the first trimester.

IV. HEMOLYTIC ANEMIAS OF IMMUNOLOGIC PATHOGENESIS

A. Autoimmune Hemolytic Anemia (Warm Antibody Type)

The warm antibody type is the most common form of autoimmune hemolytic anemia. It can be idiopathic (often following overt or subclinical viral infection) or secondary, as shown in Table 20.5.

Diagnosis relies on the demonstration of antibodies coating the red cells or circulating in the serum. RBC-fixed antibodies are detected by the direct antiglobulin (Coombs) test. The test can be done using anti-IgG antiglobulin, anticomplement, or polyspecific antiglobulin serum that has both anti-IgG and anticomplement. The polyspecific or broad spectrum antiglobulin sera produce positive results in higher numbers of patients, as shown in Table 20.6. IgG antibody usually can be eluted from the cells of patients with warm-type autoimmune hemolytic anemia.

The search for antibodies in serum is carried out by the indirect antiglobulin test. Circulating antibodies are present only when the red cells have been maximally coated, and the test is positive in only 40% of the cases tested with un-

TABLE 20.5 Immune Hemolytic Anemias

Autoimmune hemolytic anemias (AIHA)
    Warm antibody AIHA
        Idiopathic (unassociated with another disease)
        Secondary (associated with chronic lymphocytic leukemia, lymphomas,
           systemic lupus erythematosus, etc.)
    Cold antibody AIHA
        Idiopathic cold hemagglutinin disease
        Secondary cold hemagglutinin syndrome
           Associated with *M. pneumoniae* infection
           Associated with chronic lymphocytic leukemia, lymphomas, etc.
    Paroxysmal cold hemoglobinuria
    Idiopathic
    Secondary to syphilis

Immune drug-induced hemolytic anemia

Alloantibody-induced immune hemolytic anemia
    Hemolytic transfusion reactions
    Hemolytic disease of the newborn

Source: Modifed from Petz, L. D. and Garraty, G. Laboratory correlations in immune hemolytic anemias, In *Laboratory Diagnosis of Immunologic Disorders*, G. N. Vyas, D. P. Stites, and G. Brechter (Eds.). Grune & Stratton, 1974.

TABLE 20.6 Typical Results of Serological Investigations in Patients with Autoimmune Hemolytic Anemia

	Cells			Serum	
	Direct Coombs test				
	Antibody to	Positivity rate	Antibody isotype	Serologic characteristics	Ab specificity
Warm AIHA	IgG	30%	IgG	Positive indirect Coombs test (40%)	Rh system antigens ("public")
	IgG + C′	50%		Agglutination of enzyme-treated	
	C′	20%		RBC (80%)	
Cold agglutinin disease	C′		IgM	Monoclonal IgMκ agglutinates RBC to titers >1024 at 4°C	I antigen

Source: Modified from Petz, L. D. and Garraty, G. Laboratory correlations in immune hemolytic anemias. In *Laboratory Diagnosis of Immunologic Disorders*, G. N. Vyas, D. P. Stites and G. Brechter (Eds.). Grune & Stratton, 1974.

treated red cells. A higher positivity rate (up to 80%) can be achieved by using red cells treated with enzymes such as trypsin, papain, ficin, and bromelin in the agglutination assays. The treatment of red cells with these enzymes increases their agglutinability either by increasing the exposure of antigenic determinants or by reducing the surface charge of the red cells. In the investigation of warm-type AIHA all tests are carried out at $37°C$.

By adsorption experiments, the antibodies involved in this type of hemolytic anemia can be shown to react to determinants of the Rh complex and with uncharacterized specificities common to almost all normal red cells ("public" antigens, thought to be the core of the Rh substance). In many patients, one can find antibodies of more than one specificity. The result is that the serum from patients with autoimmune hemolytic anemia of the warm type is likely to react with most, if not all, of the red cells tested.

B. Cold Agglutinin Disease and Cold Agglutinin Syndromes

Cold antibody AIHA can also be idiopathic (cold agglutinin disease) or secondary (cold agglutinin syndromes). Hemolysis, although severe in some cases, is usually mild and the clinical picture is often dominated by symptoms of cold sensitivity (Raynaud's phenomenon, vascular purpura, tissue necrosis in exposed extremities).

The cold agglutinins are classically IgM (very rarely IgA or IgG), and they react with red cells at temperatures below normal body temperature. The range of thermal reactivity of cold agglutinins may reach up to $35°C$. Such temperatures are not difficult to experience in exposed parts of the body during the winter. Cold-induced intravascular agglutination and hemolysis are the main pathogenic mechanisms in cold agglutinin disease.

Testing for cold agglutinins is usually done by incubating at $4°C$ a series of dilutions of the patient's serum (obtained by clotting and centrifuging the blood at $37°C$ immediately after drawing) to which we add normal group O RBC (to avoid false positive results due to anti-A and anti-B isohemagglutinins). Titers up to the thousands or even millions can be observed in patients with cold agglutinin disease; lower titers (below 1000) can be found in patients with postinfectious cold agglutinins, and titers of 10-20 can be found in normal asymptomatic individuals.

In chronic, idiopathic, cold agglutinin diseases, 95% or more of the antibodies, which are IgM kappa, react with the I antigen. This is the adult specificity of the I, i system: The fetus expresses the i antigen, common to primates and other mammalians, which is the precursor of the I specificity. The newborn expresses i predominantly over I; in the adult, the situation is reversed. In postinfectious cold agglutinin disease the antibodies are also predominantly IgM, but these contain both kappa and lambda light chains, suggesting their polyclonal

TABLE 20.7 Correlation Between Mechanisms of Red Cell Sensitization and Laboratory Features in Drug-Induced Immunohematological Abnormalities

Mechanism	Prototype drugs	Clinical findings	Serologic evaluation	
			Direct Coombs	In vitro tests and Ab identification
Immune complex formation	Quinidine Phenacetin	Intravascular hemolysis; renal failure; thrombocytopenia	C' usually IgG rarely	Drug + serum + RBC Ab is often IgM
Drug adsorption to RBC	Penicillins	Extravascular hemolysis ass. with high doses of penicillin i.v.	Strongly positive with anti-IgG[a]	Drug-coated RBC + serum. Antibody is IgG
Membrane modif. causing non-immunological adsorption of proteins	Cephalosporins	Asymptomatic	Positive with a variety of antisera	Drug-coated RBC + serum. No specific antibody involved
Autoimmune	α-methyldopa	Hemolysis in 0.8% of patients taking this medication	Strongly positive with anti-IgG[a]	Normal RBC + serum. Autoantibody to RBC identical to Ab in warm AIHA

[a]When hemolytic anemia is present.
Source: Modifed from Garraty, G. and Petz, L. D. *Amer. J. Med., 58*:398, 1975.

origin. The cold agglutinins that appear in patients with *Mycoplasma pneumoniae* infections are usually reactive with the I antigen, whereas those that appear in association with infectious mononucleosis usually react with the i antigen.

C. Drug-Induced Hemolytic Anemia

Immune mechanisms may play a role in many drug-induced hemolytic anemias, as summarized in Table 20.7.

The first mechanism, formation of soluble immune complexes between the drug and the corresponding antibodies, followed by nonspecific adsorption to red cells, complement activation, and red cell lysis, leads to intravascular hemolysis and appears to involve predominantly IgM antibodies. The direct Coombs test is usually positive if anticomplement antibodies are used. IgG antibodies can also form immune complexes with different types of antigens and be adsorbed onto red cells and platelets. In vitro, such adsorption is not followed by hemolysis or by phagocytosis of red cells, but in vivo it has been reported to be associated with intravascular hemolysis. The absorption of IgG-containing immune complexes to platelets is also the cause of drug-induced thrombocytopenia. Quinine, quinidine, digitoxin, gold, meprobamate, chlorothiazide, rifampin, and the sulphonamides have been reported to cause this type of drug-induced thrombocytopenia.

A second mechanism consists of the adsorption of the drug onto the red cells. The drug then functions as hapten and the RBC as carrier, and an immune response against the drug will be possible. If so, the antibodies, usually IgG, will be present in high titers, and they may activate complement after binding to the drug adsorbed to the red cells, inducing hemolysis (Fig. 20.3) or phagocytosis.

Cephalothin has been shown to modify the red cell membrane, which becomes able to adsorb proteins nonspecifically, a fact that can lead to a positive direct Coombs test but not to hemolytic anemia. Immune hemolytic anemia may, however, result from the reactivity of anticephalosporin antibodies to cephalosporin adsorbed to the cell membrane or to the binding of cross-reactive antipenicillin antibodies (see drug adsorption mechanism).

The anemia induced by α-methyldopa (Aldomet) is particularly interesting in that it is indistinguishable from a true autoimmune hemolytic anemia. It is also the most frequent type of drug-induced hemolytic anemia. 10-15% of the patients receiving the drug will have a positive Coombs test, and 0.8% of the

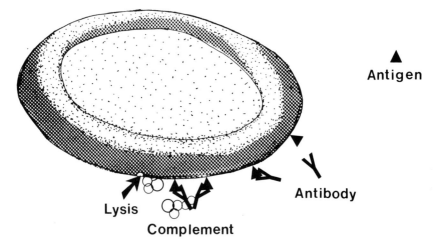

FIGURE 20.3 Diagrammatic representation of the pathogenesis of drug-induced hemolytic anemia as a consequence of adsorption of a drug to the red-cell membrane.

patients develop clinically hemolytic evident anemia. Although the administration of α-methyldopa is unquestionably the trigger for this type of anemia, the produced antibodies are IgG1, complement-fixing, and react with Rh antigens. Once formed, the anti-red-cell antibodies will react in the absence of the drug, as true autoantibodies. L-dopa, a related drug used for the treatment of Parkinson's disease, can also cause autoimmune hemolytic anemia. Both α-methyldopa and L-dopa also stimulate the production of antinuclear antibodies.

D. Paroxysmal Cold Hemoglobinuria

Paroxysmal cold hemoglobinuria is a rare disease, sometimes idiopathic, other times secondary to syphilis or viral infections. Hemolysis occurs after local or general exposure to cold. This is because of the presence of the biphasic Donath-Landsteiner antibody, an IgG antibody that binds (sensitizes) the cells in the cold (usually below 15°C), fixing complement (a direct antiglobulin test will be positive using an anticomplement reagent after rewarming). Complete complement activation occurs at higher temperatures (37°C), resulting in hemolysis.

SELF EVALUATION

Questions

Choose the one best answer.

20.1 A direct Coombs test using antisera to IgG is virtually always positive in
  A. Females with circulating anti-D antibodies.
  B. Newborns with Rh hemolytic disease.
  C. Patients with warm-type autoimmune hemolytic anemia.
  D. Patients with paroxysmal cold hemoglobinuria.
  E. Patients with cold hemagglutinin disease.

20.2 Penicillin-induced hemolytic anemia is usually due to
  A. Drug adsorption to red cells and reaction with antipenicillin antibodies.
  B. Nonspecific adsorption and activation of complement components.
  C. Emergence of a neoantigen on the red cell membrane.
  D. Formation of soluble IC, adsorption to red-cell membranes, and complement activation or phagocytosis.
  E. None of the above.

20.3 The drug that causes a true autoimmune hemolytic anemia is
  A. Procainamide.
  B. Quinidine
  C. Cephalosporin.
  D. α-Methyldopa.
  E. Phenacetin.

20.4 The destruction of Rh positive erythrocytes after exposure to IgG anti-D
antibodies is due to
A. Complement activation.
B. Fc-mediated phagocytosis.
C. C3b-mediated phagocytosis.
D. C3d-mediated phagocytosis.
E. A combination of Fc-mediated and C3b-mediated phagocytosis.

20.5 In a patient with penicillin-induced hemolytic anemia you should be
concerned with the induction of a similar situation if prescribing
A. Aspirin.
B. Quinidine.
C. Cephalosporins.
D. Aminoglycosides.
E. Sulfonamides.

20.6 An A, Rh negative mother will not be sensitized by a first Rh positive
baby if
A. The baby is B, Rh positive.
B. The baby is A, Rh positive.
C. The baby is O, Rh positive.
D. The father is A, Rh positive.
E. The father is B, Rh positive.

20.7 The major crossmatch is used to detect
A. Antibodies in the donor's red cells.
B. Antibodies in the donor's serum.
C. Antibodies in the recipient's cells.
D. Antibodies in the recipient's serum.
E. Antibodies in both the donor's and the recipient's sera.

20.8 The Coombs test is not useful for the investigation of
A. Hemolytic disease of the newborn.
B. Allotype incompatibility.
C. Autoimmune hemolytic anemia.
D. Drug-induced hemolytic anemia.
E. Hemolytic transfusion reaction.

20.9 The highest frequency of positive results in the serological investigation of
autoimmune hemolytic anemia is obtained with
A. A direct Coombs test using anti-IgG.
B. A direct Coombs test using anti-IgG and complement.
C. An indirect Coombs test using patient's serum and normal red cells.
D. A cold agglutinin test.
E. A direct agglutination test using the patient's sera and enzyme-treated
normal red cells.

20.10 The Donath-Landsteiner antibody is also known as biphasic because it
  A. Is responsible for a disease with two distinct phases.
  B. Binds to red cells better at 30°C but maximal agglutination is seen at low temperatures.
  C. Binds to red cells better below 15°C but activates complement more efficiently at 37°C.
  D. Activates complement in two phases, the first at 37°C and the second at lower temperatures.
  E. Is an incomplete antibody requiring a second anti-IgG antibody for the second phase of complement activation to occur.

Answers

20.1 (B) Rh Hemolytic disease is, by definition, due to IgG antibodies that cross the placenta and bind to the newborn's erythrocytes, where they will be easily detected by a direct Coombs test using anti-IgG antibodies.

20.2 (A)

20.3 (D) α-methyldopa (Aldomet) induces a unique type of hemolytic anemia in which the antibodies are directed to red-cell antigens and not to the drug itself.

20.4 (B) IgG anti-D antibodies do not cause complement fixation after binding to red cell membrane.

20.5 (C) There is marked cross-reaction between penicillin and the cephalosporins.

20.6 (A) The maternal anti-B isoagglutinins will function as a natural anti-D antibody by destroying the fetal red cells before there is an opportunity to induce the anti-D immune response.

20.7 (D)

20.8 (B) Transfusion reactions due to antiallotype antibodies are investigated by techniques involving inhibition of passive hemagglutination that are unrelated to the Coombs test (see Chapter 14).

20.9 (E)

20.10 (C)

BIBLIOGRAPHY

Brown, D. L. Immunological aspects of blood disease. In *Pediatric Immunology*, J. F. Soothill, A. R. Hayward, and C. B. S. Wood (Eds.). Blackwell Scientific, Oxford,1983, p. 368.

Issitt, P. D. *Applied Blood Group Serology*, 3rd Ed. Montgomery Scientific, Miami, Florida, 1985.

Like, Y. W. *Immunology and Immunopathology of the Human Fetal-Maternal Interaction*. Elsevier/North Holland, Amsterdam, 1978.

Mollison, P. L. *Blood Transfusion in Clinical Medicine*, 8th Ed. Blackwell Scientific, Oxford, 1987.

Petz, L. D. and Garraty, G. *Acquired Immune Hemolytic Anemias*. Churchill/ Livingston, New York, 1980.

Race, R. R. and Sanger, R. *Blood Groups in Man*, 6th Ed. Blackwell Scientific, Oxford, 1975.

Salmon, C. Blood groups and Autoimmune hemolytic anemia. In *Immunology*, 2nd Ed., J. F. Bach (Ed.). John Wiley, New York, 1982.

Wells, J. V. and Isbister, J. P. Hematologic diseases. In *Basic and Clinical Immunology*, 6th Ed., D. P. Stites, J. D. Stobo, and J. V. Wells (Eds.). Lange Medical, Los Altos, 1987, p. 386.

21

Immune Complex Diseases

GABRIEL VIRELLA

The formation of circulating antigen-antibody (Ag-Ab) complexes is one of the natural events that characterize the immunologic response against soluble antigens. Normally, immune complexes (IC) formed by soluble proteins and their respective antibodies are promptly phagocytized and eliminated from circulation without any detectable adverse effects on the host. However, pathogenic consequences of the formation of Ag-Ab complexes were recognized early in this century (although incorrectly interpreted) by von Pirquet, in his early studies of serum sickness in humans.

In the late 1800s and early 1900s passive immunization with equine antisera was a common therapy for severe bacterial infections. It was often noted that one to two weeks after administration of the horse antisera, when the symptoms of acute infection had often disappeared, the patient would start to complain of arthralgias and exanthematous rash and had proteinuria and an abnormal urinary sediment suggestive of glomerulonephritis. The correct interpretation of this clinical picture was possible only after the work of Germuth, Dixon, and co-workers in the 1950s. These authors carried out detailed studies in rabbits on which serum sickness was induced by injection of single doses of heterologous proteins. As summarized in Figure 21.2, after the lag time necessary for antibody production, soluble immune complexes could be detected in serum, serum complement levels decreased, and the rabbits developed glomerulonephritis, myocarditis, and arthritis. The onset of disease coincides with the disappearance

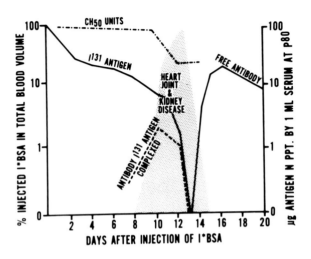

FIGURE 21.1 Diagrammatic representation of the sequence of events that takes place during the induction of acute serum sickness in rabbits. Six days after injection of radiolabeled BSA, the synthesis anti-BSA antibodies start being produced and form complexes with the antigen, which is eliminated rapidly with the circulation. The maximal concentration of immune complexes shortly precedes a decrease in complement levels and the appearance of histological abnormalities in the heart, joints, and kidney. After the antigen is totally eliminated, the antibody becomes detectable and the pathological lesions heal without permanent sequelae. (Reproduced with permission from Cochrane, C. G. and Koffler, D. *Adv. Immunol 16*:185, 1973.)

of circulating antigen, and free circulating antibody appears in circulation soon after the beginning of symptoms. Both the experimental one-shot serum sickness and human serum sickness are usually transient and will leave no permanent sequelae. However, if the organism is chronically exposed to antigen (as in chronic serum sickness), irreversible lesions will develop.

I. PHYSIOPATHOLOGY OF IMMUNE COMPLEX DISEASE

The formation of an immune complex does not have direct pathological consequences. The pathogenic consequences of immune complex formation depend on the ability of those immune complexes (1) to become fixed at some anatomical structure, (2) to activate the complement system, and (3) to interact with cells able to release enzymes and mediators involved in inflammation. All these properties are related to the physicochemical characteristics of immune complexes, such as size, affinity of the Ag-Ab reaction, and class and subclass of antibodies involved in immune complex formation.

A. Immobilization of Immune Complexes

The interaction of IC with cells able to release mediators of inflammation appears to be considerably enhanced if the IC are surface-bound rather than soluble. This immobilization of immune complexes is likely to be mediated by C3 receptors (glomerular epithelium), by C1q receptors (endothelial cells), by Fc receptors (renal interstitium, damaged endothelium), and by the affinity of some antigen moieties in IC for specific tissues, such as that of DNA for glomerular basement membrane and collagen. Immune complexes can also bind to platelets and red cells. The binding to human platelets involves a cellular Fc receptor specific for all IgG subclasses. The binding to red cells may involve a C3b binding site, but some early observations on the absorption of drug-antibody complexes and aggregated IgG, and experimental work carried out in our laboratory, have clearly demonstrated that complement is not required for the binding. Clinically, the pathological significance of IC binding to peripheral blood cells has been thought to be restricted to the thrombocytopenic purpura often associated to serum sickness and to some forms of drug-induced hemolytic anemia. Considering the enormous mass of red cells in the organism, the binding of IC to red cells may have a wider biological significance as a mechanism of presentation of IC to other cells. Experimental work in primates and metabolic studies of labeled IC in humans suggest that binding to RBC may be one of the important mechanisms for clearance of soluble IC from the systemic circulation, probably through presentation to phagocytic cells that remove the IC from the RBC membrane without causing red-cell damage.

B. Capacity to Activate Complement

The capacity to interact with complement may be closely related to the pathogenic potential of soluble IC. Part of this potential will result from the added capacity to interact with cell membranes, as outlined previously, and part will result from the activation of the complement cascade, leading to the release of factors like C3a and C5a that have chemotactic and anaphylactic activities. As a consequence of the chemotactic activity of C5a, neutrophils will be brought to the area of IC deposition. On the other hand, C5a and C3a will be able to exert its anaphylatoxic effect, leading to the release of histamine and vasoactive amines from basophils and mast cells, which will enhance the extravascular deposition of IC and the inflammatory response at the area where IC are deposited. C5a is also able to induce the aggregation and release of constitutents from neutrophils and causes an increase in vascular permeability independent of the release of histamine. This increase in vascular permeability is an essential first step in creating the necessary conditions for the interaction of IC with extra-vascular structures such as the C3b receptors of the renal epithelial cells, the Fc receptors in the renal interstitium, and the interaction between DNA and the glomerular basement membrane. From the point of view of complement activa-tion, IC involving IgM, IgG1, and IgG3 are those with the highest pathogenic potential.

C. Interactions with Cells Able to Release Enzymes and Mediators of Inflammation

The IC-cell interactions we will first consider are those involving cells potentially able to release vasoactive amines, such as basophils, mast cells, and platelets. In some animal species, it is believed that these interactions require the synthe-sis of homocytotrophic antibodies (IgE) of the same specificity as those involved in the formation of soluble IC (most IgG). The IgE antibodies, bound to the membrane of circulating basophils, would react with free antigen (or with un-blocked determinants of the antigen included in soluble IC), and as a conse-quence of this reaction the basophils would release their intracellular contents, including histamine, serotonin, and platelet-activating factor (PAF) that can lead to further release of vasoactive amines from platelets. In humans, direct interac-tion of IC with basophils and mast cells does not appear to play a very signifi-cant role, because there is no evidence for the production of reaginic antibodies with the same specificity as those involved in soluble IC formation in most pa-tients with IC disease. A more significant role is probably played by platelets that can interact with IgG-containing IC through their Fc receptors and as a result undergo aggregation and release their mediators. Among such mediators are included vasoactive amines that may lead to increased vascular permeability. An alternative way to lead to the release of vasoactive amines from platelets has been suggested by studies showing that rabbit neutrophils can release their intracellular contents after interaction with insoluble antigen-antibody aggre-gates and surface-bound immune complexes. Among those intracellular contents there are some poorly characterized cationic protein(s) that can induce the de-granulation of basophils and mastocytes, leading to the release of vasoactive amines and PAF. In man, the release of PAF must follow a different pathway, because human basophils do not synthesize this compound. However, human neutrophils and monocytes have also been shown to be able to release at least some of their intracellular contents after interaction with insoluble IC or with cell-bound IC, including PAF (in case of the neutrophils) and interleukin 1 (in the case of the monocytes). The role of polymorphonuclear leukocytes also ap-pears extremely important in the late stages of IC deposition, when they reach the tissues where IC deposition has taken place, releasing intracellular enzymes

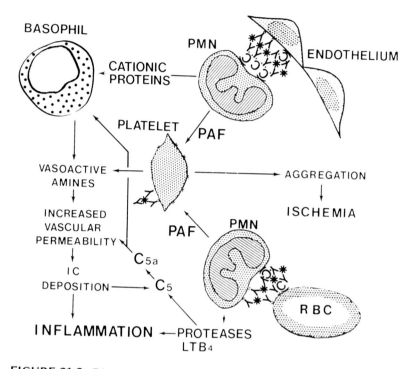

FIGURE 21.2 Diagram illustrating the IC-cell interactions that may play a
significant role in IC deposition and subsequent inflammation. The first step
is likely to be the immobilization of soluble IC on cell membranes, such as
those of the endothelial cells (believed to have Fc and C3b receptors) and those
of the red cells (which have Fc and C3b binding sites). PMN leukocytes, also
having membrane receptors for C3b and Fc, will recognize the cell-bound IC
and be stimulated to release soluble mediators including platelet activating factor
(PAF), which will in turn trigger the release of vasoactive amines from platelets.
The release reaction from platelets could also be induced directly by the binding
of IC to their Fc receptor. An alternative pathway for vasoactive amine release
could be mediated by cationic proteins released by the PMN leukocytes, which
will induce basophil degranulation. After extravascular deposition, chemotactic
factors (such as C5a) are generated, and PMN leukocytes are attracted to the site
where they release proteases, which cause tissue damage and cleave C5, generating additional C5a, which will amplify the inflammatory response.

such as proteases and collagenase. These enzymes are believed to be ultimately
responsible for most of the tissue damage in IC disease Also, C5 can be directly
split by those proteases, and the C5a fragment generated in this way will be able
to amplify the inflammatory reaction.

A brief graphic summary of the interactions between IC and different types of cells that are likely to play significant roles in the pathways that lead to IC deposition and later to tissue inflammation in man is shown in Figure 21.2.

II. HOST FACTORS THAT WILL INFLUENCE THE DEVELOPMENT OF IMMUNE COMPLEX DISEASE

The development of immune complex disease in experimental animals is clearly dependent on host factors. For example, if several rabbits of the same strain, age, weight, and sex are immunized with identical amounts of heterologous proteins by the same route, only a variable proportion of animals will respond to the protein, and of those that respond not all will develop immune complex disease. This may depend on the general characteristics of the antibodies produced (such as affinity and the ability to bind complement and to interact with cell receptors) and, probably, on the functional state of the reticuloendothelial system of the animal. In experimental animals, it appears that the induction of glomerular damage is more common when the immune response is somewhat weak and when small-sized immune complexes in antigen excess are produced. Such IC are not efficiently bound by red cells and tend to persist in circulation for longer periods of time. Larger IC, formed close to equivalence, appear to be quickly removed from the circulation by phagocytic cells, and the importance of this removal has been demonstrated by studies showing that if the RES is blocked by a massive injection of colloidal carbon, the clearance of immune complexes deposited on the glomerular capillaries is considerably slowed. The longer IC persist in and around the glomerular basement membrane, the higher will be the risk of developing inflammatory lesions as a consequence of complement activation and direct interaction with PMN leukocytes.

III. DETECTION OF SOLUBLE IMMUNE COMPLEXES

Many techniques have been proposed for the detection of soluble immune complexes. Table 2.1 lists those assays that have achieved wider use and that deserve to be considered in some detail.

A. Detection of Cryoglobulins

The detection of cryoglobulins is the simplest technique. Blood is drawn and clotted at 37°C, serum is immediately separated, without cooling, and immediately after centrifugation, 5-10 ml of serum are placed in a refrigerator at 4-8°C. The serum will be examined daily for 72 hr for the appearance of a precipitate (Fig. 21.3). Characteristically, this precipitate will resuspend if the serum is warmed to 37°C. A positive screening test should be followed by washing of

TABLE 21.1   Most Commonly Used Screening Tests for Soluble IC

Based on thermosolubility
    Cryoprecipitation

Based on differential PEG solubility
    PEG-total protein
    PEG-IgG

Based on interactions with complement
    ^{125}I-labeled C1q binding assay
    Solid-phase C1q binding assay

Based on interactions with rheumatoid factor

Based on IC-cell interactions
    Raji cell assay

Specific tests
    For DNA-anti-DNA IC
    For HBsAg-Ab IC
    For insulin-antiinsulin Ab IC

the precipitate (to eliminate contaminant proteins), redissolution, and immuno-chemical characterization of the proteins contained in the precipitate (Fig. 21.4). Cryoglobulins can be classified in two major types according to their constitution: (1) monoclonal cryoglobulins (type I) and (2) mixed cryoglobulins, with one monoclonal component and at least one other population of polyclonal immunoglobulins (type II) or with more than one immunoglobulin class, but all immunoglobulins in the precipitate being polyclonal (type III).

Monoclonal cryoglobulins are usually detected in patients with plasma cell malignancies and in some cases of idiopathic cryoglobulinemia. Essentially this type of cryoglobulin corresponds to monoclonal proteins with abnormal thermal behavior and has no correlation with immune-complex formation.

Mixed cryoglobulins, on the contrary, represent cold-precipitated immune complexes (low temperatures increase the stability of Ag-Ab reactions and enhance precipitation). One of the immunoglobulins present in the precipitate (the monoclonal one in type II cryoglobulinemia) is an antibody that reacts with the other immunoglobulin(s) that constitute the cryoglobulin. The most frequent type of mixed cryoglobulin is IgM-IgG, in which IgM is a "rheumatoid factor." It is believed that, at least in some cases, the IgM antibody is directed to determinants expressed by IgG antibodies bound to their corresponding antigens (Fig. 21.5). Evidence favoring this mechanism has been obtained by identifying antigens and/or antibodies in cryoprecipitates. Viral antigens and corresponding antibodies (for example, HbsAg and anti-HBsAg) are fequently found

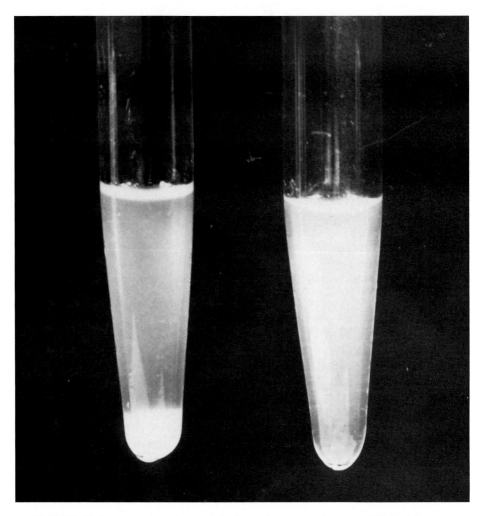

FIGURE 21.3   Screening of cryoglobulins. Two test tubes were filled with sera from a patient (left) and a healthy volunteer (right). After 48 h at 4°C a precipitate is obvious in the patient's serum but is not present in the control.

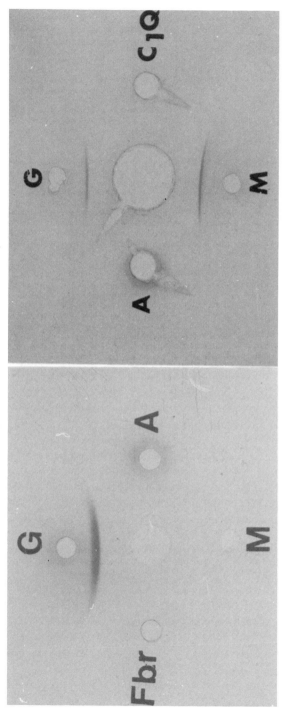

FIGURE 21.4 Characterization of two washed cryoglobulins. In both studies the washed and redissolved cryoglobulin was placed on the center well, and four different antisera were placed in the surrounding wells. The cryoglobulin studied on the left reacted with anti-IgG (G) only and was classified as a monoclonal cryoglobulin; the one studied on the right reacted with anti-IgG (G) and anti-IgM (M) and was classified as a mixed cryoglobulin.

403

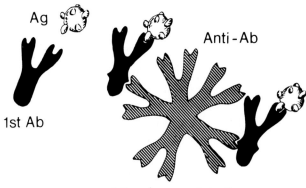

Mixed cryoglobulin

FIGURE 21.5   Diagrammatic representation of the pathogenesis of mixed cryoglobulins. Initially, an antimicrobial antibody (for example) of the IgG class is
produced. This antibody, a consequence of binding to the antigen, exposes a
new antigenic determinant, which is recognized by an IgM antiglobulin. The
combination of this IgM with the first IgG antibody and the microbial antigen
constitutes the mixed cryoglobulin.

in the cryoprecipitates from patients with mixed cryoglobulins, both with and
without a history of previous viral infections. It is believed that this mechanism—antiviral IgG combined with an IgM antibody—accounts for over 50% of the
cases of essential or idiopathic mixed cryoglobulinemia (mixed cryoglobulins
are often detected in patients with autoimmune disorders or with chronic infections).

The main limitation of this technique lies in its low positivity frequency; perhaps less than 5% of the sera positive for IC by general screening techniques are
found positive in cryoglobulin screening.

B.   Techniques Based on the Precipitation of Soluble Immune Complexes
     with Polyethylene Glycol

These owed their popularity to their relative simplicity. Small concentrations
of PEG (3-4%) cause preferential precipitation of IC relative to monomeric immunoglobulins. In the simplest versions, a dilution of patient's serum and PEG
are mixed and the turbidity of the sample is measured after adequate incubation;
a direct correlation can be established between the degree of turbidity and the
concentration of IC in the serum. In other assays, mixtures of PEG and sera are
incubated overnight, until a precipitate is obtained, and then total protein, IgG,
of C1q are measured in the precipitate.

C. Assays Based on Interactions with Complement

One of the most widely used techniques for general screening of IC is based on the binding of C1q. Two main variants of this technique have been described. In the original method, C1q was purified and labeled with ^{125}I and a small amount added to a serum supposed to contain soluble IC. If IgM or IgG-containing IC were present, the radiolabeled C1q would attach to the IC. Finally, a substance known to promote the precipitation of IC (such as PEG) was added to the mixture of serum and ^{125}I-C1q in a concentration that would not affect unbound C1q but would cause precipitation of IC; if these IC had complement-fixing capacity, radiolabeled C1q would also be precipitated and would be quantitated by measuring the amount of radiation contained in the precipitate.

A solid-phase technique was later introduced that proved to be equally simple but considerably more precise and reproducible. Purified C1q is immobilized in the wells of a microtiter plate, and when an adequate dilution of an IC-containing sample is added to the well, the IC will be bound to the immobilized C1q. To determine whether IC are bound to C1q, enzyme-labeled antihuman IgG antibodies are added to the wells; their fixation indicates a positive result (Figure 21.6).

D. The Raji Cell Assay

The Raji cell assay is another popular technique for IC detection. Raji cells (a lymphoblastoid cell line that can be indefinitely grown in culture) have receptors for C3b, C1q, and the Fc fragment of IgG (these last ones are quantitatively the least important) through which IC can be bound to their surface. The cells are incubated with IC-containing samples, and ^{125}I-labeled anti-immunoglobulin antiserum (reacting with all major Ig classes) is used to detect cell-bound IgG, which usually will correspond to complement-binding IC (Fig. 21.7). In spite of its popularity, the Raji cell assay has not been successfully introduced into clinical diagnostic laboratories for two main reasons: (1) to set up the assay requires the availability of tissue culture facilities and technical expertise to keep a cell line in continuous culture and to check the expression of surface receptors on the cells, and (2) antilymphocyte antibodies are a recognized cause of false positive results, and unfortunately these antibodies and soluble IC do often coexist in patients with autoimmune disorders.

E. Specific Immune-Complex Screening Tests

All the IC screening tests discussed above are nonspecific. The possibility of using specific tests, based on the detection of IC through their antigen or antibody moieties, is conceptually very attractive. Indeed, the probability of obtaining false positive results is greatly minimized by the use of specific tests,

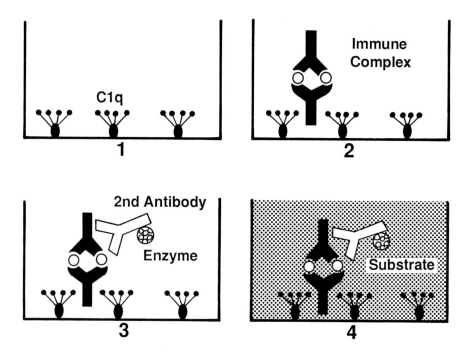

FIGURE 21.6 Diagrammatic representation of the principle of the C1q binding assay. Radiolabeled C1q will bind to IC containing IgG antibodies, and if those antigen-antibody complexes are precipitated (wth polyethylene glycol) the amount of coprecipitated C1q will be proportional to the IC concentration.

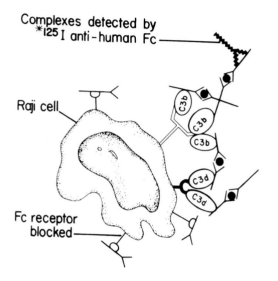

Complexes detected by
*125I anti-human Fc

Raji cell

C3b
C3b
C3b
C3d
C3d

Fc receptor
blocked

FIGURE 21.7 Diagrammatic representation of the Raji cell radioimmunoassay. The Raji cell has receptors for the Fc fragment and for C3b and C3d (predominant in number). The former account for a background binding and can be blocked with nonhuman IgG. Soluble IC will be bound by the cells through complement components and be detected using a radiolabeled antihuman Fc. (Reproduced with permission from Williams, R. C. *Immune Complexes in Clinical and Experimental Medicine.* Harvard Univ. Press, Cambridge, Massachusetts, 1980.)

which also have the advantage of measuring a parameter directly related to the pathogenesis of the disease. The main difficulty with this approach is the lack of knowledge concerning the antigen-antibody systems involved in a wide variety of immune complex diseases. However, if all the relevant antigen-antibody systems were to be identified, this would create a considerable problem for the use of specific tests, because the number of different tests required would be beyond practicality.

IV. THE ROLE OF IMMUNE COMPLEXES IN HUMAN DISEASE

Immune complexes have been implicated in human disease either through demonstration in serum or through identification in the tissues where lesions are found. Most often the antibody moiety of the immune complex is detected, and knowledge about the antigens involved is still very fragmentary. The World

Health Organization proposed a classification of IC disease according to the
nature of the antigens involved, but the classification was based on scanty documentation or on controversial data; however, this classification was one of the
first attempts to bring some order into a field whose rapid expansion has led to
a considerable degree of confusion. According to this classification, immune
complex diseases (ICD) are divided into the following groups according to the
identity of the antigens involved.

1. ICD *involving endogenous antigens*
   a. Immunoglobulin antigens, e.g., rheumatoid arthritis, Sjogren's syn-
      drome, hypergammaglobulinemic purpura
   b. Nuclear antigens, e.g., systemic lupus erythematosus
   c. Specific cellular antigens, e.g., tumors, autoimmune diseases
2. ICD *involving exogenous antigens*
   a. Iatrogenic antigens, e.g., serum sickness, drug allergy
   b. Environmental antigens (inhaled, e.g., extrinsic alveolitis;
      ingested, e.g., dermatitis herpetiformes)
   c. Antigens from infectious organisms
      1) Viral, e.g., hepatitis B, HIV infection, dengue hemorrhagic fever,
         essential cryoglobulinemia
      2) Bacterial, e.g., poststreptococcal glomerulonepthritis, leprosy,
         syphilis
      3) Protozoan, e.g., malaria, trypanosomiasis
      4) Helminthic, e.g., schistosomiasis, onchocerciasis
3. ICD *involving unknown antigens*
   In this category are included most forms of chronic immune-complex
   glomerulonephritis, vasculitis with or without eosinophilia, and many
   cases of mixed cryoglobulinemia.

The clinical expression of ICD varies according to the target organs where the
deposition of IC predominates (see Chapters 24 and 25). The kidney is very
frequently affected (systemic lupus erythematosus, mixed cryoglobulinemia,
chronic infections, chronic glomerulonephritis, Sjogren's syndrome, purpura
hypergammaglobulinemica, serum sickness, etc.), usually with glomerular damage as a predominating feature; the joints are predominantly affected in rheumatoid arthritis; the skin is affected in cases of serum sickness, mixed cryoglobulinemia and vasculitis; the lungs are affected in extrinsic alveolitis. The reasons
why the target organs can vary from disease to disease are not very clear. In
some cases it can be related to the exposure route (extrinsic alveolitis). The
kidneys, on the other hand, because of their physiological role and existence of
C3 and Fc receptors in different anatomical structures, appear to be an ideal
organ for IC trapping. In rheumatoid arthritis, IC appear to be present not only
in the circulation but also (and presumably formed) in and around the joints,

and although they do not appear to be the initiating factor for the disease, their potential for perpetuating the inflammatory lesions is unquestionable. The reasons why some IC are trapped in the skin and lead to vasculitis and, in some cases, ulcerative necrosis, are unknown.

V. THERAPEUTIC APPROACHES TO IMMUNE COMPLEX DISEASE

Basically, three types of therapeutic measures can be taken in cases of immune complex disease: removal of the antigen source (infections, tumors), suppression of antibody production (by using immunosuppressive drugs such as cyclophosphamide, azathioprine, or corticosteroids), and removal of IC by plasmapheresis.

Plasmapheresis consists of the removal of blood (up to 5 liters), separation and reinfusion of red cells, and replacement of the patient's plasma by normal plasma or plasma-replacing solutions. It has been found to be efficient in many IC diseases, hyperviscosity syndrome, autoimmune diseases, intoxications, etc. (see Table 21.2). In situations such as SLE and rheumatoid arthritis, plasmapheresis appears most beneficial when associated with immunosuppressive drugs; by itself it can even induce severe clinical deterioration perhaps related to changes in the immunoregulatory circuits. But we have found that, in conditions such as chronic vasculitis, plasmapheresis can be efficient by itself in reducing IC levels (Fig. 21.8), which is often associated with clinical improvement. The main drawbacks of plasmapheresis are its high cost (derived from the sophisticated equiment used and from the cost of plasma and plasma-replacing products) and the necessity of its being performed in a well-equipped medical center.

TABLE 21.2 Pathological Situations in Which Several Groups Have Reported Favorable Therapeutic Results with Plasmapheresis

Immune complex diseases
   SLE
   Rheumatoid arthritis
   Glomerulonephritis
Autoimmune diseases
   Myasthenia gravis
   Goodpasture's syndrome
Hypersensitivity states (nonautoimmune)
   Kidney transplant rejection
   Hemolytic disease of newborn
Excessive levels of normal substances
   Hyperviscosity syndromes
   Hyperlipemias
Intoxications
   Mushroom and methyl parathion poisoning

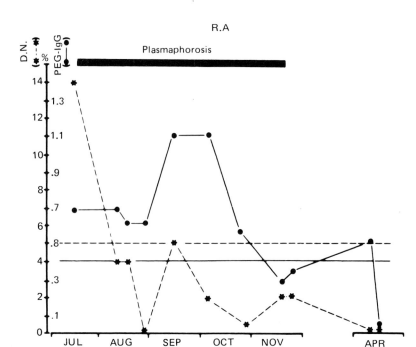

FIGURE 21.8   Plasmapheresis in a patient with chronic necrotizing vasculitis.
The patient has elevated levels of IC by two techniques, direct nephelometry
(DN) and PEG-IgG, upper normal levels for DN being indicated by broken horizontal line and for PEG-IgG by a horizontal solid line. After four months of
regular plasmapheresis, IC levels had normalized. A few months later a short
plasmapheresis course was sufficient to normalize the PEG-IgG test. The patient
improved clinically with the healing of ulcerative lesions in the dorsal aspect of
both feet.

SELF-EVALUATION

Questions

21.1   A patient injected with horse antirattlesnake venom serum complains of
general weakness, headaches, and muscular and joint pains and notices
that his urine is darker in color 10 days after the injection. A urine test
shows increased elimination of proteins. Laboratory tests show normal
immunoglobulin levels and low serum C4 and C3. The most likely cause
for this clinical situation is

A. Systemic reaction to snake venom released after the effects of the anti-toxin have disappeared.
B. Deposition of antigen-antibody complexes made of snake venom proteins and horse antibody.
C. Delayed hypersensitivity to horse proteins.
D. Anaphylactic reaction (type I) to snake venom.
E. Deposition of antigen-antibody complexes made of horse proteins and human immunoglobulins.

21.2 An IC screening test that will detect exclusively those complexes containing complement-fixing antibodies is
A. Platelet sedimentation test.
B. Raji cell assay.
C. PEG-protein A radioimmunoassay.
D. PEG-IgG test.
E. Cryoprecipitation.

21.3 Polymorphonuclear leukocytes may contribute to the development of inflammatory reactions by the release of all of the following except
A. Proteases.
B. Platelet activating factor.
C. Serotonin.
D. Cationic proteins.
E. Collagenase.

21.4 A frequent finding in the mixed cryoglobulins isolated from patients with essential mixed cryoglobulinemia is
A. DNA and/or anti-DNA antibodies.
B. Anti-insulin antibodies.
C. IgG "rheumatoid factor."
D. HBsAg and/or anti-HBsAg antibodies.
E. Streptococcal antigens.

21.5 C5a can have all of the following actions contributing to the development of inflammation except
A. Direct vasoactive properties.
B. Ability to degranulate basophils and mast cells.
C. Chemotactic capacity.
D. Induction of PMN aggregation.
E. Stimulation of serotonin release by platelets.

21.6 In humans, the increased vascular permeability that precedes extravascular deposition of IC may be a consequence of all of the following except
A. Direct effect of C5a.

412   Virella

B. Degranulation of basophils induced by C5a.
C. Release of PAF by basophils recognizing the antigen involved in IC formation through IgE antibodies.
D. Release of PAF by PMN leukocytes recognizing cell-bound IC.
E. Direct aggregation and stimulation of platelets by IC.

21.7 All of the following are considered as possible manifestations of IC disease except
A. Immune hemolytic anemia.
B. Glomerulonephritis.
C. Type I cryoglobulinemia.
D. Extrinsic alveolitis.
E. Vasculitis.

21.8 All of the following are true statements about cryoglobulins except
A. "Mixed" cryoglobulins usually correspond to cold-insoluble antigen-antibody complexes.
B. A positive cryoglobulin screening test can be considered as evidence for the presence of soluble circulating immune complexes.
C. IgG is found in virtually all mixed cryoglobulins.
D. C1q and/or C3 may be found in cryoprecipitates.
E. In a mixed cryoglobulin containing IgM and IgG, IgM usually is an anti-IgG antibody.

21.9 Factors associated with increased risk of development of immune complex disease include all of the following except
A. Strong immune response against the offending antigen.
B. Formation of immune complexes at antigen excess.
C. Blockade of RES.
D. Involvement of IgG1 and IgG3 in the formation of IC.
E. Release of vasoactive substances.

21.10 The Raji cell assay for soluble IC requires all of the following except
A. Raji cells in continuous culture.
B. Radiolabeled antihuman immunoglobulin antibodies.
C. A method to check the expression of C3b receptors on the cell surface.
D. Polyethylene glycol to separate cell-bound IC from cell-free aggregates.
E. Tissue-culture facilities.

Answers

21.1 (E)   This is a classical example of serum sickness. The horse antisnake venom serum will initially neutralize the poison, but enough horse serum proteins will be left in circulation to induce an immune response. As soon as antihorse protein antibodies are secreted, antigen-antibody complexes will be formed and their deposition will cause pathological symptoms, namely glomerulonephritis reflected by hematuria and proteinuria.

21.2 (B) The tests based on insolubilization of IC by cold temperatures or PEG are not specific for complement-fixing IC. Platelets interact with IC through an Fc receptor to which all IgG subclasses can bind, including IgG4, which does not activate complement. The Raji cell assay detects IC mainly through the C3b receptor.

21.3 (C) Serotonin is released by platelets.

21.4 (D)

21.5 (E) This is an action attributed to platelet activating factor (PAF).

21.6 (C) Human basophils do not synthesize PAF, and there is no evidence that IgE antibodies are produced as part of the sensitization process that result in the formation of soluble IC.

21.7 (C) Type I cryoglobulins are monoclonal proteins that precipitate at cold temperature and do not represent cold-insoluble IC.

21.8 (B) Only mixed cryoglobulins are considered to correspond to IC; a positive screening test for cryoglobulins has to be followed by the immunochemical characterization of the precipitated immunoglobulins before we can know whether the patient has a monoclonal or a mixed cryoglobulin.

21.9 (A) A strong immune response is usually associated with rapid elimination of the antigen without apparent consequences for the animal.

21.10(D) The separation of bound complement-fixing IC from free IgG and noncomplement-fixing IC is done by simple centrifugation and washing of the cells.

BIBLIOGRAPHY

Bielory, L., Gascon, P., Lawley, T. J., Young, N. S., and Frank, M. M. Human serum sickness: A prospective analysis of 35 patients treated with equine antithymocyte globulin for bone marrow failure. *Medicine 67*:40, 1988.
Cochrane, C. G. and Koffler, D. Immune complex disease in experimental animals and man. *Adv. Immunol. 16*:185, 1973.
Fearon, D. T. Complement, C receptors, and immune complex disease. *Hospital Practice 23*:63, 1988.

Germuth, F. G., Senterfit, L. B., and Pollack, A. D. Immune complex disease.
   I. Experimental acute and chronic glomerulonephritis. *Johns Hopkins Med.*
   J. 120:225, 1967.
Kimberly, R. P. Immune complexes in the rheumatic disease. *Rheum. Dis.*
   Clin. North. Am. 13:583, 1987.
Ng, Y. C. and Schifferli, J. A. Clearance of cryoglobulin in man. *Springer*
   Semin. Immunopathol. 10:75, 1988.
WHO Scientific Report No. 606: *The Pathological Role of Immune Complexes.*
   WHO, Geneva, 1977.
Williams, R. C. *Immune Complexes in Clinical and Experimental Medicine.*
   Harvard Univ. Press, Cambridge, Massachusetts, 1980.
Wilson, C. B. Immune aspects of renal disease. *J. Amer. Med. Assoc. 258*:2957,
   1987.
Virella, G. and Glassman, A. B. Apheresis, exchange, adsorption and filtration
   of plasma: Four approaches to the removal of undesirable circulating sub-
   stances. *Biomed. & Pharmacotherapy 40*:286, 1986.

22

Tolerance and Autoimmunity

CHRISTIAN C. PATRICK, JEAN-MICHEL GOUST, and GABRIEL VIRELLA

The understanding of how living organisms with fully developed immune systems differentiate between self and nonself is perhaps the most important issue of immunology. Paul Erlich in 1901 postulated that individuals tolerate their own tissues by not developing an immune response against the corresponding antigens, and coined the term *horror autotoxicus* to describe the innate state of unresponsiveness of any immunocompetent being against his own tissues. Erlich's hypothesis was apparently supported by the later definition of autoimmune disorders, in which a postulated breakdown or alteration of the immunoregulatory networks leads to the development of an antiself immune response that would be the cause of disease.

I. TOLERANCE

Tolerance can be best defined as a state of immunological unresponsiveness to a specific antigen consequent to the elimination or down-regulation of the immune cells able to recognize it. The first experimental observation of tolerance was made by Felton in 1942 when he showed that mice that could mount an immune response to small amounts of pneumococcal polysaccharide, with subsequent protection against a corresponding *Streptococcus pneumoniae* infection, would not be protected if amounts of pneumococcal polysaccharide in great excess of those required for immunization were injected.

One important point that must be made at the onset of this discussion is that tolerance is not synonymous with generalized immunosuppression. Tolerance is antigen-specific and causes no impairment of the immune response to other antigens, whereas in generalized immunosuppression there is a depression of the immune response to a wide array of different antigens. Tolerance may be transient or permanent, while immunosuppression is usually transient.

A. Natural and Acquired Tolerance: Tolerogenic Conditions

Tolerance may be natural or acquired. Natural tolerance is present at birth and has been classically explained by the clonal deletion theory and its modern revisions, whereby immune reactive clones to self antigens are eliminated or down-regulated during embryonic life. Acquired tolerance is observed mainly in adult animals. In acquired tolerance, the ability to achieve tolerance is related to several factors, including (1) the degree of structural homology or molecular mimicry between the antigen and the host, (2) the immunocompetence of the host, (3) the structure and configuration of the antigen, (4) the amount of the antigen used, (5) the route of antigen administration, and (6) the immunogenicity of the antigen.

The immunocompetence of the host varies physiologically according to age. In original experiments in 1945, Owen observed that bovine dizygotic twins could tolerate blood cells from each other even though they bore different serological specificities on their own red cells. In the bovine species, the fetuses share placentas, even if dizygotic. Thus the intermixing of blood groups between twins in utero leads to tolerance of each others' blood type. This condition of having two sets of genetically dissimilar cell types in one single animal is termed *chimerism*. These findings by Owen led Burnet along with Fenner and Medawar, in the 1940s, to hypothesize that self tolerance is achieved by the elimination of autoreactive clones as they develop. In 1953, Medawar showed that this type of tolerance could be experimentally induced. Using inbred mice with known genetic compositions, he injected lymphoid cells from one genetic strain of mice (strain A) into immunologically immature newborn mice of another genetic strain (CBA). He observed that CBA mice upon reaching adulthood and becoming immunologically mature could tolerate a skin graft from stain A. The major conclusion was that exposure to a given antigen during embryonic differentiation results in acquisition of long-lasting tolerance. A later extension of this concept relates to the observation that tolerance is easier to induce in animals whose degree of immunocompetence is artificially lowered (e.g., by drug-induced immunosuppression).

The general structure and configuration of the antigen is another important factor in the induction of a tolerant state. An antigen that induces tolerance is termed a *tolerogen*, and it has been observed that large or complex antigens are usually not tolerogenic, because they are phagocytosed and processed by macrophages, with subsequent presentation to immune cells in a form that is highly immunogenic. On the other hand, small soluble antigens may not be taken up by the macrophages and thus induce a state of tolerance more easily. A good example is shown by comparing the response to aggregates versus soluble monomers of a given protein. When aggregated proteins are injected, one usually elicits an active immune response. If, instead, all protein aggregates are removed from the suspension by high-speed centrifigation and only soluble protein monomers are injected, it is easier to achieve a state of tolerance. Finally, the greater the structural homology between the antigen and any endogenous protein of the host, the easier it is to induce tolerance.

The route of antigen administration is also crucial for the induction of a state of tolerance. Tolerance is achieved more easily when antigens are injected intravenously rather than intramuscularly or subcutaneously.

The immunogenicity of the antigen also plays an important role in the induction of tolerance. As a rule, it is extremely difficult or impossible to induce tolerance against a strong immunogen. This fact is obviously related to the degree of homology and chemical complexity of the antigen, but it is also related to the genetic constitution of the animal (some antigens are strongly immunogenic in a given species or strain and not in another).

B. High-Zone and Low-Zone Tolerance

In trying to induce tolerance in experimental animals it became evident that two broad types of tolerant states could be induced, according to antigen dosage (Table 22.1). Low-zone tolerance is induced with small amounts of antigen and appears to affect exclusively T cells. This T-cell tolerance is established quickly, is long-lasting, and is restricted to T-dependent antigens. Tolerance to self antigens is probably a form of low-zone tolerance. High-zone tolerance ("immune paralysis") is induced with any type of antigen given in very high dosage, and it affects both T and B cells.High-zone tolerance has a slow onset and a short duration._

TABLE 22.1 Main Characteristics of Low- and High-Zone Tolerance

	Low-zone tolerance	High-zone tolerance
Cells affected	T cells	T and B cells
Onset	Immediate	Delayed
Duration	Long	Brief
Antigen	T-dependent	Any type

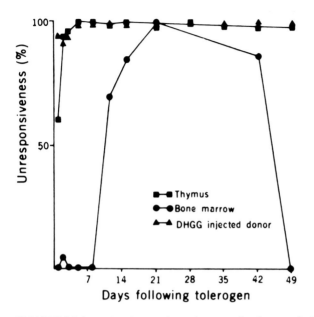

FIGURE 22.1 Induction and persistence of tolerance in B- and T-cell populations. Thymus (T) and bone marrow (B) cells were removed at various times
from mice rendered tolerant with 2.5 mg of deaggregated human globulin (HGG,
the tolerogen) and were tested, with complementary cells from normal donors,
for the ability to cooperate in Ab formation when transferred to irradiated syngeneic mice subsequently challenged with 0.4 mg of aggregated HGG. Results
are given as percentages of antibody levels obtained in controls using untreated
donors as cell sources. Tolerance appeared sooner and lasted longer in T than in
B cells. (Reproduced with permission from Chiller, J. M., Habicht, A. S., and
Weigle, W. O. *Science 171*:813, 1971.)

The basic differences between low- and high-zone tolerance are illustrated by
the classic studies of Weigle and co-workers. They injected various doses of
monomeric human or bovine gamma globulin into adult mice. Thymic tissue
(T-cells) and bone marrow (B-cells) were obtained both from HGG-injected mice
(at specific time intervals following the injections) and from noninjected mice,
mixed in various combinations, and transfused into irradiated (immunoincompetent) recipients. The reconstituted mice were then challenged with the corresponding antigen on the same day of the cell transfusion and boosted again with
the same antigen on day 10. A few days after the boost, the mice were sacri-
ficed and their spleens observed for antibody-producing cells by a plaque-form-
ing cell procedure. Both T- and B-cell tolerance could be demonstrated, with the
difference that T-cell tolerance was induced at lower antigen concentrations than

B-cell tolerance and, as shown in Figure 22.1, becomes apparent faster and lasted longer.

C. Theories Concerning the Induction of Tolerance

Many theories have been postulated to explain the induction of tolerance. The most well-accepted include

(1)   Clonal deletion or inactivation,
(2)   Effector-cell blockade,
(3)   Production of blocking antibodies, and
(4)   Anti-idiotypic down-regulation.

The clonal deletion theory is based on the principle described by Burnet as outlined earlier in this chapter. In its original version, the theory proposed that the autoreactive clones were actually eliminated during embryonic differentiation.

This theory had the advantage of simplicity, but it was discredited by the findings of low levels of autoreactive antibodies in almost all healthy individuals and by the demonstration of the existence of many autoreactive clones in adult experimental animals. Still, the fact remains that no autoimmunity to the ABO system or the major circulating serum proteins (with the exception of immunoglobulins) has ever been reported, and this could be interpreted as meaning that for some major antigens clonal deletion may actually be operative. This possibility finds experimental support in studies suggesting that clonal deletion is not an all-or-nothing phenomenon but rather affects predominantly clones of cells interacting with self determinants with high avidity, while sparing low avidity cells, which in normal conditions may be down-regulated as a consequence of antigen recognition.

It is however unquestionable that autoreactive clones persist after embryonic differentiation. One of the best-studied examples is the persistence in normal adults of the sets of immunoglobulin V region genes encoding the antigen-binding sites of autoantibodies reacting with autologous IgG (discussed in more detail in Chapter 25). This led to the emergence of a variety of theories concerning clonal inactivation or down-regulation. The most popular among these are based on the activity of antigen-specific suppressor T cells. These theories assume that any antigen has the potential of specifically activating suppressor cell clones that will suppress the immune response to that specific antigen. Experimental animal studies have suggested that the suppression of contact sensitivity is mediated by one or more soluble substances released by suppressor T cells, which are not immunoglobulins but can bind to an antigen, preventing the stimulation of delayed hypersensitivity. However, none of these substances has ever been purified to homogeneity, nor have their genes been isolated. The lack of contrasuppressor T cells has also been suggested as a possible cause for the hyperactivity of suppressor T cells in tolerance. Finally, some authors have proposed that tolerance is a consequence of the inactivation of helper T cells by exposure to unprocessed self antigens not associated to MHC molecules. Under these conditions the signal provided by the interaction between the T cell receptor and the self antigen would be weak, and rather than trigger activation it would down-regulate the reactive T cell. The major problems with these theories stem from the lack of absolute proof for existence of some of these cell populations (particularly the suppressor and contrasuppressor subpopulations) and the difficulty in devising adequate experiments to test them in humans.

The effector cell blockade theory is based on the need for optimal conditions in the interaction between surface immunoglobulins on B cells and the corresponding antigens for B cells to be properly stimulated. The normal B-cell activation sequence starts with the reaction of an immunogenic molecule with specific membrane immunoglobulins. As a result of the interaction, the membrane immunoglobulin molecules are cross-linked and form aggregates that appear as patches by immunofluorescence. These aggregates then migrate to the pole of the cell surface, forming caps, and are finally internalized. This progression of events causes the cell to undergo differentiation. The B-cell receptor blockade theory postulates that large amounts of antigens with repetitive subunits (such as polysaccharides) bind to the membrane immunoglobulin but inhibit capping; in the absence of capping the immune response is not efficiently triggered. This theory explains some forms of experimentally induced tolerance, but it is difficult to generalize to physiological tolerance.

A third theory favors the production of blocking factors. This theory, which evolves from tumor immunology studies, is based on three separate theories, (1) the formation of antigen-antibody complexes blocking antigen receptors of immune cells or leading to the rapid elimination of the antigen, (2) the blocking of antigenic sites on target tissues, thereby not allowing the antigen to react with T cells, and/or (3) the activation and proliferation of suppressor T cells as a consequence of the formation of soluble immune complexes with the corresponding antigen. These theories are not mutually exclusive, but like the effector cell blockade theory they seem better suited to explain special cases of tolerance (or unresponsiveness) than the broader problem of physiological tolerance.

The fourth theory is based on the possible regulatory effects of anti-idiotypic immune responses. When an immunogen is introduced into a host it stimulates specific T and B cells whose antigen receptors have specific idiotypic determinants (here designated as X) associated with the particular structure of the hypervariable regions. This stimulation induces the proliferation of T- and B-cell clones carrying idiotype X, which in turn may induce the response of lymphocytes able to recognize specifically idiotype X. B-cell clones will produce anti-X-idiotypic antibody (against idiotype X), and such antibody can in turn depress the activity of B cells producing antibody with idiotype X or even "delete" such B-cell clones. T-cell clones stimulated by idiotype X may include specific suppressor cells able to turn off the response of cells carrying this idiotype in their antigen receptors. Both mechanisms have, at least theoretically, the capacity to down-regulate the immune response, tolerance being an extreme manifestation of such down-regulation. This theory is intellectually very attractive, but in the absence of good experimental evidence to support it or disprove it, its supporters and detractors use arguments based on concepts rather than on facts.

There is no question that a state of physiological tolerance is established during embryonic differentiation towards self antigens (including any nonself antigens to which the animal might be exposed at that crucial stage, which will in fact be handled as self), but the mechanisms remain unexplained. First of all, the exposure of the immune system of the developing embryo follows most of the rules that would be expected to result in tolerance, i.e., constant exposure to small concentrations of soluble or cellular antigens, which are, for the most part, structurally similar to antigens present in the immunocyte itself. The process of tolerance induction, nevertheless, appears to involve the recognition of antigenic differences in self tissues. Newborn mice of some strains, for example, appear to be actively involved in autoimmune processes; however, the outcome of the response is not disease but rather the control of autoreactive clones. Such control is likely to be achieved by a variety of mechanisms. Clonal deletion may eliminate a number of potentially dangerous clones, and other down-regulating mechanisms may control the nondeleted clones. Anti-idiotypic responses (both cellular and humoral), lack of help, and specific suppression may all play important roles. Actually, the different theories concerning the generation of physiological tolerance do not need to be mutually exclusive. It may be that tolerance to self, being such a crucial requirement for the survival of the individual, is established and maintained by a variety of mechanisms. The importance of understanding as much as possible about the mechanisms leading to physiological tolerance to self is obvious, given the potential applications of this type of knowledge to the management of organ transplants and of autoimmune disorders.

D. Termination of Tolerance

Experimentally induced tolerance can often be terminated as a consequence of (1) a prolonged lack of stimulation with the tolerogen or (2) immunization with a cross-reacting antigen. In the first case, since new B and T cells are constantly being produced from stem cells, if a tolerogenic dose of antigen is not maintained, the immune system will eventually recover the ability to mount an immune response. In the second case, T helper cells specific for the cross-reacting antigen are activated and help B cells to respond against the tolerogen.

A transient break of tolerance can be induced by transfusion of cells from a normal donor to a syngeneic tolerant recipient, but tolerance will reappear when the responding cells reach the end of their lifespan.

II. AUTOIMMUNITY

A. Theoretical Background

Autoimmunity is defined as an immune response directed against self antigens. In other words, autoimmunity appears to be due to a breakdown in self tolerance. Six main theories have been advanced to explain the origin of autoimmunity. These theories are

1. The sequestered antigen theory,
2. The forbidden clone theory,
3. The altered antigen theory,
4. The cross-reaction theory,
5. The viral infection theory, and
6. The polyclonal B-cell activation theory.

The premise of the sequestered antigen theory is that certain antigens are not accessible to the immune system because of their anatomical distribution. Thus no opportunity is given for these antigens to establish tolerance in fetal life. Antigens on tissues such as the CNS, the thyroid, spermatozoa, and the lens of the eye were thought to be sequestered, normally not exposed to immunocompetent cells. If during a disease process these tissues release antigens into the blood stream an immune reaction would occur. By its very nature, this theory can account for only some specific and individualized types of tolerance, and the true sequestered nature of many of these antigens can be questioned. Thyroglobulin, for example, can be detected in very small concentrations in the serum of normal individuals.

The forbidden clone theory, part of the clonal selection theory of Burnet, postulates that normally, autoreactive clones are eliminated (or down-regulated by a variety of mechanisms, according to modern revisions of the theory) during differentiation. If these clones are not eliminated, or if the down-regulating mechanisms fail, self-reactive clones can mount an autoimmune response. An example of this theory is the current explanation for tolerance to thyroglobulin. As stated previously, small amounts of this protein are released into the circulation, leading to low-zone tolerance. An autoimmune reaction to thyroglobulin could take place if the balance of suppressor/helper cells were disturbed as a consequence of some exogenous factor (e.g., bacterial or viral infection) leading to activation of autoreactive clones.

Tolerance can be abrogated by altering the antigenic structure of a tolerogen, which would allow an autoimmune reaction to occur. Such a mechanism has been proposed as the cause of autoimmune hemolytic anemia in patients treated with α-methyldopa. This drug (or its metabolic products) is believed to alter the configuration of red-cell antigens in a manner not fully understood, but which elicits an autoimmune response. However, the resulting antibodies react with red-cell antigens in the absence of the drug, behaving as true autoantibodies (see Chapter 20). In other words, the drug must change the red-cell antigens to the extent that the immune response is triggered, but the resulting antibodies cross-react with unmodified red-cell antigens. Similar mechanisms may explain the onset of autoimmune diseases after viral infections. The virus directly or indirectly may modify surface antigens of the infected cells, with a resulting immune response that is cross-reactive with the antigens expressed by normal, uninfected cells.

The possibility that some autoimmune diseases may result from cross-reacting immune responses appears as most likely. As discussed earlier, cross-reactions may result from the modification of an endogenous antigen. In other cases, the cross-reaction may be fortuitous, a result of the sharing of chemical structures between human cells and common pathogens. Two well-known examples of this latter possibility may be mentioned. One is the cross-reaction observed between certain strains of group A *Streptococcus* and myocardium, responsible for the carditis associated to rheumatic fever. Another is the enteropathy that develops in some individuals who become sensitized to gluten; the immune response originally directed to gluten eventually affects the intenstinal cells, which have an antigen sharing an eight-amino acid oligopeptide with gluten. In experimental animals, the induction of arthritis in rats using complete Freund's adjuvant (adjuvant arthritis) is believed to result from an immune response primarily directed against a particular epitope of *Mycobacterium tuberculosis* that cross-reacts with the cartilage's proteoglycan; the induction of experimental autoimmune encephalomyletis by injecting heterologous brain tissue homogenates emulsified in Freund's adjuvant elicits cross-reactive antibodies against myelin basic protein.

This "molecular mimicry" could be more frequent than initially suspected and is accessible to direct testing. With the accumuation of amino acid sequence data for many viral and bacterial antigens it is possible to compare their primary structure to that of many known self antigens and to test the hypothesis that an autoimmune response may develop in individuals who are high responders to shared oligopeptides.

Studies in animals that develop spontaneous autoimmunity have shown that the appearance of autoantibodies coincides with a state of generalized B-cell hyperactivity involving both autoreactive clones and clones recognizing heterologous antigens. Thus it has been proposed that autoimmunity may develop as a consequence of uncontrolled polyclonal B-cell activation. The mechanism of this B-cell hyperactivity is not known but may involve a biased ontogeny (1) favoring B-cell subsets particularly prone to the production of autoantibodies, (2) deleting subsets involved in maintaining tolerance, or (3) preserving subsets able to respond strongly to the association with class II MHC. Human parallels can be found in systemic lupus erythematosus (see Chapter 24) and the graft-vs.-host disease (see Chapter 26). In both situations there is evidence of polyclonal B-cell activation and autoimmunity, usually associated with increased helper-T-cell activity.

B. Viral Infections and Autoimmunity

Viral infections are believed to be the basis of at least some autoimmune diseases, and the proposed mchanisms may be divided into two groups according to the effect of the virus on the host cell.

1. The Viral Infection Causes Cell Death

As a consequence of cell death, normally sequestered intracellular antigens are released and induce an immune response. One of the few examples in which this mechanism may be operative is autoimmune myocarditis associated with coxsackie B3 virus. The viral infection leads to myocardial cell necrosis, the release of intracellular constituents, and the development of autoantibodies reactive with sarcolemma and myofibril antigens, which are associated to the development of persistent myocarditis. In this group one should also include the occurrence of molecular mimicry between the envelope of some viruses and the myelin of the peripheral nerves, which may explain the association of the Guillain-Barre syndrome with specific viral infections. Since the autoimmune manifestations in these two examples occur only in some of the infected individuals, it is necessary to postulate that genetic factors may control the extent to which cross-reacting antigens are recognized.

2. The Viral Infection is Nonlytic

Latent viral infections, associated with undetectable cytotoxicity and minimal or nonexistent clinical symptoms directly attributable to the infection, are thought to be responsible for the development of many autoimmune disorders. Latent infection is commonly associated to integration of the viral genome into the host chromosomes, and while integrated viruses very seldom enter a full replicative cycle, they can interfere, directly or indirectly, with the structure or expression of self antigens. For example, T-cell activation by an unknown nonlytic virus has been proposed to explain the onset of autoimmune thyroiditis. The infection would lead to T-cell activation and, as a consequence, to the release of interferon γ and tumor necrosis factor, which are known to be potent inducers of class II MHC antigen expression. The increased expression of class II MHC antigens in the thyroid gland could favor the onset of an autoimmune response, because the autoantigens would be expressed by cells with high densities of MHC II molecules that can function very effectively as antigen-presenting cells.

Finally, it has been postulated that anti-idiotypic immune responses may play an important role in autoimmunity (Fig. 22.2). A first possibility is that during a normal immune response to a virus (for example) antibodies against the viral structures mediating attachment to its target cell are formed. As the immune response evolves, anti-idiotypic antibodies reacting with the antigen-binding site of the antiviral antibodies will develop. These anti-idiotypes, by recognizing the "internal image of the antigen" (which is the configuration of the binding site of the first antibody) yield antibodies whose configuration is similar to the viral structure recognized by the first antibody. Therefore, the anti-idiotype may be able to combine with the virus receptor protein in the cell. If the membrane protein recognized by the virus happens to be a receptor with important physiological functions, the synthesis of anti-idiotypic antibodies may have adverse effects. For example, if the anti-idiotypes react with the acetylcholine receptor or the TSH receptor, they may cause either cell death or cell stimulation, depending upon the isotype of the anti-idiotype and the epitopes recognized by the anti-idiotype antibody on the receptor (Fig. 22.2). Another way in which anti-idiotypes could promote the emergence of autoimmune responses is by depleting suppressor cells involved in the control of autoreactive clones. It has also been postulated, as a third alternative, that autoantibodies could be derived from the stimulation of autoreactive immunocompetent cells whose membrane immunoglobulines or TcR shared idiotypes with an antibody originally directed against an infectious agent (cross-reactive idiotypes).

C. The Pathogenesis of Tissue Damage in Experimental Models of Autoimmunity

Animal models of autoimmune diseases offer opportunities to investigate the relative roles of humoral and cellular immunity in the pathogenesis of tissue damage. It is now established beyond doubt that the passive transfer of autoantibodies can, at best, cause very transient pathological changes. To reproduce the disease in a normal animal, it is necessary passively to transfer syngeneic sensitized T cells; the cellular population responsible has been identified as antigen-activated $CD4^+$ T cells (which can induce disease even when the number of transferred cells is very small). One of the first abnormalities seen after T-cell transfer is an increased expression of Ia antigen by the vascular endothelium or by cells of the target organ itself. This is rapidly followed by the appearance of a T-cell infiltrate in the target organ. The obvious interpretation is that

I=Production of Anti-Virus Antibodies

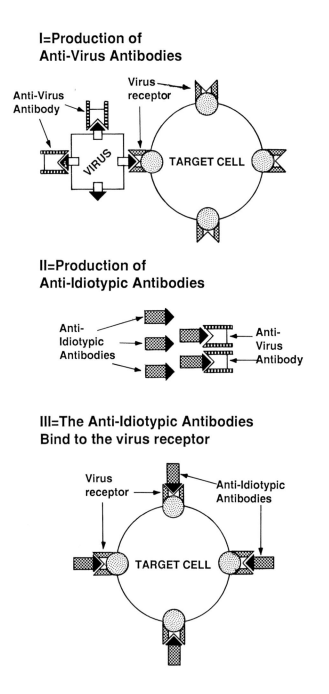

II=Production of Anti-Idiotypic Antibodies

III=The Anti-Idiotypic Antibodies Bind to the virus receptor

antigen-activated T cells lead to the increased expression of MHC II antigens, favoring the onset of an autoimmunity in the normal recipient of the T-cell transfer. This interpretation is supported by the successful prevention of the disease by preadministering monoclonal antibodies against Ia antigens to the recipient animals. Pretreatment with monoclonal antibodies against the CD4 antigen have similar effects, which is not surprising if MHC II and CD4 have to interact in order for helper T cells to be properly activated. Finally, in experimental animals it has been possible to prevent the onset of experimental autoimmune encephalomyelitis by passive transfer of suppressor T cells harvested from in-vitro-grown suppressor T-cell lines. This last approach could find application in humans if human suppressor-cell lines were successfully established.

D. Autoimmunity in Humans

A wide variety of diseases, some of which will be discussed in the following chapters, have been classified as having an autoimmune etiology. This assumption is usually based on the finding of autoreactive antibodies absent in the majority of healthy controls.

1. Induction of Autoimmune Responses in Humans

How are autoantibodies generated in humans? It is impossible to answer with certainty or to encompass all autoimmune diseases within a single theory. Some theories, however, are better fitted to our factual knowledge than others.

The deletion of autoreactive clones, for example, would appear as a most likely mechanism to explain why autoimmunity directed against the ABO antigens or the majority of the circulating serum proteins (with the exception of immunoglobulins) has never been reported. However, there are many examples of autoantibodies found in low titers in healthy individuals (such as anti-immunoglobulin antibodies and antinuclear antibodies) without obvious patho-

---

FIGURE 22.2 Schematic representation of the mechanisms responsible for the development of autoimmunity as a consequence of the synthesis of anti-idiotypic antibodies. Panel I: during an immune response to a virus, antibodies are produced that react with the viral structures that mediate binding to target cells. Panel II: later during the immune response, antidiotypic antibodies directed against the antigen-binding site of the first antibody are synthesized. Panel III: the anti-idiotypic antibodies recognize an "internal image" of the antigenic site recognized by the first antibody, which is the virus receptor in the target cell. As a consequence of the structural homology, the anti-idiotypic antibody can bind to the same structure as the virus.

logical consequences. Thus, clonal deletion, if it exists, does not eliminate all autoreactive clones, many of which will persist during adult life.

If one accepts that autoreactive clones are always present, but their activity controlled, the key to understanding autoimmunity is to elucidate the mechanisms whereby autoreactive clones are activated. For many years it was believed that most antigens recognized in autoimmune responses were *sequestered antigens*, normally shielded from the immune system. Most sequestered antigens have been shown to be accessible to the immune system in normal healthy individuals. However, the uveal structures of the eye and the spermatozoa are still held by some as examples of sequestered antigens. In the case of uveal antigens, it is known that after a penetrating injury to one eye an acute uveal inflammation of the uninjured eye may develop (sympathetic ophthalmia), and although classically this has been considered as an example of autoimmunity triggered by the exposure of normally sequestered antigens, by no means is there unanimity concerning this disease. In the case of spermatozoa it has been proposed that the appearnce of antispermatozoa antibodies after vasectomy is triggered by surgical trauma, exposing these normally sequestered cells to the immune system. Given how few of the diseases classified as autoimmune can be explained as a result of the release of sequestered antigens, it is obvious that other pathogenic mechanisms are involved in the vast majority of those diseases.

Three basic mechanisms (not mutually exclusive) have been proposed to explain the onset of most autoimmune diseases; (1) immune responses primarily directed against altered self that are triggered by abnormally increased expression of class II MHC antigens in the target tissues; (2) immune responses against microbial antigens, resulting in the stimulation of autoreactive clones as a consequence of cross-reactivities between self and microbial antigens and between self and altered self, and (3) inordinate proliferation of autoreactive clones (perhaps triggered by microbial antigens and mitogens) in patients with unbalanced help/suppression (as a consequence of either helper-cell hyperactivity or suppressor-cell hypoactivity).

2. Pathogenic Role of Autoimmune Responses

From a general standpoint of autoimmunity it is useful to separate acute from chronic diseases. In the first case a chance encounter with a pathogen inducing a cross-reacting immune response may have very damaging consequences, but if the patient survives and the infectious agent is eliminated, the manifestations of autoimmunity will also disappear (for example, the production of cold anti-red-cell antibodies in patients with infections by *Mycoplasma pneumoniae* will cease once the infectious agent is eliminated). The development of a chronic autoimmune disease that will last for the rest of the patient's life requires a more complex set of preexisting abnormalities, such as the expression of specific

HLA antigens or the existence of abnormalities in the T- or B-cell repertoires that lead to the development of permanent autoimmunity.

3. The Role of Autoantibodies

The detection of autoantibodies does not necessarily mean that they are responsible for pathological changes in the patient. Autoantibodies are obviously of primary importance in autoimmune hemolytic anemia, in which they are primarily responsible for the disease. In other circumstances, such as in myasthenia gravis, the autoantibodies may mediate the symptoms. For example, the transplacental transfer of autoantibodies to the acetylcholine receptor from a myasthenic mother to her newborn induces transient myasthenia in a relatively small percentage of the newborns. The symptoms in the newborn last only as long as the antibodies, the children do not become myasthenic. In other cases, the pathogenic role of autoanitbodies is open to question. For example, it is unquestionable that clinically identical forms of rheumatoid arthritis can be found in patients with and without rhematoid factor, and even in agammaglobulinemic patients. It is also difficult to interpret the meaning of autoantibodies found in asymptomatic relatives of patients with autoimmune diseases and of autoantibodies apparently unrelated to clinical symptoms in patients with multiple autoantibodies.

However, even if the direct pathogenic role of an autoantibody is ambiguous, an indirect pathogenic role is possible. The best example of indirect pathogenic effects of autoantibodies is provided by lupus glomerulonephritis, which has been proven to be caused by the deposition of immune complexes formed by nucleic acids and the corresponding autoantibodies. It is also possible that immune complexes involving autoantibodies may play a significant role in inducing alterations in immunoregulatory circuits that could result in intensification of autoimmune responses.

4. The Role of Cell-Mediated Immune Responses

Mononuclear cell infiltrates characteristic of a CMI reaction are frequently observed in many autoimmune diseases such as thyroiditis and pernicious anemia. In most instances, the infiltrates contain a large majority of $CD4^+$ cells, but the presence of $CD8^+$ cells suggests that cytotoxic T cells play a pathogenic role. Since it is necessary to study their possible role by testing cells obtained from tissue biopsies, their contribution to the development of the lesions is difficult to establish. However, the presence of IL2 receptors on a large percentage of the $CD4^+$ cells can be interpreted as direct evidence of their activation in situ, which should be associated with interferon γ secretion and increased expression of class II HLA antigens. Whether this postulated sequence of events actually occurs is under investigation.

SELF-EVALUATION

Questions

Choose the one best answer.

22.1 In low zone tolerance,
A. T lymphocytes are predominantly affected.
B. Both T and B lymphocytes are unresponsive.
C. Only B lymphocytes are unresponsive.
D. The duration of the tolerant state is relatively short.
E. A, B, and D are correct.

22.2 To induce tolerance, you would prefer to immunize with
A. Aggregated antigens, intradermally.
B. Aggregated antigens, intramuscularly.
C. Aggregated antigens, intravenously.
D. Deaggregated antigens, intramuscularly.
E. Deaggregated antigens, intravenously.

22.3 Tolerance due to clonal inactivation is likely to be
A. Reversible, if suppressor function becomes deficient.
B. Irreversible, due to the elimination of autoreactive clones.
C. Irreversible, due to lack of antigen processing.
D. Irreversible, due to antigen-specific helper-T-cell deficiency.
E. Irrelevant in human autoimmunity.

22.4 In an animal made tolerant to low doses of dinitrophenyl (DNP)-BGG, the injection of an immunogenic dose of nitrophenyl acetyl (NP)-BGG will be followed by
A. No apparent response to either NP or BGG.
B. Antibody response to NP only.
C. Antibody response to BGG only.
D. Antibody response to NP and BGG.
E. Antibody response to NP, DNP, and BGG.

22.5 Tolerance to self antigens is favored by all of the following factors except
A. Continuous exposure to low doses of circulating antigen.
B. Soluble nature of noncellular endogenous antigens.
C. Exposure to endogenous antigens during the differentiation of the immune system.
D. Cross-reaction with microbial antigens.
E. Adequate suppressor-T-cell function.

22.6 Carditis associated with rheumatic fever is believed to be caused by
A. High titers of rheumatoid factor

B. Anti-HLA antibodies.

C. Antibodies to group A *Streptococcus* that cross-react with heart structures.

D. Deposition of immune complexes.

E. NK cells reacting with the myocardium.

22.7 An animal injected with 2 μg of DNP-BSA intravenously while immunosuppressed with cyclophosphamide fails to show antibody responses to either DNP or BSA. Cyclophosphamide is stopped and two weeks later the animal is challenged with 2 mg of DNP-HGG mixed with complete Freund's adjuvant intramuscularly. Ten days later you are able to detect antibodies to HGG but not to DNP. The best interpretation for this would be that

A. The B cells of this animal are tolerant to DNP.

B. The animal is congenitally unresponsive to DNP.

C. The animal is still immunosuppressed.

D. The helper T cells of this animal are tolerant to DNP.

E. There is no memory for DNP in the animal.

In Questions 22.8-22.10, match the numbered phase with the letter heading that is most closely related to it. The same heading may be used once, more than once, or not at all.

(A) Anti-idiotype antibodies;

(B) Anti-isotype antibodies;

(C) Cross-reactive antibodies;

(D) Sequestered antigens;

(E) Modified antigenicity.

22.8 α-methyldopa-induced hemolytic anemia.

22.9 Sympathetic ophthalmia.

22.10 Guillain-Barre syndrome.

Answers

22.1 (A) Low-zone tolerance (induced with small concentrations of antigen) affects predominantly T cells and is of long duration.

22.2 (E)

22.3 (A) Modern theories for clonal inactivation postulate that suppressor-cell activity predominates over helper-T-cell activity, turning off the immune response. If suppressor function becomes deficient (through a variety of mechanisms), autoimmune clones may become activated. Lack of processing of a given antigen may be an important factor leading to tolerance; however, this is not an inherent deficiency but rather a consequence of the characteristic of the antigen.

22.4   (A)   The animal is tolerant to BGG, and its T cells will not assist the NP-responding B cells.

22.5   (D)   The cross-reactivity with microbial antigens is actually believed to be an important factor leading to loss of tolerance.

22.6   (C)   Rheumatic fever is believed to be an example of cross-reactive autoimmunity. Some strains of group A *Streptococcus* elicit antibodies that cross-react with heart tissues, leading to the development of the cardiac lesions characteristic of the disease. The arthritis component is more likely to be due to the deposition of immune complexes.

22.7   (B)   B-cell tolerance is of shorter duration than T-cell tolerance and is unlikely to be involved in the situation described. The help from helper T cells is not specific and can assist any carrier-responding T cells. Memory is not a factor in this experiment, because there was also no priming with HGG and a response was obtained. Similarly, the fact that a response to HGG was obtained argues against persistence of an immunosuppressed state. Therefore, if the animal could respond to the carrier, there is no reason why an antihapten response should not be elicited unless the animal was genetically unable to respond to DNP.

22.8   (E)   α-methyldopa is believed to modify the antigenicity of red cells and lead to the formation of antibodies that actually react very well with unmodified red cells, so that the reaction will persist even when the patient is off the medication.

22.9   (D)

22.10 (E)   The Guillain-Barre syndrome is believed to result from an autoimmune response triggered by the cross-reactivity between viral envelope antigens and neuronal cells.

BIBLIOGRAPHY

Ada, G. L. and Rose, N. R. The initiation and early development of autoimmune diseases. *Clinical Immunology and Immunopathology 41*:3, 1988.

Ciba Foundation Symposium 129. *Autoimmunity and Autoimmune Disease*. John Wiley & Sons, New York, 1987. (The proceedings of an excellent conference with many outstanding contributions and discussion transcripts.)

Cohen, I. R. The self, the world and autoimmunity. *Scientific American*, April 1988, p. 52.

Klein, J. *Immunology: The Science of Self-Nonself Discrimination.* John Wiley & Sons, New York, 1982.

Moller, G. (Ed). Mechanisms of B lymphocyte tolerance. *Immunological Reviews*, Vol. 43, 1979.

Waldman, T. A., Blaese, R., Broder, S. and Krakauer, R. S. NIH conference: Disorders of suppressive immunoregulatory cells in the pathogenesis of immunodeficiency and autoimmunity. *Ann. Intern. Med. 88*:226, 1978.

Weigle, W. O. Immunologic tolerance and immunopathology. In *The Biology of Immunologic Disease*, F. J. Dixon and D. W. Fisher (Eds.). Sinauer, Sunderland, Massachusetts, 1983, p. 107.

23

Organ-Specific Autoimmune Diseases

CHRISTIAN C. PATRICK

Autoimmune diseases can be divided into organ-specific and systemic, based both on the extent of their involvement and on the type of autoantibodies present in the patients. The systemic forms of autoimmune diseases are best exemplified by systemic lupus erythematosus (SLE) and rheumatoid arthritis (RA), which will be discussed in later chapters. The major autoimmune diseases, their target organs, and their associated autoantibodies are listed in Table 23.1. It is obvious from the table that autoimmune processes may affect virtually every organ system; in many instances only certain cell types within an organ system will be affected in a particular disease, e.g., gastric parietal cells in pernicious anemia.

In this chapter we shall restrict our discussion to the major autoimmune diseases that affect specific organs, and the associated autoantibodies, with the understanding that it is not clear whether these antibodies are the cause of the disease or just secondary manifestations. Whatever the role of autoantibodies might be, the basis of many autoimmune diseases appears to be an aberration of some aspect of immune regulation apparently resulting in excessive production of autoantibodies. In this perspective, autoimmune disease are truly diseases of immunologic aberration, probably determined genetically (by immune response genes?), as suggested by the associations between several autoimmune diseases and specific HLA haplotypes, often involving class II antigens.

TABLE 23.1   Representative Examples of Organ-Specific and Systemic Autoimmune Diseases

Disease	Tissue	Antibodies mainly against
Organ-specific diseases		
Graves' Disease	Thyroid	TSH receptor
Hashimoto's thyroiditis	Thyroid	Thyroglobulin
Myasthenia gravis	Muscle	Acetylcholine receptors
Pernicious anemia	Gastric parietal cells	Gastric parietal cells, Intrinsic factor (IF), B_{12}-IF complex
Addison's disease	Adrenals	Adrenal cells
Insulin-dependent diabetes mellitus	Pancreas	Pancreatic islet cells
Primary biliary cirrhosis	Liver	Mitochondrial antigens
Pemphigus	Skin and mucosae	Intercellular matrix of skin and mucosae
Bullous pemphigoid skin	Skin and mucosae	Basement membranes of skin and mucosae
Autoimmune hemolytic anemia	RBC	RBCs
Idiopathic thrombocytopenic purpura	Platelets	Platelets
Systemic diseases		
Systemic lupus erythematosus	Kidney, skin,	Nuclear antigens, microsomes
Rheumatoid arthritis	Joints	IgG, nuclear antigens
Sjogren's syndrome	Salivary and lacrimal glands	Nucleolar mitochondria,
Goodpasture's syndrome	Lungs, kidneys	Basement membranes

I. THYROID GLAND

Autoimmune factors have been implicated in a hyperthyroid disease, Graves'
disease, and a hypothyroid state, Hashimoto's disease. Graves' disease, also
known as diffuse toxic goiter and exophthalmic goiter, is the result of the
production of thyroid-stimulating antibodies. Such antibodies, of which the
long-acting thyroid stimulator (LATS) was the first described, are some of the
best examples of antireceptor antibodies; they are found in 80-90% of patients
with the disease. The nomenclature and definition of those antibodies is somewhat confusing, because in most cases it is based on a given assay method developed for their detection rather than on a proper structural and functional

evaluation, but it appears well established that true thryoid stimulating anti-bodies (TSI) have the capacity to stimulate the production of thryoid hormones by activating the adenylate cyclase system after binding to the thyrotrophic hormone (TSH) receptor. These antibodies are usually IgG.

Graves' disease presents with diffuse goiter and, in 60-70% of patients, with ocular disturbances. It has its peak incidence in the third or fourth decade and has a female-to-male ratio of 4-8:1. Patients have symptoms of hyperthyroid-ism, e.g., increased metabolic rate with weight loss, nervousness, weakness, sweating, heat intolerance, and loose stools. Signs include tachycardia, warm, moist skin, and tremor. The ophthalmopathy can be unilateral or bilateral and may be associated with proptosis, conjunctivitis, and/or periorbital edema. These ophthalmic findings are mainly related to the increased volume of extra-ocular tissues due to edema and/or to deposition of mucopolysaccharides. Pathologically, the thyroid gland shows diffuse enlargment with infiltration of lymphocytes and plasma cells.

Laboratory data shows an increase in the levels of thyroid hormones (triiodo-thyronine or T_3 and thyroxine or T_4) and in the uptake of T_3. Two basic types of assays can be used to demonstrate thyroid-stimulating antibodies: those that are based on the inhibition of TSH binding by TSI antibodies, and those that are based on the functional consequences of TSI antibody binding to TSH. This last group of assays includes (1) tests in which the accumulation of intra-cellular colloid droplets or the penetration of thrombogenic substrates into lysosomal membranes is measured, (2) tests in which the activation of adenylate cyclase is measured, and (3) tests in which cAMP accumulation is measured. The functional assays correlate better with disease activity, but they are difficult to calibrate and reproduce, and when heterologous thyroid is used as substrate, there is always the possibility that some human TSI antibodies might not react across species. The TSH-binding-inhibition assay is relatively simple and precise, but the results obtained with it do not always correlate with disease activity, because nonstimulating antibodies can also block TSH binding.

Therapy can be surgical (subtotal thyroidectomy) or pharmacological, in-cluding administration of radioactive iodine (^{131}I), which is difficult to dose, or the use of antithyroid drugs such as propyluracil and methimazole, which are useful but slow-acting.

Hashimoto's thyroiditis (autoimmune thyroiditis) is a chronic illness with maximal incidence during the third to fifth decades and with a female-to-male ratio of 10:1. It is functionally characterized by a slow progression to hypo-thyroidism. This is the most common form of thyroiditis. Autoantibodies directed against thyroglobulin and microsomal antigens are clinically the most important for diagnosis, but autoantibodies are also found against thyroxine (T_4), triiodothyronine (T_3) and nonthyroglobulin colloid component.

Although these autoantibodies correlate well with disease activity, two findings have shown that cell-mediated immunity (CMI) appears to cause the resulting pathology. First, thyroiditis in experimental animals cannot be passively transferred with serum; there must be lymphocyte transfer to produce the disease. Second, infants of mothers with active disease carrying IgG antibodies are unaffected. These two findings, added to the finding of increased lymphokine production by T cells during the disease, point to a CMI mechanism, autoantibodies probably being formed secondarily to the tissue damage caused by CMI. However, T lymphocytes from these patients appear not to be cytotoxic against thyroid cells, and it has been postulated that antibody-dependent cellular cytotoxicity plays a major role. Antibodies or antigen-antibody complexes would bind to follicular cells, and those cells would in turn be destroyed by killer cells recognizing the Fc fragments of the bound antibodies.

Another point that deserves comment is the close association between Graves' disease and Hashimoto's thyroiditis. Both have been shown to be associated with HLA-B8, and it is believed that Graves' disease may progress to Hashimoto's thyroiditis.

The symptoms of Hashimoto's thyroiditis are insidious, and patients often present with dysphagia or a complaint that their clothes are too tight around the neck. Most patients become hypothyroid with symptoms of malaise, fatigue, cold intolerance, and constipation. Signs include diffuse enlarged goiter, usually not tender, with dry, coarse hair. Pathologically, the architecture of the gland is disturbed with heavy lymphocytic infiltrates in which numerous plasma cells can be seen.

The diagnosis is usually confirmed by the detection of antithyroglobulin antibodies; 60-75% of patients show a positive reaction by passive hemagglutination using thyroglobulin-coated erythrocytes (titers higher than 25, while normals usually have titers up to 5). Although these antibodies are also found in other autoimmune disorders such as pernicious anemia, Sjogren's syndrome, and in 3-18% of normal individuals, the titer of these autoantibodies is lower in all other groups with the exception of patients with Sjogren's syndrome. In patients with hypothyroidism, T_3 and T_4 levels and T_3 uptake are low, and TSH is increased.

Surgery and administration of radioactive iodine are not usually indicated. Thyroxine and triiodothyronine may reduce the size of the thyroid gland. Corticosteroids may be used as mild immunosuppressants, with the aim of reducing the autoimmune response.

II. ADRENAL GLANDS

Addison's disease (chronic primary hypoadrenalism) is either caused by exogenous agents (e.g., infection of the adrenal glands by *Mycobacterium tuber-*

culosis) or idiopathic. The idiopathic form is believed to have an immune basis, since 50% of patients have been found to have antibodies to the microsomes of adrenal cells (as compared to 5% in the general population) by immunofluorescence. Localization of these antibodies is usually in the zona glomerulosa, the zona fasciculata, and the zona reticularis. Hence the adrenal atrophy that characterizes idiopathic Addison's disease may be due to an autoimmune aggression against the adrenal cortex. This autoimmune form of Addison's disease is found frequently in association with other autoimmune diseases, such as thyroiditis, pernicious anemia, and diabetes mellitus; autoantibodies to the adrenal cortex are not found in Addison's disease caused by tuberculosis of the adrenal glands.

The pathology of Addison's disease is nonspecific. The adrenal glands show marked cortical atrophy with an unaltered medulla. Abundant lymphocytes are seen between the residual islands of epithelial cells.

Symptoms of Addison's disease or adrenal insufficiency include weakness, fatigability, anorexia, nausea, vomiting, weight loss, and diarrhea. Signs include increased skin pigmentation and vascular collapse and hypotension. Addison's disease is most commonly found in the fourth and fifth decades of life and is two to three times more frequent in females.

Laboratory tests show metabolic acidosis, hyperkalemia, hyponatremia and low levels of chloride and bicarbonate. Hypoglycemia is also frequently seen. Blood counts show lymphocytosis with eosinophilia. Plasma cortisol levels are low and urine 17-ketosteroids and 17-hydroxycorticoids are also low.

Therapy consists of replacement of glucocorticoids and mineralocorticoids.

III. PANCREAS

Diabetes mellitus (DM) is a multiorgan disease, perhaps with multiple etiologies, and certainly with more than one basic abnormality. In insulin-dependent or type I diabetes, the basic defect is a decreased or absent production of insulin, while in non-insulin-dependent or type II diabetes there is a decrease of the effect of insulin at the target-cell level.

Many different types of autoantibodies have been detected in patients with DM, but a considerable degree of uncertainty remains as to their precise pathogenic role. In type I DM, anti-islet-cell antibodies (ICA) have been observed in almost all newly diagnosed patients and have been suggested as being involved in the pathogenesis of islet-cell damage. Many of these patients develop islet-cell antibodies, usually of the IgG2 and/or IgG4 subclasses, months or years before the appearance of clinical symptoms. At the time of diagnosis, ICA are detected in as many as 90% of type I diabetic patients, but they diminish in frequency to 5-10% in patients with long-standing type I DM. There is also evidence that certain HLA class I and class II serotypes are unusually frequent in patients with type I DM; many patients are positive for DR-3 and DR-4 (MHC class II antigens). It has been speculated that the MHC class II genes coding for these highly represented specificities may be linked to immune response genes whose presence may predispose towards autoimmune responses and thus account for the increased risk of developing diabetes in individuals who express them. In type II diabetic patients, the coexistence of DR3/DR4 heterozygosity and ICA positivity is associated with significant impairment of β-cell function, suggesting that both genetic and immune factors are synergistically involved in the process that leads to β-cell destruction. More recently, McDevitt and collaborators have established that individuals homozygous for an Asp-negative allele of HLA-DQβ are susceptible to type I diabetes, and it has been postulated that the gene in question may control the extent and specificity of the immune response directed against islet-cell antigens.

Anti-insulin antibodies are found in a large majority of patients (of both types of DM) treated with heterologous insulin and are basically induced by the repeated injection of bovine or porcine insulin, particularly when not very pure. In this group of patients the antibodies appear to be predominantly of the IgG2 and IgG4 isotypes, which do not activate complement very efficiently. In the last few years it has been found that as many as one third of non-insulin-treated patients with type I diabetes have anti-insulin antibodies at the time of diagnosis, which appear to be true autoantibodies (in contrast to the antibodies seen after insulin therapy). The pathogenic significance of insulin autoantibodies is not clear, but in patients with organ-specific autoimmune diseases the coexistence of anti-insulin antibodies and ICA has a strong predictive value for the future development of diabetes. The mechanism responsible for the producton of auto-antibodies to insulin has been the subject of some speculation. It has been proposed that during destruction of the islet cells insulin may be exposed to the immune system in a form that may be recognized as foreign. This could explain the development of anti-insulin antibodies in type I patients with insulitis (islet-cell inflammation). A recent finding of antigenic mimicry between insulin and a retroviral antigen, apparently leading to the spontaneous emergence of anti-insulin antibodies in nonobese diabetes-prone mice, supports the alternative possibility that anti-insulin antibodies may be triggered as a result of infection with an agent expressing cross-reactive antigen(s).

Antibodies against insulin receptors may be seen in type I and type II DM as well as in *acanthosis nigricans*, a rare syndrome in which patients develop a particularly labile form of diabetes associated with antibodies directed against the insulin receptor. In this disease, which received its name because of thickening and hyperpigmentation of the skin in the flexural and intertriginous areas, it is believed that the antibodies to the insulin receptor play the primary role in the development of diabetes by blocking the binding of insulin to its receptor. At the same time, the antireceptor antibodies may induce some of the cellular metabolic effects usually triggered by insulin, albeit in an abnormal and unregulated fashion.

It seems highly questionable that either ICA or anti-insulin antibodies may represent the initial pathogenic mechanism in DM. Most authors believe that cell-mediated mechanisms are probably more important in causing islet-cell damage. Current data, based on in vitro experiments and on observations made in animal models of the disease, suggest that a direct cytotoxic effect of T cells is highly unlikely, whereas NK cells and IL1 have been shown to be cytotoxic for islet cells in different experimental systems. The role of T cells is more likely to be related to altered regulation of the autoimmune response. This is supported by the finding of a transient diminution of suppressor/cytotoxic $CD8^+$ cells in the early stages of diabetes; such imbalance would create favorable conditions for the development of an autoimmune response. Activated $CD4^+$ T cells could also play an important role by releasing IFNγ, which can up-regulate the expression of MHC II antigens in a variety of cells and enhance the release of IL1 by monocytes and monocyte-derived cells. Of crucial importance to our understanding of the pathogenesis of DM is the definition of the insult(s) that may activate autoreactive T cells and trigger the disease. Viral infections have been suspected for a number of years, but the epidemiological data is inconclusive.

The general consensus favoring a crucial role of immune mechanisms in the pathogenesis of DM has led several groups to use immunosuppressive drugs in the treatment of recently diagnosed diabetics. The drug most often used has been cyclosporine A (CsA), and its use appears to result in a higher rate of remission and enhancement of β-cell function. However, CsA has considerable toxicity (as discussed in Chapter 28), and in most cases the patients suffer remission soon after therapy is discontinued. But the results are considered encouraging by many, and it is likely that efforts in this direction will continue in the future.

IV. GASTROINTESTINAL TRACT

A. Pernicious Anemia

Two major abnormalities characterize pernicious anemia: chronic atrophic gastritis and failure of production of intrinsic factor, which is required for the absorption of vitamin B_{12}. Although the evidence is indirect, it is believed that immunologic mechanisms play an important pathogenic role, based on the detection of three autoantibodies present in most but not all patients. The type I antibody, termed *blocking* antibody, is present in 75% of patients; it binds to intrinsic factor (IF) and prevents its binding to vitamin B_{12}. These antibodies are mainly IgG in serum but are IgA in gastric secretions. The type II or *binding* antibody reacts with the IF-vitamin B_{12} complex inhibiting IF action. The type II antibody is found in 50% of patients, and it does not occur in the absence of antibody I. A third antibody, termed *parietal canalicular antibody*, is present in the microvilli of the canalicular system of the gastric mucosa. It is found in 85-90% of patients and reacts against the parietal cell, inhibiting the secretion of IF. In 10-15% of patients with pernicious anemia no antibody can be detected with currently available techniques; perhaps those patients have a disease with a different pathogenesis. Other autoimmune diseases such as thyroiditis and Addison's disease are diagnosed with abnormally high frequency in patients with pernicious anemia.

The symptoms of pernicious anemia are insidious in onset. Most striking are the neurological symptoms. The patient may experience weakness and numbing of the extremities. Signs consist of loss of vibratory sense, ataxia, incoordination, and impaired mentation. These signs and symptoms are due to loss of myelin on the dorsal and lateral spinal tracts. Vitamin B_{12} is an essential coenzyme for the metabolism of homocysteine, which is the metabolic precursor of methionine and choline. Choline is required for the synthesis of choline-containing phospholipids, and methionine is also needed for the methylation of basic myelin. The synthesis of fatty acids is also abnormal, and these abnormal fatty acids are incorporated into neural tissues. Therefore, the metabolism of myelin is abnormal in patients with vitamin B_{12} deficiency resulting in demyelination and nervous tissue damage. Vitamin B_{12} is also required for the normal cellular metabolism of tetrahydrofolate; if tetrahydrofolate is not properly synthesized, folate will not be properly conjugated and a tissue folate deficiency will ensue. In turn, purine metabolism will be impaired, DNA metabolism abnormal, and hemopoiesis altered.

Pathologically, changes are seen in the central nervous system, the gastrointestinal tracts, and the bone marrow. The CNS effects, as have been stated, are due to myelin degeneration. The gastrointestinal tract reveals an atrophic glossitis and gastritis. Additionally the stomach undergoes metaplasia with the appearance of goblet cells (termed *intestinalization*). The bone marrow shows hypercellularity with numerous megaloblasts (megaloblastic anemia).

Laboratory studies show a megaloblastic anemia with hypersegmented neutrophils and a mild to moderate thrombocytopenia. There is decreased vitamin B_{12} absorption, so there are low levels of B_{12}. A histamine stimulation test of the gastric cells shows achlorhydria. If vitamin B_{12} is given parentally a marked increase in the reticulocyte count will result.

Treatment is by intramuscular injection of vitamin B_{12}.

B. Primary Biliary Cirrhosis

Primary biliary cirrhosis is a chronic granulomatous inflammatory liver disease that results in the destruction of the intrahepatic biliary tree. This disease is associated with other autoimmune diseases such as Sjogren's syndrome. Although the true pathogenic process is not known, over 99% of patients have detectable antimitochondrial antibodies and circulating serum immune complexes that fix complement by both the classical and the alternative pathway. Other immunological abnormalities include a decrease in suppressor-T-cell activity, increased concentrations of monomeric and polymeric IgM, and a deficient switch from IgM to IgG production during immune responses.

The disease is mainly a disease of middle-aged women. The onset is insidious and heralded by pruritus and symptoms of cholestasis. Jaundice is a late sign. The patients have a large, nontender liver.

Laboratory tests show an increase in serum alkaline phosphatase with normal transaminases and bilirubin and positive antimitochondrial antibodies. Penicillamine, a heavy metal chelating agent, has been used therapeutically in this disease. By unknown mechanisms this drug is known to reduce the ratio of helper to suppressor cells, which is reflected in a depression of humoral immune responses both in experimental animals and in man. However, penicillamine is nephrotoxic, and its use may create considerable problems.

V. MUSCULOSKELETAL SYSTEM

Myasthenia gravis (MG) is a chronic neuromuscular disorder caused by a disorder of neuromuscular transmission. The proposed pathogenic mechanism is the production of antiacetylcholine-receptor antibodies, which can be detected in 85-90% of the patients. Probably more significant is that there is a 70-90% reduction in the receptors for acetylcholine in patients. This could be a consequence of direct cytotoxicity by complement, opsonization, ADCC, activation of phagocytic cells, or CMI mechanisms. Cell-mediated immunity has been suggested as playing a role due to the lymphocytic infiltration that is often seen at the neuromuscular junction level, given that blast transformation can be achieved in vitro by stimulating T cells from patients with MG with acetylcholine receptor protein. Thymic abnormalities occur in 75% of MG patients.

Symptoms of MG are increased muscular fatigability and weakness, especially with exercise. Weakness is usually first detected in extraocular muscles resulting in diplopia or ptosis. The face, tongue, and upper extremities are also frequently involved. Skeletal muscle involvement is usually proximal. The disease is usually marked by spontaneous remission periods.

The pathological studies in MG patients are inconsistent. A few patients have a lymphocytic infiltrate within the muscles, whereas others appear normal. Concerning the thymic abnormalities, 10% of the patients have true thymoma and 70% have increased numbers of B-cell germinal centers within the thymus, which some authors have suggested to be the source of autoantibodies. No laboratory tests are significant for MG, except for the finding of antiacetylcholine receptor antibodies.

Treatment consists of anticholinesterase drugs such as neostigmine and pyridostigmine (Mestinon) in combination with atropine. Adrenocorticoids have shown good results in 60-100% of patient studies. Plasmapheresis and thoracic duct drainage are also effective to remove antibodies. Thymectomy is undertaken with improvement in 75% of patients and remission in 25%, although it may be several months after surgery when clinical improvement starts to be obvious.

VI. SKIN DISEASES

A. Pemphigus

Pemphigus refers to a group of diseases with autoantibodies against antigens in the intercellular zones of the epidermis. In patients with pemiphigus there is a direct correlation between antibody titers and the severity of the disease. Immunofluorescence studies have shown immunoglobulins and complement deposited in the intercellular matrix of the patient's skin. The true nature of the antigen is unknown.

There are four clinical forms of pemphigus: pemphigus vulgaris, pemphigus vegetans, pemphigus foliaceus and pemphigus erythematosus; pemphigus vulgaris is the most frequent, and it is the only one that we are considering in this discussion. It occurs usually between the ages of 40 to 60 and presents with a vesicular eruption on the oral and nasal mucosa. These lesions then spread in random fashion to other areas of the body. The vesicles lead to bullae which are very fragile. Histological sections show edema in the intercellular area early with acantholysis (loss of cohesion between epidermal cells) occurring later.

Treatment consists of supportive skin care, and corticosteroids have been administered in an attempt to reduce the autoimmune response.

B. Bullous Pemphigoid

Bullous pemphigoid is a blistering disease in which autoantibodies to the skin basement membrane are detected in 80% of the patients. Immunofluorescence shows immunoglobulins and complement deposited in a linear pattern at the dermoepithelial junction of affected skin. The autoantibody is an IgG, but no correlation is observed between antibody titers and the severity of the disease, and passive transfer of the antibody does no cause disease.

Bullous pemphigoid is a self-limiting disease occurring mainly in people over 60 years of age who present with a tense bullae on an erythematosus base, mainly located on flexor surfaces. In one-third of the patients the mouth is involved, although mucous membranes are not usually involved. The disease follows a chronic course with remissions and exacerbations.

Histologically, vacuolization is seen early at the dermoepidermal junction with subsequent coalescing of these vacuoles to form bullae. Acantholysis is not a feature of this disease. Immunofluorescence shows a linear pattern of IgG and complement along the dermoepithelial junction.

Therapy is basically identical to that of pemphigus, including supportive measures and administration of corticosteroids.

VII. BLOOD DISEASES

Autoimmune hemolytic anemia (AHA) is a term used for a collection of diseases that have as a basis the production of anti-red-cell antibodies; it is discussed in detail in Chapter 20.

Idiopathic thrombocytopenic purpura (ITP) is an autoimmune purpura caused by antiplatelet antibodies. Antibodies have been detected in 60-70% of patients with the "immunoinjury" technique, which relies on the release of platelet factors such as serotonin following exposure to autoantibodies. Competitive binding assays and antiglobulin assays can also be used to demonstrate antiplatelet antibodies.

Idiopathic thrombocytopenic purpura can present as an acute or as a chronic form. *Acute ITP* is seen mainly in children, often in the phase of recovery after a viral exanthem or an upper respiratory infection, and it is usually self-limited. The thrombocytopenia is due to the formation of immune complexes containing viral antigens that become adsorbed to the platelets or to antiviral antibodies that cross-react with platelets. Platelet destruction can be due to a variety of mechanisms, including irreversible aggregation caused by immune complexes or, when antiplatelet antibodies are involved, complement activation or phagocytosis. *Chronic ITP* is an adult disease due to the formation of autoantibodies that react with platelets and lead to their destruction by phagocytosis. Chronic ITP is often associated with other autoimmune diseases.

Patients with ITP usually present with petechiae, ecchymosis, epistaxis, and gingival, genitourinary, and gastrointestinal tract bleeding. The platelet count in the acute form is usually less than 20,000 platelets per microliter, whereas the chronic form has platelet counts between 30,000 and 100,000 platelets per microliter. The white-cell count is usually normal. The bone marrow is also usually normal, but in some cases an increase in megakaryocytes may be seen. The spleen may be enlarged due to platelet sequestration by phagocytic cells.

The treatment of ITP is usually supportive. Steroids have been used but are usually not necessary, and their efficiency in severe cases is questionable. In the last few years considerable interest has been given to the use of large doses of intravenous gamma globulin, which cause a prolongation of platelet survival. Two mechanisms have been postulated to explain the action of intravenous gamma globulin in ITP: (1) a competition with immune complexes for the binding to platelets (immune complexes would cause irreversible aggregation or complement-mediated cytolysis, and intravenous gamma globulin would not) and (2)

competitive inhibition of Fc-receptor-mediated binding of platelets by phagocytes (for which there is experimental documentation). As a last resort, in
severe cases, splenectomy may be performed in the hope of prolonging platelet
survival by removing the major site of destruction.

SELF-EVALUATION

Questions

Choose the one best answer.

23.1 Thyroid-stimulating antibodies
   A. Stimulate the production of thyroid hormones by binding to the thy-
   roglobulin receptor.
   B. Compete with TSH in binding to the corresponding receptor.
   C. Are measured by a variety of assays that give equivalent results.
   D. Are frequently found in autoimmune thyroiditis.
   E. Can be identified, in most cases, as IgM immunoglobulins.

23.2 The autoimmune nature of insulin-dependent (type I) diabetes mellitus is
   suggested by all of the following except
   A. The frequent finding of anti-islet-cell antibodies early in the disease.
   B. The frequent finding of anti-insulin antibodies after prolonged insulin
   therapy.
   C. The association with DR3 and DR4 HLA antigens.
   D. The finding of anti-insulin antibodies in newly diagnosed patients.
   E. The evidence of CMI or ADCC obtained with peripheral lymphocytes
   from patients with type I diabetes when cultured with insulinoma cells.

23.3 Splenectomy in idiopathic thrombocytopenic purpura may be beneficial
   because
   A. It eliminates a major source of platelet destruction.
   B. It leads to significant depression of antiplatelet antibody levels.
   C. Splenectomy leads to generalized immunosuppression.
   D. The spleen is often autodestroyed and does not play any functional
   role.
   E. The spleen is enlarged and causes discomfort to the patient.

23.4 Pernicious anemia is associated with
   A. Gastric hyperchlorydria.
   B. Good response to immunosuppressive therapy.
   C. Sjogren's syndrome.
   D. Microcytic anemia.
   E. Abnormal myelin metabolism.

In Questions 23.5-23.10, match each numbered word or phase with the one lettered heading that is most closely related to it. The same heading may be selected once, more than once, or not at all.

(A) Anti-islet cell antibodies;
(B) Antimicrosomal antibodies;
(C) Antibodies to the skin basement membrane;
(D) Frequent mucosal lesions;
(E) Anti-insulin receptor antibodies.

23.5 Addison's disease.

23.6 Hashimoto's thyroiditis.

23.7 Bullous pemphigoid.

23.8 Pemphigus vulgaris.

23.9 Insulin-dependent diabetes mellitus.

23.10 Non-insulin-dependent diabetes mellitus.

Answers

23.1 (B) TSI antibodies can be considered as *stimulating* anti-TSH receptor antibodies.

23.2 (B) Anti-insulin antibodies emerging after prolonged insulin therapy are a result of antigenic stimulation by heterologous insulin.

23.3 (A) Antibody-coated cells (including platelets) tend to be sequestered, phagocytized, and destroyed in organs such as the spleen and the liver (reticuloendothelial system).

23.4 (E) Demyelination and neurological symptoms are prominent in patients with pernicious anemia.

23.5 (B)

23.6 (B)

23.7 (C)

23.8 (D)

23.9 (A)

23.10 (E) Anti-insulin receptor antibodies are found in rare cases of non-insulin-dependent diabetes, often associated with *acanthosis nigricans*, which characteristically show a marked clinical instability.

..

BIBLIOGRAPHY

Bach, J. F. Mechanism of autoimmunity in insulin-dependent diabetes mellitus. *Clin. Exp. Immunol.* 72:7, 1988.

Betterie, C., Presotto, F., Pedini, B., Moro, L., Slack, R. S., Zanette, F., and Zanchetta, R. Islet cell and insulin autoantibodies in organ-specific autoimmune patients. Their behavior an predictive value for the development of type I (insulin-dependent) diabetes mellitus. A 10-year follow-up study. *Diabetologia 30*:292, 1987.

Burman, K. D. and Baker, J. R., Jr. Immune mechanisms in Graves disease. *Endocr. Rev.* 6:183, 1985.

Dotta, F. and Eisenbarth, G. S. Type I diabetes mellitus: A predictable autoimmune disease with interindividual variation in the rate of β cell destruction. *Clin. Immunol. Immunopath.* 50:s85, 1989.

Fisher, D. A., Pandian, M. R., and Carlton, E. Autoimmune thyroid disease: An expanding spectrum. *Pediatr. Clinics of N.A.* 34:907, 1987.

Holborow, E. J. and Reeves, W. G. (Eds.). *Immunology in Medicine*, 2nd Ed. Grune & Stratton, London/New York, 1983. (Includes several chapters on systemic disorders, including some of autoimmune etiology.)

Karpatkin, S. Autoimmune thrombocytopenic purpura. *Blood 56*:329, 1980.

Lachmann, P. J. and Peters, D. K. (Eds.). *Clinical Aspects of Immunology*, 4th Ed., 2nd Vol. Blackwell Scientific, Oxford, 1982. (Includes the section on "Organ based immunology," in which most organ-specific autoimmune disorders are discussed.)

Levinson, A. I., Zweiman, B., and Lisak, R. P. Immunopathogenesis and treatment of myasthenia gravis. *J. Clin. Immunol.* 7:187, 1987.

Mariotti, S., Chiovato, L., Vitti, P., Marcocci, C., Fenzi, G. F., Del Prete, G. F., Tiri, A., Romagnani, S., Ricci, M., and Pinchera, A. Recent advances in the understanding of humoral and cellular mechanisms implicated in thyroid autoimmune disorders. *Clin. Immunol. Immunopath.* 50;S73, 1989.

Marx, J. L. Cytokines are two-edged swords in disease. *Science 239*:257, 1988.

Morell, A. and Mydegger, U. E. (Eds.). *Clinical Use of Intravenous Immunoglobulins*. Academic Press, Orlando, Florida, 1986. (Includes several chapters on intravenous immunoglobulin therapy in idiopathic thrombocytopenic purpura.)

Rose, N. R., Lorenz, M., and Lewis, M. Endocrine diseases. In *Basic and Clinical Immunology*, D. P. Stites, J. D. Stobo, and J. V. Wells (Eds.), 6th Ed. Lange Medical, Los Altos, California, 1987, p. 582-597.

Todd, J. A., Bell, J. I., and McDevitt, H. O. HLA-DQβ gene contributes to the susceptibility and resistance to insulin-dependent diabetes mellitus. *Nature 329*:599, 1987.

Volpé, R. (Ed.). *Autoimmunity in the Endocrine System. Monographs in Endocrinology*, Vol. 20. Springer-Verlag, New York, 1981.

24

Systemic Lupus Erythematosus

JEAN-MICHEL GOUST

Systemic lupus erythematosus (SLE) is a generalized disorder that expresses itself predominantly as a systemic vasculitis of unknown cause. It is most common in young females (15 to 35 years of age), and the diagnosis is usually based on the verification that any four of the manifestations listed in Table 24.1 are present serially or simultaneously during a period of observation. Given the multisystemic nature of the disease, the clinical diagnosis must be based on features that reflect involvement of more than one organ or system.

The clinical manifestations that may be observed during the entire course of SLE, and the frequency of their occurrence, are shown in Table 24.2. Exacerbations and remissions, heralded by the appearance of new manifestations and the worsening of preexisting symptoms, give the disease its fluctuating natural history. These manifestations are so polymorphic that it is often difficult to absolutely differentiate SLE from other diseases that share similar abnormalities of the connective and vascular tissues, such as the so called mixed connective tissue disease (MCTD). It is not infrequent to observe clinical situations in which the differentiation between SLE and another connective tissue disease is difficult. In some patients the distinction may be impossible, and they are classified as having the overlap syndrome. This syndrome represents the association of SLE with another disorder such as scleroderma or rheumatoid arthritis. As a rule, however, even if many patients share some common immunologic abnormalities, particularly the presence of antinuclear antibodies or of rheumatoid

TABLE 24.1 Diagnostic Features of Systemic Lupus Erythematosus

Facial erythema (butterfly rash)
Discoid lupus
Raynaud's phenomenon
Alopecia
Photosensitivity
Oral or nasopharyngeal ulceration
Arthritis without deformity
Pleuritis or pericarditis
Psychosis or convulsions
Hemolytic anemia, leukopenia, or thrombocytopenia
Heavy proteinuria with cellular cases in the urinary sediment

TABLE 24.2 Clinical Manifestations of SLE During Entire Course of Illness

Manifestation	Percentage of patients
Musculoarticular	95
Renal disease	55
Pulmonary disease (pleurisy, pneumonitis)	60
Cutaneous disease (photosensitivity, alopecia, etc.)	80
Cardiac disease (pericarditis, endocarditis)	50
Fever of unknown origin	80
Gastrointestinal disease (hepatomegaly, ascites, ect.)	45
Hematologic/reticuloendothelial (anemia, leukopenia, splenomegaly)	85
Thrombophlebitis	9
Sicca syndrome[a]	10
Neuropsychiatric (Organic brain syndrome, seizures, peripheral neuropathy, etc.)	60

[a]Syndrome characterized by keratoconjunctivitis sicca and deficient lacrimal and salivary secretions; also seen in patients with rheumatoid arthritis (in what is then designated as Sjogren's syndrome) and sarcoidosis.

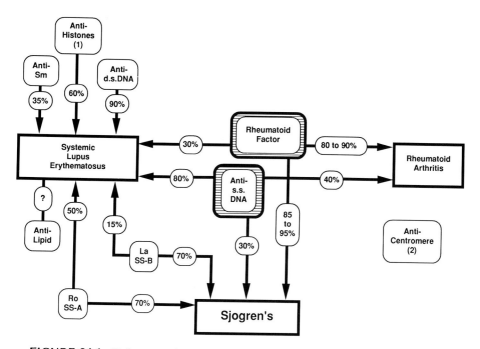

FIGURE 24.1 Daigrammatic representation of the different types of auto-antibodies detected in SLE and related diseases. The percentages over arrows refer to the positivity rate in the disease to which the arrows point. Note that antihistone antibodies are frequently found as the only serological abnormality in cases of SLE-like syndromes, and that anticentromere antibodies are characteristically associated to the CREST syndrome (the association of calcinosis, Raynaud's syndrome, scleroderma involving the skin and the esophagus, and telangiectasia).

factor, specific disorders can usually be individualized by the presence of a specific set of autoantibodies, as illustrated diagrammatically in Figure 24.1. Therefore even if thepathogenic role of autoantibodies remains unclear, their presence is diagnostically significant. Also, the existence of defined patterns of autoreactivity in specific disorders suggests that the immune abnormality is antigen-driven.

I. HUMORAL ABNORMALITIES IN SLE

A. The Discovery of Antinuclear Antibodies (ANAs)

The original observation that led to the discovery of antinuclear antibodies was reported in 1948 by Hargraves, who described the presence of what he named an LE cell in a clot of the patient's blood. This peculiar-looking cell is a poly-morphonuclear leukocyte that has ingested nuclear material. It was possible to reproduce this phenomenon in vitro by incubating normal neutrophils with damaged luekocytes preincubated with sera obtained from SLE patients. This suggested the presence of antibodies directed against the cells' nuclear components in the sera. Indeed, it was unquestionably proven that normal phago-cytic cells ingest antibody-coated nuclear material, forming the LE cell. The antibodies responsible for LE-cell formation were originally designated as *LE factor*. Investigation of the reactivity of LE factors from different patients led to the definition of the now very heterogeneous group of anti-nuclear antibodies (ANAs).

B. Anti-DNA Antibodies in SLE

Nowadays antinuclear antibodies are detected by indirect immunofluorescence, and this is the technique most often used as a first screening assay by the diagnostic laboratories. A negative result virtually excludes the diagnosis of SLE, while high titers are strongly suggestive of SLE but not confirmatory, because ANAs can be detected in other conditions. At first the idea that there could be an association between a naturally occurring disease and the production of antibodies to DNA or RNA met with considerable skepticism, because purified nucleic acids are extremely poor immunogens in experimental conditions and it is almost impossible to induce an immune response to these molecules in most animal species. However, once the existence of antinuclear antibodies was accepted, it was shown that the epitopes recognized by them were not on the nucleic acids themselves but on proteins associated to the nucleic acids (forming nucleoproteins). Thus the association of nucleic acid and protein renders the protein immunogenic, but normally the immune system is not stimulated by these intracellular complexes. When there is extensive cell death, the nucleo-proteins are released into the extracellular compartment and stimulate antibody production.

Three types of relatively common anti-DNA antibodies have been described. Those that react with *single stranded (ss) DNA* and with *denatured double-stranded (ds) DNA* are not SLE-specific. These antibodies are very frequently found in many connective tissue diseases (see Chapter 25). However, their detection in high titers should lead one to perform a confirmatory test for the diagnosis of SLE, which involves the detection of antibodies to native, double-stranded DNA. In contrast to other anti-DNA antibodies, those that react with native DNA recognize a conformation epitope that depends on the helical structure of DNA molecules. These antibodies discriminate SLE from all other connective tissue disorders and are detected by immunofluorescence using as a substrate a noninfectious flagellate, *Chritidia luciliae*, which has a kinetoplast packed with double-stranded DNA. This test is very sensitive and can be semiquantitated by titration of the last serum dilution still giving positive fluorescence. If the clinical context warrants it, every positive ANA (even when the titer is relatively low) should be followed by the more definitive test for anti-native dsDNA. The test is positive in about 80% of SLE patients and negative in virtually all other situation in which antinuclear antibodies are present.

One of the characteristics of the abnormal immune response in SLE is that it is directed against many cellular autoantigens. Anti-DNA antibodies are only an example of the wide variety of autoantibodies found in these patients. It is accepted as a clinical rule that the usual SLE patient has an average of three different circulating autoantibodies present simultaneously.

C. Response to Other Cellular Autoantigens in SLE

Emphasis has recently been placed on the detection of antibodies against soluble cellular antigens that can be detected by double immunodiffusion using calf or rabbit thymus extracts as antigens. In some cases this type of antibody can be extremely specific to a given disease. For example, the anti-Sm antibody is detected almost exclusively in SLE patients (the term Sm corresponding to the initials of the patient in whom the antibody was first detected). The Sm antigen is a uridine-rich RNA-protein complex; treatment with ribonuclease destroys the RNA part of the antigen but does not affect reactivity with anti-Sm antibodies, which recognize the protein part of the complex (not affected by ribonuclease treatment). Though highly specific for SLE, anti-Sm antibodies are found in only 30 to 40% of the patients. When detected in association to anti-dsDNA antibodies the diagnosis of SLE is virtually established.

Other frequently observed antiribonucleoprotein antibodies are directed against the so-called SS-A and SS-B antigens, where SS stands for *Sjogren's syndrome* and A and B designate 2 distinct antigens (Figure 24.1).

D. The Pathogenic Role of Autoantibodies in SLE

Some remarkable associations between autoantibodies and clinical symptoms suggest that these antibodies may be involved in the pathogenesis of some of the lesions associated with the disease. This is the case with anti-Sm antibodies, for instance, which are often the only autoantibodies detected in SLE patients with symptoms of isolated central nervous system involvement. Other examples are the presence of anti-SS-A antibodies during pregnancy, which has been associated to the presence of congenital heart block or to the development of neonatal lupus in the newborn. Anticardiolipin antibodies, which are the basis for false positive results in serological tests for syphilis, are frequently observed in patients with SLE but may also be found as the only serologic abnormality in patients with chorea, repeated miscarriages, and coagulopathies. Other pathological manifestations in SLE patients directly caused by autoantibodies include hemolytic anemia (due to anti-red-cell antibodies) and thrombocytopenia (due to antiplatelet antibodies). In addition, autoantibodies directed against striated muscle or central nervous system antigens may be detected in patients with SLE. Less frequently, antiorgan antibodies such as antithyroid, antiliver, and antigastric tissue antibodies may be found with or without obvious abnormalities of the target organ(s).

E. Immune Complex Formation in SLE

The antibodies most frequently associated with tissue damage in SLE are the anti-dsDNA antibodies. The presence of these antibodies is closely associated with the development of glomerulonephritis. Anti-DNA antibodies are usually present in the circulation of patients with SLE, but if their levels are followed up longitudinally, a precipitous drop can be seen before the appearance of symptoms suggestive of renal involvement. The reduction in circulating levels of anti-DNA coincides with the very transient presence of free native double-stranded DNA in the serum. Thus it appears that the drop in antibody levels corresponds to the formation of soluble complexes in slight antigen excess, too small to be quickly bound by RBC and presented to phagocytic cells but large enough to activate complement and cause tissue damage. Marked elevations in the levels of circulating immune complexes can be detected in patients with SLE sera during acute episodes of the disease by a variety of techniques (see Chapter 21). The pathogenic role of immune complexes is made even more likely by the fact that those patients with IgG1 and IgG3 (complement fixing) anti-DNA antibodies develop lupus nephritis more frequently than those patients in whom anti-DNA antibodies are of other isotypes. Laboratory tests can also demonstrate evidence for complement activation via the classical pathway. For instance, following the decrease in the levels of anti-dsDNA antibodies, C3 levels start to decline, coinciding with an increase in the levels of circulating immune complexes. These serological changes usually precede a clinical relapse. Antibody and complement levels return toward their pretreatment levels when the relapse has been controlled. It thus appears that a generalized abnormality of antibody production exists in SLE, that the immune system of these patients is cyclically activated, and that these activation bursts may be responsible for clinical deterioration.

It is believed that immune complexes are predominantly formed in the circulation and subsequently fixed to target tissues, where they cause inflammatory changes secondary to complement activation. However, it is possible that in some instances the reaction occurs locally. Free double-stranded DNA has a high affinity for collagen, and it can be passively adsorbed to the glomerular basement membrane, where it becomes involved in the in situ formation of im-

mune complexes by reacting with circulating anti-DNA antibodies. Glomerulonephritis, cutaneous vasculitis, arthritis, and some of the neurologic manifestations of SLE are fully explainable by the local consequences of immune complex deposition. Immunofluorescence studies indicate that the capillary tufts of
renal glomeruli in patients with lupus nephritis contain deposits of immunoglobulins and complement. Elution studies have shown that DNA and anti-DNA
antibodies are present in these deposits, confirming that they correspond to
antigen-antibody complexes. A number of studies have revealed depression of
serum factor B and properdin, which can also be found deposited in the glomeruli. Hence, both the classical and the alternative (properdin) pathway of
complement activation play a role in SLE.

In SLE patients, immune complex deposits have also been noted on the
dermoepidermal junction of both inflamed skin and normal skin, appearing
as a fluorescent "band" when a skin biopsy is studied by immunofluorescence
with antisera to immunoglobulins and complement components. This is the
basis of the band test, which is easy to perform but must be done on a biopsy
of normal-appearing skin, because nonspecific fixation of serum proteins, including Igs and complement, can be seen at the dermoepidermal junction in
many other conditions. The band test is one of a battery of tests with diagnostic value in SLE.

II. INSIGHTS FROM ANIMAL MODELS

The understanding of the pathogenic mechanisms underlying the progression
of systemic lupus erythematosus was helped by the discovery of a spontaneously occurring disease in mice that resembled SLE in many respects. During
the inbreeding of mice strains, it was observed that the F1 hybrids obtained
by mating white and black mice from New Zealand (NZBxNZW F1) spontaneously developed a systemic autoimmune disease involving a variety of
organs and systems (Table 24.3).

Throughout the course of the disease the mice are hypergammaglobulinemic,
reflecting an underlying lymphoproliferation that is initially benign. The animals have a variety of autoantibodies and manifestations of autoimmune disease and immune complex disease similar to those seen in humans with SLE.
As the disease progresses, malignant lymphomas producing monoclonal immunoglobulins very often evolve, often leading to a rapid deterioration and death.

A. Genetic Factors in Murine and Human SLE

This animal model has been extensively studied, and the data generated by these
studies has given important contributions to our understanding of the pathogenesis of SLE. The most important conclusion at present is that this SLE-like

TABLE 24.3 Natural History of Spontaneous SLE in NZB Mice and Their First-Generation Hybrids

Age (months)	Abnormalities
3	Autoantibodies to nucleic acids and T-lymphocyte subsets
5-6	Tissue lymphocytic infiltration
5-7	Immune complex glomerulonephritis
7-8	Autoimmune hemolytic anemia
10-12	Malignant lymphoma followed by monoclonal gammopathy of the IgM class

Source: Modified from Steinberg, A. D. et al. *Ann. Int. Med. 100*:174, 1984.

disease is multifactorial, its outcome representing the synergistic effects of environmental and intrinsic factors, namely immune regulatory genes and several other genetic factors. The importance of genetic factors is underlined by the observation that the parental NZB mice had a very mild and often undetectable form of the disease but that the introduction of the NZW genetic background made the disease accelerate and worsen. Genetic linkage studies showed that many of the immunologic abnormalities were under multigenic control, one set of genes controlling the animal's ability to produce anti-DNA antibodies, another the presence of antierythrocyte antibodies, and still others controlling high levels of IgM production and lymphocytic proliferation (Table 24.4).

After a controversy that lasted for several years, it has been accepted that genes linked to the MHC, or at least in linkage disequilibrium with the MHC, influence and severity of the SLE-like syndrome occurring in the NZBxNZW F1 hybrids. The identification of genetic factors that determined the disease in NZB mice led to studies of the role of genetic factors in human SLE.

TABLE 24.4 Genes Responsible for NZB Autoimmune Traits

Trait	Number of genes
Anti-T-cell antibodies	1
Hypergammaglobulinemia M	1
Anti-DNA antibodies	1
Antierythrocyte antibodies	3
Lymphocytic hyperproliferation	3

Source: Modified from Steinberg, A. D. et al. *Ann. Int. Med. 100*:174, 1984.

One argument in favor of the role of genetic factors in SLE is the finding of anti-DNA antibodies in healthy relatives of SLE patients. Also, there is a moderate degree of concordance amongst monozygotic twins. However, the degree of concordance in twins is too low to support the concept of a strong influence of genetic factors on human SLE. The genes that could play a role, probably in synergy with environmental factors, have not been identified, but the current evidence indicates that in humans, as in mice, they could be linked to the MHC. For example, the HL-DR2 haplotype is overrepresented in patients with SLE. Also, an SLE-like disease develops in patients with C4A deficiency, which occurs in linkage disequilibrium with HLA-DR3. It is known that C4 plays a critical role in the solubilization and inactivation of circulating immune complexes. Thus, a genetically determined C4A deficiency may help to create the conditions favorable to the development of SLE.

B. Immune Response Abnormalities

1. B Cell Abnormalities

The pathogenic role of spontaneous B-cell hyperactivity was first shown by crossing NZBxNZW F1 mice expressing the most severe form of murine SLE with the so-called Xid strain, which is hypogammaglobulinemic because of a genetically determined abnormal B-cell development. The resulting hybrids do not develop the SLE-like disease of the NZBxNZW F1 mice. However, the protective effect of the Xid gene in NZBxNZW/Xid hybrids is not absolute because it can be abrogated by repeated polyclonal B-cell stimulation with lipopolysaccharides. In human SLE there is also, as a rule, a persistent hypergammaglobulinemia, which seems to correlate with the finding of activated and terminally differentiated plasmablasts actively secreting IgG in the circulation. Furthermore, it is well known that any infection that would induce B-cell activation is likely to cause a clinical relapse.

2. T-Cell Abnormalities

The production of IgG anti-dsDNA antibodies in high titers, which are believed to be responsible for many of the clinical problems in patients with SLE, is dependent upon the help from CD4 helper T cells. The finding of anti-T-cell antibodies in the serum of NZBxNZW F1 mice raised the possibility that a simple explanation for the inordinate B-cell activity associated with the SLE-like disease of the mouse would be found in the deletion of a specific subset of regulatory cells. Indeed, suppressor functions are profoundly depressed in the F1 hybrids, and the depletion of suppressor cells closely follows the onset of hypergammaglobulinemia. Although similar anti-T-cell antibodies have been detected in humans, their role is far from being clear, because they are not specific for any T-cell subset. On the other hand, these antibodies may be responsible for the lymphopenia frequently seen in patients with SLE. Functional studies of cellular immunity in SLE have shown that the functions of both CD4 and CD8 subsets are altered, as is shown by a significant decrease in IL2 production during active disease. As a consequence of these functonal alterations, anergy (lack of reactivity) to common recall antigens is an early and constant finding during active phases of human SLE. This impairment of cell-mediated immunity may explain the increased risk of severe opportunistic infections.

The recent finding of extensive deletions in the T-cell repertoire of the NZW mice, in which the $C\beta2$ and $D\beta2$ genes of the T-cell antigen receptor are missing, opens some interesting questions. For example, these deletions could be associated with a faulty establishment of tolerance to self MHC during intrathymic ontogeny and be responsible, at least in part, for the B-cell hyperresponsiveness when these defective T-cell receptor genes are introduced in the special MHC background found in NZB mice. Whether similar abnormalities of the T-cell receptor gene exist in SLE patients is being investigated.

C. Nonimmune Factors Influencing the Course of SLE

1. Hormonal Effects

The expression of the genetic and immunologic abnormalities characteristic of murine lupus-like disease is influenced by female sex hormones. The disease is more severe in NZBxNZW F1 females. Administration of estrogens aggravates the evolution of the disease, which is also seen in castrated male mice but not in complete males. The extent of the hormonal involvement in human SLE cannot be proven so directly, but the large female predominance as well as the influence of puberty and pregnancies on the onset of the disease or the severity of its manifestations indicates that sex hormones play a role in the modulation of the disease.

2. Environmental Factors

The first environmental factor influencing the clinical evolution of human SLE to be identified was sunlight exposure, known to induce severe relapses. This could be related to the fact that the Langerhans cells of the skin release significant amounts of interleukin 1 upon exposure to UV light. This mediator will stimulate helper/inducer T cells, "spontaneously" initiating a CMI reaction in light-exposed areas. Infections also seem to play a role. Bacterial and viral infections may tip an immune system in precarious balance towards hyperactivity, triggering a relapse. Other important environmental factors are drugs, particularly those with DNA binding ability such as hydantoin, isoniazide, and hydralazine. ANA antibodies appear in 15 to 70% of patients treated with any of these drugs for several weeks. These ANA antibodies belong, in most cases, to the IgM class and react with histones. Only when the antibodies switch from IgM to IgG does the patient become symptomatic. These ANA usually disappear after termination of the treatment; however, full-blown SLE may develop in genetically predisposed individuals after exposure to any one of the drugs listed above.

III. TREATMENT

Even without a good understanding of the pathogenesis of SLE, there are presently enough leads about pathogenic mechanisms and risk factors to allow the establishment of reasonable therapeutic objectives. The most commonly prescribed medications for SLE are corticosteroids, which combine anti-inflammatory effects with a weak immunosuppressive capacity. The anti-inflammatory effect is probably beneficial in immune complex disease, while the immunosuppressive effect may help to curtail the activity of the B-cell system. In cases with obvious manifestations secondary to immune complex deposition (e.g., glomerulonephritis), plasmapheresis has been used to remove circulating immune

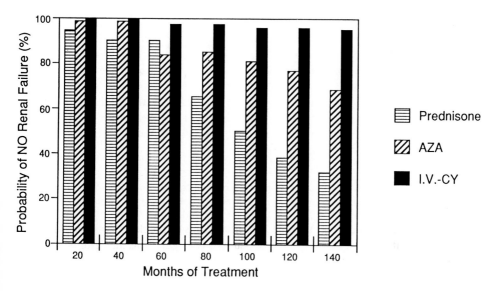

FIGURE 24.2 Graphic representation of the prevention of renal disease in SLE patients with three different types of immunosuppressive therapy: prednisone, oral azathioprine, and cyclophosphamide administered intravenously. Cyclophosphamide appears to be most successful in delaying the onset of renal failure.

complexes, but it must be used in conjunction with steroid and immunosuppressive therapy, because it causes worsening of the symptoms when used alone (probably as a result of the interference with immunoregulatory circuits resulting from the removal of immune complexes and antibodies). In severe cases, immunosuppressive drugs may be indicated. Cyclophosphamide, given intravenously, has been successfully used to prolong adequate renal function with only a few side effects (Fig. 24.2). Careful avoidance of factors implicated in the induction of relapses, such as high-risk medications, exposure to sunlight, infections, etc., is also indicated. Preventing relapses is important, because since their severity is impossible to predict and even when successfully treated they may leave irreversible sequelae such as chronic glomerulonephritis. As a collary, every effort should be made to detect a relapse early and initiate therapy before it produces irreversible damage. In spite of the limitations in our understanding of the disease and in our therapeutic approaches, the prognosis of SLE has steadily improved over the past 25 years.

SELF-EVALUATION

Questions

Choose the one best answer.

24.1 Circulating anti-dsDNA in the serum of patients who have systemic lupus erythematosus is
  A. An indication that severe membranous glomerulonephritis is likely to be present.
  B. Rarely associated with high titers of antinuclear factor.
  C. Unusual, because this antibody is generally associated with CREST.
  D. Associated with leukopenia, because the antibody reacts with neutrophil membrane antigens.
  E. Of no diagnostic value.

Questions 24.2-24,4 refer to the following case history. A 28-year old woman has a history of weight loss, intermittent fever and pains in several joints, mainly hands, wrists, and knees. The physical shows a butterfly rash on the face and enlarged, nontender lymph nodes in the axillary and inguinal regions. Laboratory tests showed anemia, a positive indirect Coombs test, and proteinuria (3 g/24 hr).

24.2 Given this history, the most likely diagnosis is
  A. Rheumatoid arthritis.
  B. Progressive systemic sclerosis (scleroderma).
  C. Systemic lupus erythematosus.
  D. Still's disease.
  E. Systemic scleroderma.

24.3 Of the following antibodies the most likely to be positive is
      A. Anti-dsDNA.
      B. Anti-Sm.
      C. Rheumatoid factor.
      D. Anti-SS-A.
      E. Anticentromere.

24.4 Of the following tests, the one that will give most specific information
      from the diagnostic point of view is
      A. Cryoglobulin determination.
      B. Anti-ssDNA.
      C. Anti-dsDNA.
      D. LE-cell phenomenon.
      E. Radiolabeled C1q binding.

24.5 The band test in SLE detects immunoglobulin and complement deposits
      at the
      A. Dermoepidermal junction of normal skin.
      B. Dermoepidermal junction of skin obtained from erythematous areas.
      C. Glomerular basement membrane.
      D. Membrane of polymorphonuclear leukocytes.
      E. Choroid plexus.

24.6 The antigen most often characterized as being involved in soluble immune
      complex formation in SLE is
      A. RNA.
      B. Sm antigen.
      C. Native double stranded DNA.
      D. Ribonucleoproteins.
      E. Histones.

24.7 Soluble immune complexes with highest potential pathogenicity are likely
      to
      A. Contain IgG1 antibodies.
      B. Be formed in antibody excess.
      C. Contain ssDNA.
      D. Contain IgM antibodies.
      E. Be of extremely large size.

24.8 Anti-Sm antibodies are detected in the absence of other autoantibodies in
      patients with
      A. Coagulopathies.
      B. Congenital heart block.
      C. Central nervous system involvement.
      D. Scleroderma.
      E. Autoimmune hemolytic anemia.

24.9   The pathogenic role of anti-DNA antibodies has best been proven in
        association to
        A. Pleurisy.
        B. Hemolytic anemia.
        C. Cutaneous vasculitis.
        D. Glomerulonephritis.
        E. Pericarditis.

24.10   The first antibodies syntehsized by NZB mice react with
        A. Cytotoxic/suppressor T cells.
        B. Red cells.
        C. Nucleic acids.
        D. Cytotoxic/suppressor T cells and nucleic acids.
        E. All of the above.

Answers

24.1   (A) Soluble IC formed at slight antigen excess between dsDNA and its
        corresponding antibody appear to play the main pathogenic role
        in SLE-associated glomerulonephritis.

24.2   (C) The diagnosis of SLE is usually based on the verification of the
        presence (simultaneously or along the course of the disease) of at
        least four diagnostic features. In this case the patient had (1)
        arthralgia, (2) butterfly rash, (3) hemolytic anemia, and (4) heavy
        proteinuria.

24.3   (A) Anti-DNA antibodies are the most frequently positive among these
        listed.

24.5   (A) The band test is always performed with normal skin, because simi-
        lar patterns of immunoglobulin and complement deposition in dis-
        eased skin may be seen in many other clinical conditions.

24.6   (C)

24.7   (A) IgG1 is complement-fixing and able to interact with the Fc receptors
        of phagocytic cells; both properties appear to be important in the
        induction of inflammatory changes secondary to IC deposition.

24.8   (C) Some atypical coagulopathies in SLE are often associated with the
        presence of anticardiolipin antibodies. The existence of a congeni-
        tal heart block is often explained by the presence of anti-Ro-SS-A in
        the mother.

24.9   (D)

24.10 (E) The antibodies to red cells, causing immune hemolytic anemia, appear later in the evolution of the disease.

BIBLIOGRAPHY

Austin, H. A., III, Klippel, J. H., Balow, J. E., Le Rich, N. G. H., Steinberg, A. D., Plotz, P. H., and Decker, J. L. Therapy of lupus nephritis. Controlled trial of prednisone and cytotoxic drugs. *N. Engl J. Med. 314*:614, 1986.

Condemi, J. J. The autoimmune diseases. *J. Amer. Med. Ass. 258*:2920, 1987.

Dixon, F. J. Murine SLE models and autoimmune disease. In *The Biology of Immunologic Disease.* Sinauer, Sunderland, Massachusetts, 1983, p. 235.

Hahn, B. H. Systemic lupus erythematosus. In *Clinical Immunology*, Vol. 1, C. W. Parker (Ed.). W. B. Saunders, Philadelphia, 1980, p. 583.

Steinberg, A. D., Raveche, E. S., Laskin, C. A., Smith, H. R., Sandoro, T., Miller, M. L., and Plotz, P. H. Systemic lupus erythematosus: Insights from animal models. *Ann. Int. Med. 100*:714, 1984.

Tan, F. J., Chan, E. K. L., Sullivan, K. F., and Rubin, R. L. Antinuclear antibodies (ANAs): Diagnostically specific immune markers and clues toward the understanding of systemic autoimmunity. *Clin. Immunol. Immunopathol. 47*:121, 1988.

25

Rheumatoid Arthritis

JEAN-MICHEL GOUST

In contrast with systemic lupus erythematosus, which has been known since Hippocratic times, the characteristic scars of this chronic disease of the joints, cartilages, and bones, which we now know as rheumatoid arthritis, are not found on English skeletons until the end of the seventeenth century. The etiology of this relatively recent disease is complex; immunologic, genetic, and hormonal factors are thought to determine its development. The role of hormonal factors is suggested by two observations: (1) the disease is three times more frequent in females than in males, and it predominantly affects women from 30 to 60 years of age; (2) pregnancy produces a remission sometimes followed by exacerbations after childbirth. It is also believed that several infectious agents with specific affinity for the joints could initiate or sustain the local and destructive inflammatory response that characterizes rheumatoid arthritis (RA).

I. CLINICAL AND PATHOLOGICAL ASPECTS OF RHEUMATOID ARTHRITIS

The most common clinical presentation of rheumatoid arthritis is the association of pain, swelling, and stiffness of the metacarpophalangeal and wrist joints, often associated with pain in the sole of the foot, indicating metatarsophalangeal involvement. The disease is initially limited to the area forming the lining

465

of the normal diarthrodial joint. The normal synovial lining is constituted by a thin membrane composed of two types of synoviocytes: the type A synoviocyte, which is a phagocytic cell of the monocyte-macrophage series with a rapid turn-over, and the type B synoviocyte, which is believed to be a specialized fibroblast. This lining sits on top of a loose acellular stroma that contains many capillaries. The earliest pathologic changes, seen at the time of the first symptoms, affect the endothelium of the microvasculature, whose permeability is increased, as judged by the development of edema and of a sparse infiltration of the edematous subsynovial space with inflammatory cells (mainly polymorphonuclear leukocytes). Several weeks later, hyperplasia of the synovial lining cells and perivascular lymphocytic infiltrates can be detected.

The disease waxes and wanes for many years but the attacks progressively run into one another, setting the stage for the chronic and well-established disease. In the chronic stage, the size and number of the lining cells increases and the synovia takes on a villous appearance. There is also subintimal hypertrophy with massive infiltration by lymphocytes and plasmablasts and granulation tissue (forming what is known as *pannus*). This thick pannus protrudes into the joint, and the synovial space becomes filled by exudative fluid that painfully limits motion. After several years of persistent and increasing local inflammation, the cartilage becomes eroded, and a progressive destruction of bones and tendons occurs, leading to more severe limitation of movement, flexion contractures, and severe mechanical deformities. The disease progresses from the distal to the proximal joints so that in the late stages joints such as the ankles, knees and elbows may become affected; this results in severe functional impairment. Thus, rheumatoid arthritis is characterized from the pathologic standpoint by the chronicity of the granulomatous reaction in the joints. However, joint involvement, an essential component of the disease, is not the only one determining the symptomatology; frequently one observes components of a more systemic nature, indicative of a generalized vasculitis. The most frequent is the formation of the rheumatoid nodules over pressure areas such as the elbows. These nodules are an important clinical feature that helps define a diagnosis of rheumatoid arthritis and generally indicates a poor prognosis. Histopathological studies show fibrinoid necrosis at the center of the nodule surrounded by histiocytes arranged in a radial palisade. The central necrotic areas are believed to be the seat of immune complex formation or deposition. When the disease has been present for some time, small brown spots may be noticed around the nail bed or associated with nodules. These indicate small areas of endarteritis. Rheumatoid patients with vasculitis usually have persistently elevated levels of circulating immune complexes and generally a worse prognosis.

In contrast, the necrotizing vasculitis associated with SLE is due almost exclusively to immune complex deposition and has little evidence of granuloma formation. However, not infrequently patients may present with an *overlap syndrome* in which both diseases are associated. This suggests that the demarcation between the diseases is not absolute and that patients with variable degrees of association of the two basic pathologic components (necrotizing vasculitides and granulomatous reaction) can be seen, so that there is a clinical continuum between the two disorders. Also, serological studies in patients with the overlap syndrome show both antibodies characteristically found in SLE (e.g., anti-dsDNA) and antibodies typical of rhematoid arthritis (rhematoid factor, see below).

II. IMMUNOLOGICAL FEATURES OF RHEUMATOID ARTHRITIS

A. Antinuclear Antibodies

Antibodies against native double-stranded DNA are conspicuously lacking in patients with classical RA, but antinuclear antibodies against single-stranded DNA can be detected in about a third of them. The epitopes recognized by anti-ssDNA antibodies belong to DNA-associated proteins. The detection of anti-ssDNA antibodies does not have diagnostic or prognostic significance, because these antibodies are not involved in immune complex formation. The reasons for their presence in RA and so many other connective tissue diseases are unknown, but they represent an indicator of immune abnormalities that may underlie an abnormal B-cell hyperactivity. This B-cell hyperactivity may be due to the persistence of abnormal B-cell clones that have escaped the repression exerted by normal tolerogenic mechanisms and that are able to produce antibodies of various types. This escape from tolerance could happen (1) spontaneously, (2) because of decreased suppressor-cell activity, or (3) as a consequence of nonspecific B-cell stimulation by microbial products (e.g., bacterial lipopolysaccharides) or infectious agents (e.g., viruses).

B. Anticollagen Antibodies

Antibodies reacting with different types of collagen have been detected with considerable frequency in connective tissue diseases such as scleroderma. In rheumatoid arthritis, considerable interest has been aroused by the finding of antibodies to type II collagen that according to some authors can induce a rheumatoid-type disease when injected together with complete Freund's adjuvant into rats. However, the frequency of these antibodies in RA patients has been recently estimated to be in the 15-20% range, which is not compatible with a primary pathogenic role. It is probable that the anticollagen antibodies arise as a response to the degradation of articular collagen, which could yield immunogenic peptides.

C. Rheumatoid Factor and Anti-Immunoglobuin Antibodies

The serological hallmark of rheumatoid arthritis is the presence of rheumatoid factor (RF) and other anti-immunoglobulin antibodies. By definition, classical RF is an IgM antibody to autologous IgG. The more encompassing designation of anti-Ig antibodies is applicable to other anti-IgG antibodies of the IgG or IgA isotypes.

1. Detection

The sera of many rheumatoid patients agglutinates sheep or human erythrocytes coated with antierythrocyte antibodies, often to high titers. This reaction is the basis of the Rose-Waaler test, the sheep cell agglutination test (SCAT), the human erythrocyte agglutination test (HEAT), and the differential agglutination test (DAT), all of which detect the classical IgM rheumatoid factors (Table 25.1). The essential feature of the reactant coating the red cells in such tests for anti-Ig antibodies is that the anti-red-cell antibody must be of the IgG class, because most anti-Ig antibodies react specifically with IgG. A particularly sensitive variant of these agglutination assays is the fraction II test, which is carried out with

TABLE 25.1 Anti-Immunoglobulin Antibodies in Healthy Controls and in Patients with Rheumatic and Nonrheumatic Diseases

	Number of patients	Age (range) (yr)	DAT titer $\geqslant 1/16$[a]	Latex titer $\geqslant 1/20$[a]	Fraction II titer $\geqslant 1/200$[a]
Control subjects					
Healthy	70	39 (17-80)	0[b]	0[b]	11[b]
Sick adults (nonrheumatic)	71	40 (16-82)	0	4	16
Chest disease (adults)	65	53 (16-76)	1.5	11	26
Degenerative joint disease	84	57 (16-76)	1.2	1.2	20
Rheumatoid arthritis					
Classic/definite	435	53 (18-84)	42	75	87
Probable/possible	69	50 (20-79	5	30	50
Ankylosing spondylitis	65	38 (15-65)	0	1	31
Gout	52	56 (31-80)	2	6	21

[a]Arbitrarily defined as cutoff for positivity.
[b]Percentage of individuals with titers exceeding the positivity cutoff.
Source: Reproduced with permission from Holborow E. J. and Swannell, A. J. *Immunology in Medicine*, 1st Ed., E. J. Holborow and W. G. Reeves (Eds.). Grune & Stratton, New York, 1979, p 541.

tannic-acid-treated sheep red cells coated with a fraction of human serum rich in IgG (Cohn's fraction II). A simpler procedure, very widely used, is the latex agglutination test, in which IgG-coated polystyrene particles are used to detect rheumatoid factors. The agglutinating titers usually considered as positive are 1:16 or more in the DAT test, 1:20 or more in the latex agglutination test, and 1:200 or more in the fraction II test.

2. Diagnostic Specificity

IgM antibodies are especially efficient as agglutinators in serological tests, such as those classically used to detect rheumatoid factor, which depend upon hemagglutination or particle agglutination; and, as noted previously, such tests selectively detect anti-Ig antibodies of the IgM class. As with many other antibodies, the titers of RF are a continuous variable within the population studied. Thus any level intending to separate the seropositive from the seronegative is arbitrarily chosen to include as many patients with clinically defined RA in the seropositive group while excluding from it as many nonrheumatoid subjects as possible.

The frequency of positivity in these different tests, as established in a survey of rheumatoid arthritis and related diseases, is shown in Table 25.1. When a line dividing negatives from positives is drawn, a minority of patients with undoubted rheumatoid disease appear persistently seronegative, whereas some patients with a variety of other diseases may have high titers of RF. Most prominent among the last are individuals suffering from Sjogren's syndrome, a disease in which the detection of anti-Ig antibodies is considered almost essential for the diagnosis. The anti-Ig antibodies in patients with Sjogren's syndrome are often specific for IgA.

3. IgG as Antigen

As a rule, the affinity of IgM rheumatoid factor for the IgG molecule is relatively low and does not reach the mean affinity of other IgM antibodies generated during an induced primary immune response. Rheumatoid factors from different individuals show different antibody specificities, reacting with different determinants of the IgG molecule. The antigenic determinants recognized by the antigen-binding sites of these IgM antibodies are located in the $C\gamma2$ and $C\gamma3$ domains of IgG; some of these determinants are allotype-related. Other RF react with determinants shared between species, a fact that explains the reactivity of human RF with rabbit IgG as well as with IgG from other mammalians. The intriguing observation of the difference in reactivity between the RF found in the serum (which react mostly with IgG1, IgG2, and IgG4) and those found in the synovial fluid (which essentially binds IgG3) could be explained by the selective homing of IgG3-producing cells to the synovium.

The finding of RF reactive with several IgG subclasses in a single patient suggests that the autoimmune response leading to the production of RF is polyclonal. This is supported by the fact the V regions of RF are heterogeneous, being obviously the product of several different V-region genes.

4. Biologic Significance of RF

Given that RF express different V-region types, it can be concluded that several sets of V genes are used to generate these autoantibodies. These V-region genes appear to be germ-line genes, and they are also expressed in normal individuals in whom anti-Ig antibodies can be detected without any clinical evidence of rheumatoid arthritis. It has been suggested that the production of anti-Ig antibodies is a normal physiologic process, perhaps assisting in the elimination of soluble immune complexes. This concept is a direct challenge to the postulate that autoantibodies emerge only as a result of the loss of tolerance to self antigens. However, the detection of anti-Ig antibodies in normal individuals seems to follow some interesting rules: (1) anti-Ig antibodies are detected *transiently* during anamnestic responses to common vaccines, and in these cases they are usually reactive with the dominant immunoglobulin isotype produced in response to antigenic stimulation; (2) the titers of vaccination-associated RF follow very closely to evolutions in titer of specific antibodies directed against the immunogen; and (3) the anti-Ig antibodies are also found in relatively high titers in diseases associated with persistent formation of antigen-antibody complexes such as subacute bacterial endocarditis, tuberculosis, leprosy, and many parasitic diseases. It has been postulated that the transient appearance of RF in normal nonrheumatoid individuals reflects a temporary down-regulation of suppressor cells, which is probably a common feature during the induction of an immune response. Later on, as suppressor circuits are activated by anti-idiotype antibodies, the production of anti-Ig antibodies is turned off.

Furthermore, the transient detection of anti-Ig antibodies in normal individuals suggest that (1) the autoreactive clones responsible for the production of autoantibodies to human immunoglobulins are not deleted during embryonic differentiation, and (2) tolerance to self IgG must be ensured by a strong negative feedback mechanism, because tolerance is broken only temporarily. A further argument in favor of the existence of autoreactive clones potentially able to synthesize anti-Ig antibodies is the observation that the bone marrow contains precursors of RF-producing B cells. Their frequency is surprisingly high in mice, where it is relatively easy to induce the production of RF in high titers after polyclonal B-cell stimulation. Similar observations were also made in humans by stimulating these bone marrow precursors with pokeweed mitogen or infecting them with Epstein-Barr virus. In both species the cell type able to differentiate into an RF-producing plasmablast has a very unusual phenotype; it expresses B-cell markers such as membrane IgM and IgD, CR2, and CD20, but also CD5, which is considered a T-cell marker. These cells represent only a very small population (less than 2%) in normal individuals in whom it would have remained undetected if not for the observation that this bizarre cell type was significantly increased in patients suffering from very active rheumatoid arthritis.

5. Pathogenic Role of Rheumatoid Factor and Anti-Immunoglobulin Antibodies

A major difference between the presence of anti-Ig antibodies in physiologic conditions and their presence in rhematoid arthritis is that RF production persists indefinitely in patients with RA, where these anti-IgG antibodies reflect an autoimmune response (either resulting from a continuous B-cell stimulation by some yet unidentified antigen or from disordered suppression).

Seropositivity for RF, especially at high titers, is associated in RA with a more rapid progression of the articular component and with systemic manifestations such as subcutaneous nodules, vasculitis, intractable skin ulcers, neuropathy, and *Felty's syndrome* (an association of rheumatoid arthritis with neuropenia). Thus the detection of RF in high titers is associated with a poor prognosis. In its reaction with human IgG, IgM RF activates complement via the classical pathway. The ability of RF to fix complement is of pathogenic significance, because it may be responsible, at least in part, for the development of rheumatoid synovitis.

Locally produced anti-Ig antibodies are likely to play an important role in causing the arthritic lesions. The joints are actually the principal site of RF production in RA patients, and it should also be noted that in some individuals the locally produced anti-Ig antibodies are of the IgG subclass. When this is the case, the joint disease is usually more severe, because anti-IgG antibodies of the IgG isotype have a higher affinity for IgG than their IgM counterparts; consequently they form stable aggregates that activate complement very efficiently. In some seronegative patients, RF and immune complexes may be detectable only in synovial fluid.

6. Seronegative Rheumatoid Arthritis

In many instances a negative result in a test for rheumatoid factor does not indicate its absence: it may be a false negative result. Two basic mechanisms may be responsible: (1) the presence of anti-Ig antibodies of isotypes other than IgM, less efficient than IgM RF in causing agglutination (particularly in tests using red cells) and therefore more likely to be overlooked; (2) the reaction between IgM RF and endogenous IgG, resulting in the formation of soluble immune complexes that, if the affinity of the reaction is high, will remain undissociated during the test for rheumatoid factor. Under these conditions, the binding sites of the rheumatoid factor are blocked, unable to react with the IgG coating indicator cell or particles. Nevertheless, true seronegative cases exist, particularly among agammaglobulinemic patients who develop a disease clinically indistinguishable from rheumatoid arthritis in spite of their inability to synthesize antibodies. This is a highly significant observation, because it argues strongly against the role of RF as the sole pathogenic insult in rheumatoid arthritis and suggests that the onset of the local inflammatory response on the rheumatoid joint could be largely cell-mediated.

D. Cellular Abnormalities in Rheumatoid Arthritis

1. T-Cell Abnormalities

All the essential cellular elements of the immune response are present in the hypertrophic synovium of the rheumatoid joints, where they are easily accessible to study by needle biopsy or by aspiration of the synovial fluid. The synovial fluid also contains many mediators and molecules synthesized by the infiltrating cells. Immunohistologic studies of the lymphocytes found in the massive lymphocytic synovial infiltrates (where they may represent up to 60% of the total net weight) indicates that in most instances $CD4^+$ helper T cells outnumber $CD8^+$ cells in a ratio of 5:1. It is not unusual to see in the inflamed synovial tissue macrophage-lymphocyte clusters, in which several T cells are in very close contact with large macrophages expressing high levels of class II HLA antigens. These $CD4^+$ lymphocytes were considered the most probable source of the helper factors needed to induce B-cell growth and differentiation, which seems to be the basis for the polyclonal B-cell activation seen at the synovial level. The synovial fluid also contains increased numbers of monocytes as well as dendritic cells. The later are nonphagocytic, but they express very high levels of class II HLA antigens and produce IL1. Thus, these dendritic cells could be functioning as antigen-presenting cells, contributing to the activation of $CD4^+$ lymphocytes.

However, the large majority of the T cells in the synovial infiltrates and in the synovial fluid do not appear to be activated. Most of them are small, do not express interleukin 2 receptors, and do not release IL2 or interferon γ. It is thus possible that the synovial T cells do not play a significant role in the pathogenesis of the joint lesions, but rather that they are attracted to the site of an ongoing inflammatory response as innocent bystanders. Alternatively, their relative idleness could result from an active down-regulation of PGE2 produced locally by activated macrophages that may be stimulated by immune complexes formed in situ. These activated macrophages actively secrete many proteolytic enzymes (such as collagenase) that play a very important pathogenic role in the joint. Therefore the macrophage could be the key cell initiating the arthritic process. A problem with this sequence of events is how to explain macrophage activation in RF-negative patients. Because the T cells found in the synovial fluid produce so little interferon γ, they cannot be responsible for macrophage activation. Thus, macrophage activation remains difficult to explain by any single theory.

2. The Monocyte Family in the Rheumatoid Joint

In this search for the initial pathogenic event that leads to the development of RA, the focus of attention has turned toward cells of the monocyte-macrophage family, such as the *dendritic cells*. These cells are found in relatively large numbers in the inflammatory lesion, where they release a variety of lymphokines, particularly IL1, which can cause an increased vascular permeability, enhance the influx of inflammatory cells, and stimulate their proliferation.

A third member of the monocyte/macrophage family that may be involved in the pathogenesis of the joint lesions is the *type A synoviocyte*. This cell is a major source of mediators that could play a major role in the formation of inflammatory granulomas. The first is platelet-derived growth factor (PDGF), a molecule with many actions, one of which is to prime fibroblasts, preparing them to react positively to the other growth factors necessary to their proliferation. The second substance is the so-called granulocyte-macrophage colony stimulating factor (GM-CSF). This mediator is a consistent inducer of HLA class II antigens on a large variety of cells including the monocyte. It is now accepted that this molecule is the inducer of class II HLA antigen expression in monocytes that infiltrate the rheumatoid joint. The effects of GM-CSF are additive to those of interferon γ. Even if interferon γ is present at low concentrations because there are only very few activated T cells producing it, GM-CSF will activate monocytes and increase HLA class II expression. In addition, activated monocytes would produce tumor necrosis factor, whose effect on HLA class II production is synergistic with that of GM-CSF. Monocytes activated by GM-CSF also produce interleukin 6, which acts on B cells and could stimulate local immunoglobulin production. This sequence of events is schematically depicted in Figure 25.1.

3. Genetic Factors

Even though the incidence of familial rheumatoid arthritis is rather low, it has been known for several years that 50 to 70% of Caucasians with rheumatoid arthritis express the HLA DRw4 antigen, which is found in no more than 15 to 25% of the normal population. Individuals expressing this antigen are 6 to 12 times more at risk of having RA than those who do not have it, and this antigen is found in 96% of the patients with Felty's syndrome. Studies at the DNA level have confirmed this observation, and with adequate DNA probes the existence of many different subtypes of DR4 has been revealed; some of those subtypes

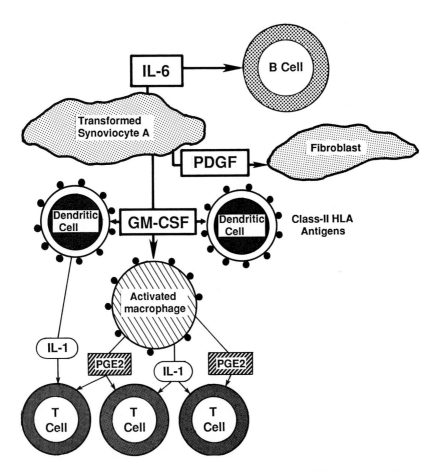

FIGURE 25.1 Diagrammatic representation of the possible immunopathology of rheumatoid arthritis. The initial event is the transformation (by an environmental factor) of a type A synoviocyte, which starts to release large levels of several cytokines. One of the released cytokines is IL6, which stimulates polyclonal B-cell activation, which may lead to the synthesis of rheumatoid factor. A second cytokine released by the synoviocyte is platelet-derived growth factor (PDGF), which promotes the proliferation of synovial fibroblasts. Finally, the synoviocyte also releases GM-CSF, which is responsible for activation and increased expression of class II MHC antigens (which favor the onset of autoimmune responses) on macrophages and dendritic cells. The activated macrophage can also release IL6 and in addition releases IL1 and PGE2, which have conflicting effects at the T-cell level.

appear to be more strongly associated with the disease than the serologically defined DRw4 antigen. However, none of these associations is so strong that it can be considered as the cause of the disease.

What is more plausible is that the overrepresentation of some class II antigens, which are linked to genes controlling the magnitude of the immune response, may reflect the genetic predisposition of the bearers to develop responses of abnormal magnitude to some pathogen that is eliminated without problems by most individuals who carry other sets of class II antigens. On the other hand this association could have a very different significance, pointing toward the possibility of a close linkage between the MHC type II genes on chromosome 6 and some other non-HLA gene that, when expressed on some synovial cell such as the synoviocyte type A, would favor the development of rheumatoid arthritis. Thus the role of the HLA complex would be only coincidental, the first abnormality being a modification of synovial cells by unidentified pathogens.

4. Infectious Agents and Rheumatoid Arthritis

Lyme disease is a transmissible disease caused by a spirochete, *Borrelia burgdorferi*. Among a variety of symptoms, patients with this disease may present monoarticular or polyarticular arthritis. The pathology of the inflamed joints in patients with Lyme disease strikingly resembles that seen in RA. However, infection with this pathogen is extremely rare in patients suffering from classical rheumatoid arthritis. Another infectious agent that could be involved is the Epstein-Barr virus (EBV), because the serum of 71% of RA patients (vs. 6% of sera from normal controls) contains an unusual type of antibody that reacts with a nuclear antigen extracted from an EBV-infected lymphoblastoid cell line. Because of the high frequency of antibodies detected in patients with rheumatoid arthritis, the antigen is designated as RA-associated nuclear antigen or RANA. The significance of the RANA antibody in RA is not clear, and the role of EBV infection in the pathogenesis of RA remains speculative, because anti-RANA and RF titers are not related in individual patients, and also because high titers of anti-RANA may be found in normal individuals.

Considering the crucial role that seems to be played by abnormally activated cells of the monocyte-macrophage series, it has been hypothesized that a yet unidentified slow virus could be involved in the pathogenesis of RA. The possibility that a hitherto unidentified human retrovirus may cause RA is suggested by the existence of a disease in goats and sheep, caused by a retrovirus of the lentiviridae family, that resembles RA in many aspects. These retroviruses cause a latent infection of monocyte precursors that, after differentiating into circulating monocytes, home predominantly in the joints. The virus replicates very slowly in the infected cells, without causing cell lysis, but a very pronounced inflammatory reaction develops in the joints. The macrophages within the inflamed tissue express large amounts of Ia antigen to which viral antigens are closely associated. Furthermore, it is known that viral infection of any cell can lead to functional changes, sometimes down-regulating important functions, sometimes up-regulating the synthesis of cell products. Thus an infection with a slow virus, leading to increased secretion of macrophage mediators, could be the basis for the development of rheumatoid arthritis. A contributing factor could be the activation of T cells by the association of viral antigens and MHC molecules. Further work is still needed to determine whether a retrovirus is involved in RA. If it is, it will open the way to the prevention of the disease by vaccination of susceptible individuals.

III. THERAPY

It is not surprising that our incomplete knowledge of rheumatoid arthritis is reflected at the therapeutic level. Most of our current therapeutic approaches are symptomatic, aiming to reduce joint inflammation and tissue damage. Given the importance of prostaglandins as mediators of inflammation, it is not surprising that drugs that inhibit the cyclooxygenase pathway (e.g., aspirin, ibuprofen, naproxen, and indomethacin) are beneficial in patients with rheumatoid arthritis. In more severe cases, in which the cyclooxygenase inhibitors may not be effective, glucocorticoids may be required. Corticosteroids are a two-edged sword in RA, however, because in most instances their administration masks the inflammatory component only as long as they are given. Thus corticosteroid therapy needs to be maintained for long periods of time, and side effects, including muscle and bone loss, may become more devastating than the original arthritis. Immunosuppression by drugs such as azathioprine or by total lymphoid irradiation may be considerably more efficient than the use of antiinflammatory drugs in the most severe cases.

The treatment of rheumatoid arthritis is based on empirical assumptions and clinical experience, and it is often a frustrating experience for patients and physicians. The rationale for our choice of therapeutic approaches is based on our current postulates about the pathogenesis of the disease. If future research shows that the role of immune disturbances is secondary and relatively negligible, it is possible that totally new approaches will emerge. Definitive progress will be achieved when the cause of the disease is elucidated and curative or preventive therapies can be devised.

SELF-EVALUATION

Questions

Choose the one best answer.

25.1 The classic rheumatoid factor is
   A. An IgG anti-IgG antibody.
   B. An IgA anti-IgM antibody.
   C. An IgG anti-IgM antibody.
   D. An IgM anti-IgG antibody.
   E. Any one of those listed.

25.2 The test that detects a higher frequency of antiglobulin antibodies in
   rheumatoid arthritis patients is the
   A. Latex agglutination test.
   B. Differential agglutination test.
   C. Fraction II test.
   D. C1q-binding assay.
   E. ANA test by immunofluorescence.

25.3 All of the following antibodies have been detected in patients with rheu-
   matoid arthritis except
   A. Anti-Sm antibodies.
   B. Antinuclear antibodies.
   C. Anticollagen type II antibodies.
   D. Antinuclear antigen (RANA).
   E. Anti-EB virus nuclear antigen (EBNA).

25.4 A latex agglutination titer of 20 in an asymptomatic individual is con-
   sidered as
   A. Indicative of silent rheumatoid arthritis.
   B. Predictive of future development of rheumatoid arthritis.
   C. A technical error.
   D. Without special meaning.
   E. None of the above.

25.5 Most patients with seronegative rheumatoid arthritis have
   A. A disease different from classical rheumatoid arthritis.
   B. IgM antiglobulin antibodies.
   C. RF with blocked binding sites.
   D. Total absence of antiglobulin antibodies.
   E. Agammaglobulinemia.

25.6 A high titer of rheumatoid factor
   A. Has no special meaning.
   B. Is likely to be associated with a nonrheumatoid disease.
   C. Is frequently seen in patients with systemic complications.
   D. Can be considered as evidence for the existence of large concentrations
      of circulating immune complexes.
   E. Is more often seen with the DAT test than with a fraction II test.

25.7   The antigen(s) recognized by rheumatoid factor is (are)
   A.   EB virus nuclear antigen.
   B.   RA-associated nuclear antigen.
   C.   IgG immunoglobulins.
   D.   IgA immunoglobulins.
   E.   Immunoglobulins of all classes except IgM.

25.8   Concerning lymphocytic abnormalities in rheumatoid arthritis, it is not
        correct to say that
   A.   B lymphocytes from RA patients are very easy to immortalize.
   B.   Synovial CD8$^+$ cells are hyperactive.
   C.   Synovial CD4$^+$ cells from clusters around macrophages.
   D.   Hyperactive CD4$^+$ cells may be responsible for B-cell hyperactivity.
   E.   The CD8$^+$ lymphocyte population is hypoactive.

25.9   The strongest argument against the role of rheumatoid factor as the ini-
        tial pathogenic insult in rheumatoid arthritis is the
   A.   Very similar clinical pictures in seronegative and seropositive rheu-
        matoid arthritis.
   B.   Development of rheumatoid arthritis in agammaglobulinemic pa-
        tients.
   C.   Non-complement-fixing nature of the antigen-antibody complexes
        formed in rheumatoid arthritis.
   D.   Presence of rheumatoid factor in normal individuals.
   E.   Lack of animal models in which passive administration of rheuma-
        toid factor reproduces the disease.

25.10   Aspirin and indomethacin are effective in rheumatoid arthritis because
        these drugs
   A.   Are immunosuppressant.
   B.   Inhibit platelet aggregation.
   C.   Reduce the synthesis and release of prostaglandins.
   D.   Depress phagocytic function.
   E.   Depress the release of interleukins by macrophages and lympho-
        cytes.

Answers

25.1   (D)

25.2   (C)

25.3   (A) Anti-Sm antibodies are virtually exclusive of patients with systemic
        lupus erythematosus.

25.4 (D) Many normal, asymptomatic individuals have low titers of autoantibodies, including RF. Those low titers are not necessarily associated
with future evolution toward clinically evident rheumatoid arthritis.

25.5 (C) True seronegative rheumatoid arthritis is rare and found among
agammaglobulinemic individuals.

25.6 (C) The detection of rheumatoid factor cannot be considered a direct
index of the concentration of soluble immune complexes, because
a positive test is dependent upon the existence of free binding sites
for IgG, and it is not practical to measure the ratio of free to bound
binding sites.

25.7 (C)

25.8 (B) Actually, $CD8^+$ cells are hypoactive, unable to control the B-cell
proliferation.

25.9 (B) Agammaglobulinemic patients are truly seronegative, and they still
develop a disease that clinically cannot be distinguished from rheumatoid arthritis.

25.10 (C) Aspirin and indomethacin inhibit the cyclooxygenase pathway of
arachidonic acid metabolism that leads to the synthesis of prostaglandins E2 and F2.

REFERENCES

Zvaifler, N. J. New perspectives on the pathogenesis of rheumatoid arthritis.
Am. J. Med. *85*(sup. 4A):12-16, 1988.

Carsons, S. Newer diagnostic parameters for the diagnosis of rheumatic disease.
Am. J. Med. *85*(sup. 4A):34-38, 1988.

Theofilopoulos, A., Kofler, R., Singer, P. A., Noonan, D. J., and Dixon, F. J.
Genomic organization and expression of B and T cell antigen receptor genes
in murine lupus. In *Rheumatic Diseases Clinics of North America 13*(3):
511-530, 1987.

Chen, P. P., Fong, S., and Carson, D. A. Rheumatoid factor. In *Rheumatic
Diseases Clinics of North America 13*(3):545-568, 1987.

Kennedy-Stoskopf, S., Zink, M. C., Jolly, P. E., and Narayan, O. Lentivirus-
induced arthritis chronic disease caused by a covert pathogen. In *Rheumatic
Diseases Clinics of North America 13*(2):235-247, 1987.

McDermott, M. and McDevitt, H. The immunogenetics of rheumatic diseases.
Bull. Rheum. Dis. 38:1, 1988.

26

Immunosuppression and Immunomodulation

JEAN-MICHEL GOUST, HENRY C. STEVENSON, ROBERT M. GALBRAITH, and GABRIEL VIRELLA

I. IMMUNOSUPPRESSION

Suppression of the immune response is at the present time the only efficient therapy in most autoimmune diseases and in the control of transplant rejection and other situations in which the immune system plays a significant pathogenic role. In recent years it has become apparent that a large number of clinically useful drugs affect immune responses. Most of these agents suppress some part of the immune response, usually in a nonspecific fashion. Some newer immunosuppressants have effects practically limited to one or another component of the immune system, but they still lead to generalized immunodepression. More recently, a variety of new biological agents have been tried in different immunosuppressive regimens, including monoclonal antibodies to T cells and their subsets, immunotoxins, IL2-toxin conjugates, anti-idiotypic antibodies, etc. In many cases these agents are still in the early stages of evaluation and it is too early to issue definitive judgments about their usefulness. It is, however, unquestionable that they are the prototypes of approaches that will be more and more used in the near future.

A. Immunosuppressive Drugs: Pharmacological and Immunological Aspects

Most cytotoxic drugs used in cancer chemotherapy have been shown to have immunosuppressive properties. While many of these drugs are loosely termed

481

immunosuppressive, they differ widely in their mechanisms of action, toxicity and efficacy for treatment of nonneoplastic diseases.

The exact mechanisms of action of immunosuppressive drugs are difficult to determine partly because the physiology of the immune response has not yet been completely elucidated. Possible target sites are: (1) phagocytosis and anti-gen-processing by macrophages; (2) antigen recognition by lymphocytes; (3) differentiation of lymphocytes; (4) proliferation of T and B lymphocytes; (5) production of interleukins, and (6) the effector mechanisms that include production and release of antibodies and/or delayed hypersensitivity mediators.

1. Alkylating Agents and Antimetabolites

The concept that some of these drugs are *cycle-active* and other *non-cycle-active* is helpful in understanding their actions. Alkylating agents (and also x-rays) can cause cellular death irrespective of whether the cells are in cycle, i.e., in the process of replicating; in contrast, other agents, primarily antimetabolites, are not able to kill if the cells are not in cycle.

The cell division cycle is conventionally divided into a G_1 (gap 1) or presynthetic phase, an S (DNA synthesizing) phase, or G_2 (gap 2) or premitotic resting phase, and an M phase (mitosis). Cycle-active agents may kill by acting at different parts of the cycle; antimetabolites such as methotrexate, azathioprine and 6-MP appear to act only on cells in the S phase. In a nonstimulated lympho-cyte population, many of the cells are not in cycle but in a prolonged G_1 or "G_0" state. These cells are not affected by exposure to cycle-active agents but may be killed by alkylating agents such as cyclophosphamide or by x-rays (although even these agents seem to kill cells in cycle to a greater degree than cells not in cycle). Thus, methotrexate, 6-mercaptopurine (6-MP) and azathioprine (a mercaptopurine derivative), which are antimetabolites, are *cycle-specific* S-phase inhibitors, while cyclophosphamide has both *cycle-specific* and non-cycle-*specific* properties. Methotrexate, azathioprine and 6-MP kill primarily rapidly dividing cells; cyclophosphamide kills both dividing and nondividing (resting) cells.

The three major cytotoxic drugs, cyclophosphamide, azathioprine, and methotrexate, all suppress primary and secondary humoral immune responses, delayed hypersensitivity, skin graft rejection, and autoimmune disease in animals. Unfortunately, few studies have compared the effects of these three drugs under the same experimental conditions. However, some striking differences in the mechanism of action of these three agents have become apparent and are summarized below.

In studies of the effects of cyclophosphamide, methotrexate, and 6-MP on antibody production in mice, one can compare the dose that kills 5% of the animals within one week (LD_5) with the dose required to reduce the antibody

TABLE 26.1 Therapeutic Indices of Agents Inhibiting Antibody Production

Agent	$LD_5{}^a$	$ID_2{}^b$	TI^c
Cyclophosphamide	300.0	50.0	6.0
Methotrexate	6.3	1.25	5.0
6-Mercaptopurine	240.0	100.0	2.4

$^a LD_5$ dose (in mg/kg) killing 5% of animals within 1 week.
$^b ID_2$ dose (in mg/kg) lowering antibody titer to $1/2^2$.
^{c}Therapeutic index = LD/ID.

response of the mice by a factor of 2 (inhibitory dose; ID_2); a therapeutic index (TI) can be calculated that is defined as the ratio of the two doses (LD5/ID2). Cyclophosphamide has the highest therapeutic index followed by methotrexate and 6-MP (Table 26.1).

Sharply different effects of azathioprine and cyclophosphamide on humoral antibody production have been demonstrated in patients, using flagellin as test antigen. There was a significant suppression of antibody response to flagellin in cyclophosphamide-treated patients, while the responses of azathioprine-treated patients did not differ significantly from those of nontreated control patients. Several workers have also shown that cyclophosphamide can decrease the production of anti-DNA antibodies, both in NZB mice and in man. This suggests that cyclophosphamide can inhibit an ongoing immune response whereas azathioprine and 6-MP cannot. This is of course the situation that one faces in the treatment of patients with autoimmune disease, since the relevant immune responses are already established at the time that they are recognized and treated. It is of interest in this regard that in patients with systemic lupus erythematosus cyclophosphamide treatment can reverse the findings on direct immunofluorescence of the skin (which correlate with renal disease) whereas steroid therapy alone does not.

Studies of the effects of these drugs have shown that all three depress cellular immunity. However, comparative studies show a greater effect with cyclophosphamide. While both cyclophosphamide and methotrexate are more effective than 6-MP in suppressing a PPD skin test in experimental animals, only cyclophosphamide depletes thymus-dependent areas of the lymph nodes. The in vitro response of lymphocytes to PHA and other mitogens is likewise inhibited only by cyclophosphamide. In addition, tolerance induction is much easier to achieve in mice treated with cyclophosphamide than with azathioprine or methotrexate. In animals with malignant plasmocytomas, cyclophosphamide can have a true immunomodulating effect. Given in appropriate doses, cyclophosphamde will affect predominantly suppressor T cells, allowing antitumor immunity to devel-

TABLE 26.2 Summary of Effects of Drugs with Alkylating and Antimetabolite
Activity[a]

Effect	Cyclo-phosphamide	Azathioprine and 6-MP	Metho-trexate
Reduced primary immune response	++	++	++
Reduced secondary immune response	++	±	+
Reduced immune complexes	++	0	0
Anti-inflammatory effect	+	++	+
Mitostatic effect	++	++	++
Reduced delayed hypersensitivity	++	+	+
		(? Anti-inflammatory)	
Suppression of passive transfer of cellular immunity	++	±	±
Lymphopenia	++	±	±
Facilitation of tolerance induction	++	+	+

[a]On the basis of a combination of experimental and clinical data.

op. Despite the extensive clinical use of these drugs, many discrepancies can be
found in the medical literature concerning their mechanisms of action. In Table
26.2, we have attempted to summarize their known effects.

2. Cyclosporine A (CsA)

Cyclosporine A is a fungal metabolite obtained from *Tolypocladium inflatum*.
Structurally a cyclic peptide, of 11 aminoacids, CsA has a uniquely selective
effect on T lymphocytes, suppressing humoral T-dependent responses and cell-
mediated immune responses.

The mechanism of action of CsA at the cellular and subcellular level has been
the object of many detailed studies. It is known that the drug is taken up by
lymphocytes and accumulates in the cytoplasm, where it binds with high affinity
to cyclophilin, which has really been identified as a peptidyl-prolyl cis-*trans*
isomerase (PPIase), and to calmodulin, a protein whose function is related to
cyclic nucleotide activation. PPIase is responsible for the intracellular folding
of nascent proteins and may also modulate intracellular signal transduction
processes. Cyclosporin inhibits the enzymatic activity of cyclophilin in vitro,
interfering with protein synthesis. The activation of calmodulin is dependent
on Ca^{2+} binding, and cyclosporin A inhibits calmodulin activation by interfering
with Ca^{2+} binding. The lack of proper activation of calmodulin has a negative
effect on the activation of several protein kinases and phosphodiesterase and

blocks the activation sequence of the lymphocyte. The nuclear induction of ornithine decarboxylase is affected by CsA, and the lack of this enzyme prevents proper gene activation and expression, as well as mRNA and DNA synthesis. As a consequence, cell-cycle progression is arrested at the G1-S transition, and there is a general down-regulation of interleukin synthesis at the pretranscriptional level.

As a result of the intracellular effects of CsA, the production of interleukin 2 (IL2), interferon γ, and other interleukins is depressed. These interleukins are predominantly synthesized by helper (CD4$^+$) T cells, which are the chief cellular target for CsA; suppressor T cells, on the other hand, appear to proliferate at higher rates. This differential effect is reflected in humans by a reversion of the CD4/CD8 ratio rates and by a relative increase in suppressor function. The activation of cytotoxic cells is also inhibited, apparently due to both the lack of stimulatory signals provided by IL2 and to a direct inhibitory effect on cytotoxic T cell precursors. The effects of preformed lymphokines are not inhibited by this drug; furthermore, CsA appears remarkably devoid of cytotoxic effects on nonlymphoid leukocytes, although it has also been shown that interleukin 1 production and accessory cell function are depressed by this drug.

As a consequence of this selective immunosuppressant activity, CsA has a remarkable ability to prolong graft survival. In experimental animals, even short courses of CsA can result in significant prolongation of kidney graft survival, suggesting that the drug facilitates the development of low dose tolerance. In humans, used alone or in association with steroids, it reduces the number of rejection episodes in renal transplantation, even in patients with cytotoxic antibodies and receiving poorly matched organs. It also induces a substantially longer survival of kidney, liver, and especially heart transplants, and it reduces the incidence and severity of graft-vs.-host disease in bone marrow transplantation.

The main advantages of CsA are its selective effect on T lymphocytes and its excellent steroid-sparing effect. Basically, the dosages of steroids necessary to achieve effective immunosuppression are considerably lower when steroids are associated to CsA than when they are associated to other immunosuppressive drugs. As a result, the incidence of infections is substantially reduced, the most common offending agent that infects CsA-treated patients being cytomegalovirus. However, CsA can have serious side effects, the main one being nephrotoxicity, which is clearly a disadvantage in renal transplantation. The renal toxicity is apparently associated with hypertension, which in turn has a negative impact on all patients, but especially in those receiving a heart transplant. The de novo appearance of lymphproliferative disorders (particularly brain lymphomas) after CsA therapy, by itself or in combination with other immunosuppressive agents (e.g., antilymphocyte globulin), has been reported. Accelerated atherosclerosis has been observed in heart transplant recipients surviving for over 2 years, but the role played by CsA in this complication is not clear. Recent observations suggest that long term immunosuppression with associations of CsA, steroids, and azathioprine, allowing substantial reductions of CsA dosages, may be preferable to long term administration of high doses of CsA, at least in patients with kidney transplants.

3. Hormones

The major agents in this group of substances are the glucocorticosteroid hormones of the adrenal complex cortex and their synthetic analogues (prednisone and prednisolone). Corticosteroids are known to have an anti-inflammatory action and decrease the number of mononuclear phagocytes at sites of inflammation. At certain dosage levels, treatment with corticosteroids may produce a rapid and profound lymphopenia. However, there are considerable differences in susceptibility to this effect of glucocorticoids between various species. Glucocorticoid-sensitive species (including the hamster, mouse, rat, and rabbit) have cytoplasmic receptors, and the interaction of these receptors with steroids leads to the inhibition of cellular metabolism, including nucleic acid synthesis and glucose uptake. In steroid-sensitive species, both primary and secondary antibody responses are impaired, but very little inhibition occurs in steroid-resistant species, although in the latter, including man, steroids can suppress cell-mediated immunity if large dosages or prolonged treatment are used. For example, prednisone in a dosage of 40 mg per day orally will result in PPD skin tests changing from positive to negative after an average of about two weeks. Glucocorticosteroids also inhibit chemotaxis of neutrophils and have marked effects on the distribution of lymphocytes in the peripheral blood. Studies in patients show that 4 h after the administration of a single large dose of prednisone, there is a profound lymphocytopenia and monocytopenia, with a preferential depletion of T lymphocytes. The lymphocytopenia is due primarily to a transient depletion of the recirculating portion of the intravascular lymphocyte pool. All these parameters return to normal by the following day. This drug-associated cyclic and transient monocytopenia and lymphocytopenia are probably due to redistribution of recirculating mononuclear cells to other body compartments, particularly the bone marrow.

B. Use of Immunosuppressive Drugs for Immunological Disorders

1. Corticosteroids

Corticosteroid treatment can be life-saving in certain acute disorders such as bronchial asthma and autoimmune thrombocytopenic purpura. It also can bring about dramatic symptomatic improvement in a number of chronic disease states of proven immunological origin. However, a word of caution is necessary, since the use of these agents has become extremely widespread in spite of a lack of controlled studies demonstrating that corticosteroids improve prognosis. For example, corticosteroids produce a dramatic response in many patients with rheumatoid arthritis. However, the disease may persist in spite of chronic corticosteroid therapy, and the patient then has two diseases, rheumatoid arthritis and iatrogenic corticosteroid-induced complications. A second example is that of acute rheumatic fever. While many physicians use corticosteroids for treatment of the carditis, controlled studies have shown that they do not improve the prognosis. In spite of those caveats, the use of corticosteroids is believed to be beneficial in a number of immunological disorders, including chronic warm autoantibody hemolytic anemia, chronic active hepatitis, autoimmune thrombocytopenic purpura, and systemic lupus erythematosus, and they are part of most immunosuppressive regimens used for preventing the rejection of transplanted organs.

2. Cytotoxic Agents

Many nonneoplastic diseases that are either proven or presumed to be immunologically mediated have been treated with cytotoxic drugs. Results of controlled trials of azathioprine and cyclophosphamide suggest that both drugs, when given in sufficient quantity, may be capable of suppressing disease activity. Cyclophosphamide is currently the drug of choice for the treatment of lupus glomerulonephritis and other vasculitides (see Chapter 24). However, toxic effects were also observed. For example, in controlled studies of azathioprine in systemic lupus erythematosus (SLE), a number of beneficial effects were seen, i.e., an increase in creatinine clearance, a decrease in proteinuria, and a decrease in mortality. However, discontinuation of azathioprine was followed by severe exacerbations of the disease. A decrease in glomerular cell proliferation has been noted in renal biopsies of SLE patients receiving azathioprine. Cyclosporine A has not been as widely used in the treatment of autoimmune disorders as azathioprine and cyclophosphamide, with the exception of type I (insulin-dependent) diabetes and myasthenia gravis. In these situations, considerable clinical improvement may be seen while the drug is being administered, but relapses occur as soon as CsA is suspended.

   In summary, cytotoxic agents have been used in most diseases treated with corticosteroids, and although controlled trials are still required to access overall benefit, it should be strated that perhaps their major advantage is the possibility, when such drugs are added to corticosteroid therapy, of reducing the dose of steroids—the previously mentioned steroid-sparing effect.

C. Adverse Effects of Immunosuppressive Drugs

The most common type of toxicity associated to the use of immunosuppressive drugs is due to effects on the bone marrow and hemopoiesis. All immunosuppressives are capable of inducing bone marrow suppression, the degree of which is usually dose-related and can be modulated by dose changes, although in rare cases, the bone marrow failure may be irreversible. This is obviously associated with a high risk of infection, particularly when neutropenia is predominant. Infections associated with neutropenia are extremely difficult to treat, and for this reason neutropenia is considered the most serious side effect of immunosuppression. In addition, most agents produce hair loss or alopecia and major constitutional symptoms (e.g., nausea, vomiting, anorexia, malaise, etc.).

The risk of infection is increased in patients treated with these agents. The depression of cellular immunity may be responsible for the fact that viral infections, such as measles, herpes simplex, and varicella may disseminate with a fatal outcome. The incidence of herpes zoster (shingles) seems to increase, but the course of the disease is similar to that seen in otherwise normal individuals. The impairment of cell mediated immunity is also probably responsible for the severity of mycobacterial and fungal infections, which are much more likely to disseminate during immunosuppressive treatment, and for opportunistic infections with cytomegalovirus, *Pneumocystis carinii*, and fungi such as *Candida* and *Aspergillus*. When neutropenia develops, severe pyogenic infections are likely to develop; these infections are extremely difficult to treat, often being the cause of death. Continuous monitoring of white cell count is essential in patients treated with these drugs. Also, the incidence of neutropenia seems to be reduced when the drugs are administered intermittently, with short courses at high doses separated by long therapy-free intervals.

Chromosomal changes and teratogenic effects have been observed with most immunosuppressive agents, but mothers receiving these agents have also borne normal children. The appropriate delay between stopping the drug and permitting conception has not been established with certainty.

Probably the major concern in treatment with these agents is the possibility of inducing malignancy. Although the precise role of the immune system in eliminating neoplastic clones in a normal individual is not clear, the incidence of malignancies is clearly elevated in patients receiving immunosuppressive drugs. The most frequently seen malignancies in immunosuppressed patients are skin cancers and lymphoreticular neoplasias. Also, the location and pattern of spread of those malignancies is unusual. For example, intracerebral lymphoma is virtually restricted to immunosuppressed patients, where it occurs in frequencies as high as 50% of the patients that develop lymphoma. The intracerebral lymphomas have a particularly malignant evolution and are always B-cell lymphomas expressing Epstein-Barr virus. It has been postulated that they emerge in individuals carrying the virus in a latent stage as a consequence of a deficient immunosurveillance that normally would control the proliferation of viral-infected B cells.

II. IMMUNOMODULATION

Many modulators have been used in attempts to influence the immune system in conditions in which it is believed to be functionally altered. In autoimmunity, immunosuppressive drugs are used to decrease the autoreactive immune responses; several different biological products with immunoregulatory properties (biological response modifiers) have been administered to patients with the aim of boosting the functions of their T-cell system; a wide variety of agents has been found to have "adjuvant" properties in man, and a number of them have been used to boost the functional status of the immune system in cancer patients. All these types of therapeutic intervention fall under the general designation of *immunomodulation*, which can be defined as any type of therapeutic intervention aimed at restoring the normal function of the immune system. In this chapter, we shall restrict our discussion to immunomodulation in nonmalignant diseases, while the use of immunomodulators in cancer is discussed in Chapter 28.

A. The Biological Response Modifier (BRM) System

The term *biological response modifier* (BRM) designates a variety of signals that allow the various elements of the immune system to communicate with one another. This communication network allows for up-regulation and coordination of immune responses when needed and down-regulation of immune responses when no longer needed by the host. Figure 26.1 lists the most important of the BRM signals that have been studied and that appear to have some clinical applicability. All BRM are short polypeptide molecules that have a surprising degree of similarity to one another in size and amino acid content; this is felt to be reflective of an early gene reduplication that occurred as the immune system of man evolved.

The BRM appear to form a very delicate network of communication signals between the four principal mononuclear leukocyte subsets that participate in the immune response. We are still without a complete understanding as to how these interactions occur, but the release of these signals appears to be different from that of hormones. Hormones tend to act at a site far distant from the original cell that secreted the signal; in contrast, BRM appear to work in the immediate vicinity of the cell type that secretes them. The timing of the release of the BRM coupled with the intensity of their secretion appears to provide the overall balance required to orchestrate the immune response.

SECRETORY PRODUCTS OF MONONUCLEAR LEUKOCYTES: SELECTED BIOLOGICAL RESPONSE MODIFIERS (BRM).

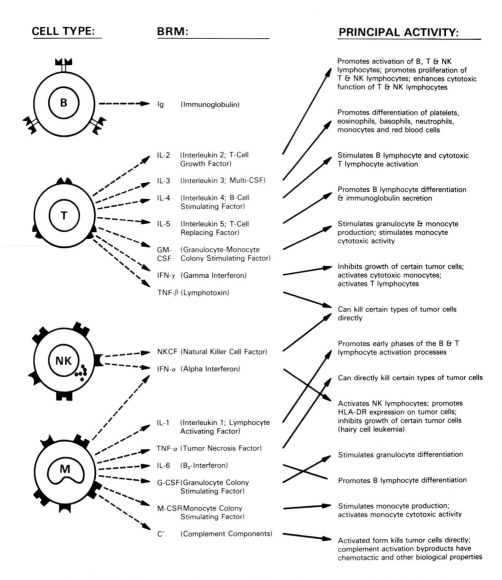

FIGURE 26.1 Diagrammatic representation of the source and principal mechanisms of action of the most important biological response modifiers secreted by mononuclear leukocytes.

As shown in Figure 26.1, the principal BRM secreted by B lymphocytes is specific antibody. Both IgM and IgG are capable of activating the complement cascade; however, only the IgG isotope is capable of activating the antibody-dependent cellular cytotoxicity (ADCC) mechanism. The T lymphocyte produces a wide range of BRM. Seven have been indicated in this figure: (1) interleukin 2 (IL2) is a factor that induces the proliferation of T lymphocytes and NK lymphocytes; this factor is also capable of up-regulating the tumor-killing capabilities of the cells whose proliferation it stimulates; (2) interleukin 3 (IL3) is a growth factor for stem cells in the bone marrow that stimulates the production of many types of leukocytes from the bone marrow when needed; (3) interleukin 4 (IL4) is a factor that stimulates B lymphocytes to proliferate; (4) interleukin 5 (IL5) promotes B-lymphocyte proliferation and differentiation into immunoglobulin secreting cells; (5) granulocyte-monocyte colony stimulating factor (GM-CSF) stimulates the bone marrow to produce both granulocytes and monocytes; it also appears capable of up-regulating the spontaneous killing capability of monocytes; (6) γ interferon (IFNγ) is a protein with moderate antiviral activity that also appears capable of stimulating both T-lymphocyte and monocyte cytotoxicity, and (7) tumor necrosis factor α (TNF-α, cachectin) is a molecule secreted by cytotoxic T lymphocytes that appears capable of killing tumor cells directly, perhaps by making their cell membranes overly permeable.

The natural killer lymphocyte also secretes a series of BRM. The two most notable are natural killer cell factor (NKCF) and α interferon (IFNα). NKCF, like lymphotoxin, appears to be capable of killing certain types of target cells by making their membranes overly permeable. Alpha interferon is an antiviral agent that also promotes the activation of NK lymphocytes. Alpha interferon appears capable of inhibiting the growth of certain types of tumor cells directly, such as in the case of hairy cell leukemia.

Mononuclear phagocytes (monocytes and macrophages) share with NK lymphocytes the ability to secrete α interferon. In addition, they secrete two types of interleukins, interleukin 1 (IL1) and interleukin 6 (IL6, β_2 interferon). IL1 promotes the early phases of the B- and T-lymphocyte activation processes. IL6 promotes B-lymphocyte differentiation and immunoglobulin secretion. Mononuclear phagocytes also secrete tumor necrosis factor β (TNFβ, lymphotoxin), which can directly kill certain types of tumor cells, and at least two types of colony stimulating factors, G-CSF and M-CSF. M-CSF promotes the production of monocytes, and G-CSF stimulates the production of granulocytes from the stem cells and the bone marrow. Like T lymphocytes, mononuclear phagocytes produce many other BRM, such as complement components.

The clinical usefulness of BRM varies widely. Passive transfer of antibodies, given as intravenous gamma globulin, is of great benefit in patients with primary humoral immunodeficiencies (see Chapter 30), and encouraging results have been obtained with several BRM in the treatment of a variety of malignancies (see Chapter 28). However, efforts to enhance cellular immunity in immunodeficient patients have often met with negative or conflicting results. This has been the case recently in efforts to correct the profound immunological dysfunction characteristic of the acquired immunodeficiency syndrome (AIDS). As discussed in detail in Chapter 30, the profound immunodepression that develops in AIDS patients is believed to be secondary to the infection of helper T lymphocytes and monocytes by the causative retrovirus HIV-1. Two basic strategies have been investigated in attempts to reconstitute the immunologic functions of AIDS patients: administration of antiviral agents and nonspecific immunostimulation. Antiviral therapies have included replication inhibitors (such as azidothymidine or AZT) and natural antiviral substances, such as α and γ interferons, as well as chemical stimulants of host interferon production, e.g., ampligen, a mismatched double-stranded RNA poly(I):poly (C_{12},U). Nonspecific efforts to restore the depressed immune function have included the administration of colony-stimulating factors (e.g., GM-CSF), to boost the production and release of uninfected leukocytes from the bone marrow; IL2 to expand the numbers and augment the function of T lymphocytes; and substances such as muramyl dipeptide, which are believed to boost nonspecifically the killing capabilities of macrophages. In vitro data suggests that immunostimulation should benefit the patients if viral replication could be simultaneously controlled, and several groups of investigators are carrying out clinical trials with different combinations of antiviral drugs and BRM, hoping to find the optimal association that will benefit the patients.

B. Dialyzable Leukocyte Extracts (Imreg) and Transfer Factor

In a series of classical experiments, Lawrence showed that the injection of an extract of lymphocytes from a tuberculin-positive donor to a tuberculin-negative recipient resulted in acquisition of tuberculin reactivity by the latter. Lawrence coined the termed *transfer factor* to designate the unknown agent responsible for the transfer of tuberculin sensitivity. Nowadays it is known that this activity is contained in the dialyzable (low-molecular-weight) fraction of a leukocyte extract, and the terms *dialyzable leukocyte extract* (DLE) and *imreg* are preferred. The term transfer factor (TF) is reserved for DLE components with antigen-specific activity of which we have limited knowledge.

In normal human subjects, injection of DLE has been shown to transfer both skin-test reactivity (delayed hypersensitivity) and the ability to produce various lymphokines in vitro in the presence of the same antigen(s) to which the donor of the leukocytes responded. Crude DLE preparations have been shown to contain approximately 160 separate moieties.

The TF activity in DLE for each antigenic specificity appears to reside in two distinct nucleopeptides of molecular weight 2000-2500, containing both RNA and protein but not DNA. Crude DLE preparations contain both nonspecific immunomodulatory (adjuvant) activity and one or more inhibitory activities in addition to the TF components.

The modes of action of the antigen-specific moieties in DLE remain undetermined. TF may act on a naive stem cell to induce specificity for an antigen or group of antigens or, alternatively, it may assist in the recruitment of specific antigen-sensitive cells. On the other hand, the adjuvant moieties in DLE appear to act nonspecifically by enhancing the preexisting reactivity of the recipient's lymphocytes. DLE is a nonantigenic substance that can be lyophilized and stored indefinitely without loss of potency. It does not transmit infectious diseases, has no HLA antigens, does not produce graft-vs.-host reactions and causes no serious side effects.

DLE has received widespread clinical use. Although few clinical trials have been double-blind, favorable results have been reported in a variety of disseminated infections such as generalized vaccinia, measles pneumonia, congenital herpes simplex, herpes zoster, cytomegalovirus infections, mucocutaneous candidiasis, coccidioidomycosis, histoplasmosis refractory to conventional antifungal therapy, miliary tuberculosis, lupus vulgaris, progressive BCG infection refractory to standard therapy, and chronic cutaneous leishmaniasis.

C. Thymic Hormones

Immunotherapeutic applications of thymic hormones have received increasing attention in recent years. Many peptides with thymic-hormone-like activity have been isolated and described, including thymosin, *facteur thymique sérique* (FTS, serum thymic factor), and thymopoietin. Thymosin is a mixture of different peptides (thymosin α_1, thymosin β_3, thymosine β_4, etc.) with different biologic activities. Thymosin α_1, the most widely studied of the thymic hormones, promotes T-cell differentiation and also may have other effects on cell-mediated immunity. Thymosins β_3 and β_4 promote early stem-cell differentiation to prothymocytes. Although animal experiments have shown little or no toxicity, reactions to thymosin α_1 have been reported in a few patients, presumably to bovine-specific antigens, since thymosin of bovine origin is used generally for immunotherapy. A number of laboratories have isolated these different thymic hormones, and some of the fractions have been purified, sequenced, and chemically synthesized. In fact, thymosin α_1 has been biologically synthesized with the use of recombinant DNA.

Thymic hormones have been used most extensively in patients with acquired or congenital T-cell defects, and dramatic improvements have been reported in some instances. In some patients with congenital T-cell deficiency, combined therapy using both thymosin and DLE appears to be beneficial, even though thymosin or DLE alone is without effect. Thymus extracts also are being tried in some autoimmune diseases such as systemic lupus erythematosus, since it appears that they can induce the proliferation and differentiation of suppressor T cells in patients with apparent deficiencies in suppressor activity and, conversely, can cause a reduction in suppressor activity (or an increase in helper activity) in some hypogammaglobulinemic patients.

D. Bacterial and Chemical Immunomodulators

1. Bacterial Immunomodulators

Killed bacteria and several substances of bacterial origin are capable of activating the immunological function of mononuclear leukocyte subset cells. *Bacillus Calmette-Guerin* (*BCG*) and *Corynebacterium parvum* have been extensively used for their adjuvant therapy in therapeutic protocols aimed at stimulating antitumoral immunologic mechanisms. At the cellular level, these bacteria appear mainly to activate macrophages. Muramyl dipeptide, a dipeptide moiety extracted from the cell walls of *Mycobacterium tuberculosis*, stimulates both monocytes and T lymphocytes.

2. Chemical Immunomodulators

a. *Levamisole*. Levamisole is an antihelminthic drug used in veterinary medicine that has been found to have immunostimulant properties. It immunopotentiates the graft-vs.-host reaction in rats, and in some animal diseases it causes an apparent increase in host resistance to tumor cells. It acts on the cellular limb of the immune system and can restore impaired cell-mediated immune responses to normal levels, but it fails to hyperstimulate the normal functioning immune system. Thus it shows true immunomodulatory activity. The primary mechanism of action of levamisole may be to facilitate the participation of monocytes in the cellular immune response, apparently by enhancing monocyte chemotaxis. In addition, it has been reported to increase DNA synthesis of T lymphocytes and to augment their proliferative responses to mitogens, as well as their production of mediators of cellular immunity in vitro.

In humans, levamisole has been reported to restore delayed hypersensitivity reactions in anergic cancer patients and to be of some benefit in the treatment of aphthous stomatitis, rheumatoid arthritis, systemic lupus erythematosus, viral diseases, chronic staphylococcal infections, and breast cancer. It has also been reported to be useful as part of the treatment of AIDS patients.

Levamisole has a variety of side-effects, and patients may complain of nausea, influenza-like malaise, or cutaneous rashes disappearing after cessation of therapy. The most serious side-effect is a granulocytopenia that is reversed upon therapy termination, but white cell counts should be monitored in patients taking the drug for prolonged periods.

b. Isoprinosine (Inosine Prabonex). Isoprinosine (ISO) is a synthetic immunomodulatory drug recently approved for clinical use in the United States. It appears to be effective in a wide variety of viral diseases. ISO increases cell-mediated immune functions in vitro, such as T-cell proliferative responses to antigens or mitogens, active T-rosette formation, and macrophage activation. It also increases active T-cell levels in vivo in patients with low levels before treatment.

In vitro experiments have shown that ISO inhibits the replication of both DNA and RNA viruses in tissue culture, including herpes simplex, adenovirus, vaccinia (DNA viruses) and poliovirus, influenza types A and B, rhinovirus, ECHO, and Eastern equine encephalitis (RNA viruses). Toxicologic, tetratogenic, and carcinogenic studies have demonstrated that ISO is safe, well tolerated, and remarkably free of side-effects, even upon prolonged administration. It contains an inosine moiety, a naturally occurring purine in lymphocytes that is metabolized via normal biochemical pathways to uric acid.

Isoprinosine potentiates cell-mediated immune responsiveness in vivo, and a major factor in its effectiveness against viral infections appears to be its ability to prevent the depression of cell-mediated immunity that has been shown to occur during viral infection and to persist for four to six weeks thereafter.

The clinical efficacy of ISO has been well documented in double-blind trials; for example, ISO produces striking decreases in both the duration of infection and the severity of symptoms in a whole host of viral diseases, including influenza virus infections, rhinovirus infections, herpes labialis and herpes progenitalis, herpes zoster, viral hepatitis, rubella, and viral otitis. Of particular interest are the results of ISO therapy in subacute sclerosing panencephalitis (SSPE), a progressive disease due to a chronic measles virus infection that results in complete debilitation and the eventual death of the patient. ISO has been reported to halt the progression of SSPE, in 80% of patients when given in stages I and II of the disease, provided it is administered for at least six months. Indeed, ISO is the only agent to date with documented beneficial effects in SSPE patients.

Isoprinosine has been considered as potentially useful in AIDS, where the combination of its immunomodulating activity with reported anti-HIV activity would appear as ideal. However, ISO does not appear to induce consistent clinical improvement in the patients to which it has been administered.

SELF-EVALUATION

Questions

26.1 Cyclosporine A
   A. Induces a decrease in the number of T lymphocytes.

  B. Has a predominant effect on helper/inducer T cells.
  C. Is cytotoxic for T4$^+$ cells.
  D. Competes at the cellular receptor level with γ interferon and IL2.
  E. Is cytotoxic for lymphoid and nonlymphoid hematopoietic elements.

26.2 The most important side effect of most immunosuppressive drugs is
  A. Neutropenia.
  B. Alopecia (loss of hair).
  C. Oral ulcers.
  D. Sterility.
  E. Cystitis.

26.3 Corticosteroid-sensitive species do not include the
  A. Mouse.
  B. Hamster.
  C. Rat.
  D. Rabbit.
  E. Man.

26.4 Transfer factor
  A. Promotes the proliferation of T cells.
  B. Induces delayed hypersensitivity to a specific antigen in a previously
     nonreactive individual.
  C. Enhances the preexisting reactivity of recipient's lymphocytes.
  D. Induces the differentiation of helper T cells.
  E. Reduces the activity of suppressor T cells.

26.5 Isoprinosine
  A. Has no immunological effects.
  B. Increases the immunoregulatory activity of monocytic cells.
  C. Reduces the activity of suppressor T cells.
  D. Enhances cell mediated immunity both in vivo and in vitro.
  E. Decreases monocyte chemotaxis.

26.6 Depression of cell-mediated immunity during immunosuppressive therapy
  can be associated with infections caused by all the agents listed except
  A. *Pneumocystis carinii.*
  B. *Aspergillus fumigatus.*
  C. *Staphylococcus aureus.*
  D. *Mycobacterium tuberculosis.*
  E. Herpes zoster virus.

26.7 Malignancies frequently seen in immunosuppressed patients include
  A. Skin neoplasias.

    B.   Lymphoreticular neoplasias.
    C.   Both A and B.
    D.   Neither A nor B.

26.8   The therapy indicated in a child with humoral immunodeficiency is
    A.   Dialyzable leukocyte extract.
    B.   Thymosin.
    C.   Interleukin 2.
    D.   Human gamma globulin.
    E. γInterferon.

26.9   The effects of corticosteroids in man do not include
    A.   Lymphocytotoxicity.
    B.   Lymphopenia.
    C.   Decreased inflammatory responses.
    D.   Depressed delayed hypersensitivity reactions.
    E.   Decreased monocyte chemotaxis.

26.10 Biological response modifiers (BRM) are
    A.   Cytolytic enzymes.
    B.   Mainly glycolipids.
    C.   Mainly polypeptides.
    D.   Immune RNA.
    E.   Equivalent to hormones.

Answers

26.1   (B) Cyclosporine A is not directly cytotoxic but inhibits the production of lymphokines by amplifier T lymphocytes and increases the proliferation of suppressor T cells.

26.2   (A)

26.3   (E) Corticosteroids are definitely able to induce immunosuppression in humans, but man is not a corticosteroid-sensitive species, and steroids are not cytotoxic for human lymphocytes.

26.4   (B) The designation *transfer factor* is reserved for the antigen-specific moieties of dialyzable leukocyte extracts that transfer the reactivity against a specific antigen from a reactive donor to a nonreactive recipient.

26.5   (D)

26.6   (C) The depression of cell-mediated immunity is associated mainly with viral and opportunistic infections, as well as with increased severity of infections by intracellular parasites such as *M. tuberculosis*. Pyogenic infections, such as those caused by *S. aureus*, will be a serious problem in the neutropenic patient.

26.7   (C)

26.8   (D) The preferred immunotherapy in a child with humoral immunodeficiency is intravenous injection of human gamma globulins, which will passively transfer antibodies to most common pathogens to the deficient child.

26.9   (A) Man is not a steroid-sensitive species.

26.10   (C)

BIBLIOGRAPHY

Currey, H. L. F. Drugs affecting the immune response. In *Immunology in Medicine*, 2nd Ed., E. J. Holborow and W. G. Reeves (Eds.). Grune & Stratton, New York, 1983.

Hess, A. D., Esa, A. H., and Colombani, P. M. Mechanisms of action of cyclosporine: Effects on cells of the immune system and subcellular events in T cell activation. *Transplant. Proc. 20*(suppl. 2):29, 1988.

Kerman, R. H. Effects of cyclosporine immunosuppression in humans. *Transplant. Proc. 20*(Suppl. 2):143, 1988.

Kirkpatrick, C. J., Burger, D. R., and Lawrence, H. S. (Eds.). *Immunobiology of Transfer Factor*. Academic Press, New York, 1982.

Rees, A. J. and Lockwood, C. M. Immunosuppressive drugs in clinical practice. In *Clinical Aspects of Immunology*, 4th Ed., P. J. Lachman and D. K. Peters (Eds.). Blackwell Scientific, Oxford, 1982.

Reeves, W. G. Therapeutic manipulation of the immune response. In *Immunology in Medicine*, 2nd Ed., E. J. Holborow and W. G. Reeves (Eds.). Grune & Stratton, New York, 1983.

Sirois, P. and Rola-Pleszczynski, M. *Immunopharmacology*. Elsevier Scientific, Amsterdam, 1982.

27

Transplantation Immunology

DOMINGOS SILVEIRA MACHADO and GABRIEL VIRELLA

The replacement of defective organs with transplants was one of the impossible dreams of medicine for many centuries. Christian legend places the first successful graft in the fourth century, in a Roman basilica dedicated to the saint-healers Cosmas and Damien, where the cancerous leg of an elderly sacristan was replaced, during his sleep, by the leg of a recently deceased Ethiopian. However, for transplantation to emerge from the realm of the miraculous into medical practice, it took the surgical techniques of vascular anastomosis, the development of a good understanding of rejection phenomena, and the introduction of drugs and antisera effective in the control of rejection. By the early 1970s, both the surgical aspects and rejection control had been achieved with considerable success; as a consequence tissue and organ transplantation emerged as a major area of interest for surgeons and physicians. According to recent statistics more than 70,000 kidney, 10,000 bone marrow, 8,000 heart, 5,000 liver, 1,600 pancreas, and 400 heart-lung transplants have been reported. Transplantation of bone, bowel, trachea, and bladder are in the phase of experimental development. Other tissues and organs will certainly follow.

The success of an organ transplant is a function of several variables. However, the major determinant of acceptance or nonacceptance of a technically perfect graft is the magnitude of the immunologically mediated rejection response. The likelihood of acceptance or rejection is closely related to the extent of genetic differences between the donor and the recipient of the graft. Transplantation of organs between animals of the same inbred strain or between homozygotic twins is usually successful. In contrast, transplants across species barriers are always rapidly rejected. In man, genetic diversity between individuals is, at this point, the main obstacle to successful transplantation.

I. DONOR-RECIPIENT MATCHING

Prevention of rejection is achieved by careful matching of donor and recipient and by manipulation of the recipient's immune response. Avoidance of antigenic differences between donor and recipient is considered a crucial factor for the success of a transplant. Although many different antigenic systems show allotypic variation, in transplantation practice only the ABO blood groups and the HLA system are routinely typed. ABO incompatibility has been considered an insurmountable obstacle to transplantation, since it leads almost always to hyperacute rejection of the graft, probably because A and B antigens are expressed in vascular endothelia. However, some groups have reported successful grafting of HLA-compatible but ABO-incompatible organs after removing anti-A and/or anti-B isohemagglutinins by plasmapheresis or by extracorporeal immunoadsorption. Matching of the HLA antigens is considered essential in most centers, since there is a positive correlation between the number of HLA antigens common to the donor and recipient and the survival of the transplanted organ or tissue. In fact, in the case of grafts from living relatives, HLA-identical sibling grafts have the best outcome, followed by haploidentical grafts, which in turn do better than two haplotype-incompatible grafts (Fig. 27.1).

Although some controversy still remains, most evidence available seems to suggest that the matching of class II MHC determinants is more important for graft survival than the matching of class I MHC specificities. The classical locus D specificities were determined by mixed lymphocyte culture, which usually requires 5 to 7 days for completion. This delay restricted the application of HLA-D typing to living related donors. With the definition of serologically defined MHC II specificities, particularly the DR locus, matching of class II MHC was extended to cadaveric donors, resulting in data suggesting that DR matching may be more significant than HLA-A, B, and C matching in determining the outcome of a transplant.

Two other approaches to avoid rejection are possible. One is to check for cytotoxic antibodies in the recipient's serum directed against the donor's lymphocytes. This is achieved by means of a cross-match test in which the recipient serum is tested against lymphocytes from several potential donors, and by screening the cytotoxicity of the recipient's serum against panels of cells of known phenotypes. In the ease of bone marrow grafting, in which there is great concern about the possibility of inducing a graft-vs.-host reaction, two-way mixed lymphocyte cultures are set, in which the recipient's lymphocytes are

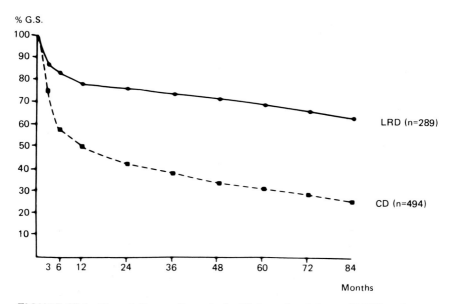

FIGURE 27.1   Cumulative graft survival of living related donor (LRD) and cadaveric donor (CD) transplants. (Reproduced with permission from Flatmark and Thorsby. *Transplant. Proc. 14*:61, 1982.)

mixed with lymphocytes from all potential donors. The best donor-recipient match is the one in which minimal blastic transformation is determined, indicating that neither the recipient's lymphocytes nor the donor's lymphocytes react strongly against each other.

II. GRAFT REJECTION

Graft rejection is the consequence of an immune response mounted by the recipient against the graft as a consequence of the incompatibility between HLA antigens of the donor and the recipient. Cells that express class II MHC antigens play a major role in sensitizing the immune system of the recipient. As a consequence, there is a clonal expansion of specific alloreactive cells from the recipient. This proliferation of sensitized cells is the cause of multiple immunological and inflammatory phenomena, some mediated by T cells and others mediated by antibodies, which eventually result in graft rejection. Clinically it is possible to classify rejection episodes as hyperacute, acute, and chronic.

A. Hyperacute (Early) Rejection

This occurs usually within the first 24 h after transplantation and is mediated by preformed antibodies against ABO or MHC antigens of the graft. It is also possible that antibodies directed against other alloantigens may play a role in this type of rejection. Once the antibodies bind to the transplanted tissues, rejection is caused either by activation of the complement system, which will result in the chemotactic attraction of granulocytes and the triggering of inflammatory circuits, or by antibody-dependent cellular cytotoxicity (ADCC). A major pathological feature of hyperacute rejection is a formation of massive intravascular platelet aggregates leading to thrombosis, ischemia, and necrosis. The formation of platelet thrombi probably results from several factors, including release of platelet activating factor (PAF) from immunologically damaged endothelial cells and/or from activated neutrophils. Hyperacute rejection episodes are usually untreatable and result in graft loss.

B. Acute Rejection

Clinically, acute rejection occurs mostly in the first month after transplantation. When it takes place in the first few days after grafting, it corresponds to a secondary (second-set) immune response, implying that the patient must have been previously sensitized to the HLA antigens present in the organ donor; this can be a consequence of a previous transplant, a pregnancy, or blood transfusions. When occurring past the first week after grafting, it may correspond to a second-set response or to a very strong first-set (primary) response. It is predominantly mediated by T lymphocytes, and considerable controversy has arisen concerning the relative importance of cytotoxic ($CD8^+$) lymphocytes vs. $CD4^+$ lymphocytes mediating a delayed-type hypersensitivity response. Helper ($CD4^+$) lymphocytes produce and release growth factors such as IL2 and IL4, which promote the expansion of $CD8^+$ lymphocytes, and interferon γ, which enhances the expression of MHC class II antigens in the graft. K and NK cells, B cells, neutrophils, and eosinophils are also present in the infiltrates of rejected tissues, but their respective roles in rejection are unclear.

The diagnosis of rejection is based on clinical suspicion. Functional deterioration of the grafted organ is usually the main basis for considering the diagnosis of acute rejection. Confirmation usually requires a biopsy of the grafted organ. There are established histological criteria for the identification of an acute rejection reaction in the most commonly transplanted organs. A hallmark finding is mononuclear cell infiltration, as it would be expected in a typical delayed hypersensitivity reaction. Recent data suggests that the measurement of elevated IL2 levels in serum (and in urine, in the case of renal transplants) may be a valuable noninvasive alternative for the diagnosis of acute rejection. A factor that limits the value of elevated IL2 levels as a diagnostic criterion for kidney rejection is that similarly elevated levels can be measured if the kidney is infected with cytomegalovirus (CMV). However, the finding of exfoliated renal cells with nuclear inclusions in the urinary sediment helps to differentiate CMV infection from rejection.

The frequency of acute rejection episodes is high—between 30 and 50% of graft recipients experiment one or several acute rejection episodes. However, in most cases acute rejection can be reversed by increasing the dosage of immunosuppressive agents (or by administering additional immunosuppressants).

C. Delayed or Chronic Rejection

Later after transplantation an insidiously progressive loss of function of the grafted organ may take place. This functional deterioration seems to be due both to immune and to nonimmune processes. The immune component of chronic rejection seems to be precipitated by antibody-mediated endothelial lesion. A variety of cells, such as PMN, monocytes, and platelets have an increased tendency to adhere to injured vascular endothelium, and the release of PAF from endothelial cells may be one of the major factors determining the adherence of neutrophils and platelets. A variety of interleukins and soluble factors are released by interacting cells under these conditions, including IL1 and platelet-derived growth factor (PDGF). The damaged endothelium is covered by a layer of platelets and fibrin, and eventually by proliferating endothelial cells. The result is a proliferative lesion in the vessels, which, as consequence of the inflammatory nature of the process, progresses towards fibrosis and occlusion. Recent data shows a positive correlation between the number of HLA incompatibilities and the progression of chronic rejection, which is difficult to control by any type of therapy.

III. IMMUNOSUPPRESSION

In principle, the ideal transplantation should take place among genetically identical individuals. This is only possible in the rare event of transplantation between identical twins. The success of clinical transplantation depends heavily on the use of nonspecific immunosuppressive agents that, by decreasing the magnitude of immunological rejection responses, prolong graft survival. Immunosuppression in transplanted patients has been achieved by a variety of means, ranging from splenectomy (virtually abandoned at the present time) to whole body irradiation, and including the use of cytotoxic/immunosuppressant drugs and biological response modifiers, such as antilymphocytic antibodies.

A. Chemical Immunosuppression

Several drugs are currently used to induce immunosuppression, including corticosteroids, azathioprine, and cyclosporine A.

Corticosteroids are used to treat and prevent rejection. They have multiple
effects on the immune system, including inhibition of antigen-driven T-cell
proliferation, inhibition of IL1 and IL2 release, and inhibition of chemotaxis.
Unfortunately, the use of corticosteroids in relatively large doses for long periods of time (as required in transplantation) is associated to severe side-effects.
Therefore, corticosteroids are usually administered together with some other
immunosuppressant drug, allowing the reduction of the steroid dosages below
the levels causing major side-effects.

Azathioprine is mostly used in the prevention of rejection episodes. Its immunosuppressant effect depends on its metabolism and conversion into 6-mer-
captopurine, which inhibits purine nucleotide synthesis and prevents lymphocyte proliferation (both T and B).

Cyclosporine A (CsA) is the newest and most effective immunosuppressant
drug used in prevention and treatment of rejection. As described in detail in
Chapter 28, the effects of CsA are mainly related to the inhibition of the release
of IL2 and other lymphokines by helper T cells, thus curtailing the onset of both
cellular and humoral immune responses. It is particularly helpful in the prevention of rejection, usually in association with corticosteroids. It has a marked
steroid-sparing effect that helps to avoid steroid side-effects, but CsA itself has
considerable toxicity. It is nephrotoxic (and this raises considerable problems in
patients receiving kidney transplants, in which it will be necessary to differentiate between acute rejection and CsA toxicity), causes hypertension, and has
been associated to accelerated atherosclerosis, particularly in heart transplants.
Whether it is advisable to keep patients under CsA therapy for long periods of
time is not quite clear. The tendency seems to be toward the use of CsA mainly
in the period immediately following transplantation or, if used in long-term
prevention of rejection, its use in association with other drugs, so that the dosage
of CsA can be reduced to safe levels. In any case, the introduction of CsA had
a marked impact on the survival of transplanted organs, which has increased by
at least 10% in the case of kidney and heart. The outburst in heart transplants
in the last few years was a direct consequence of the availability of CsA, and
the success of liver transplants is also directly related to the use of this drug.

B. Biological Response Modifiers

Antithymocyte and antilymphocyte globulins are among the earliest successful
therapeutic agents used in the prevention of graft rejection. These are gamma
globulin fractions separated from the sera of animals (usually horses) injected
with human thymic lymphocytes or human peripheral blood lymphocytes.

They are very effective in the prevention and reversal of rejection episodes, and their mechanism of action is related to the destruction of recipient lymphocytes.

Anti-T-cell monoclonal antibodies directed against T cells, particularly those reacting with the CD3 marker, have been extensively used in the prevention and treatment of rejection episodes. Their mechanism of action is similar to that of antithymocyte and antilymphocyte globulins, causing massive lymphocyte depletion in the recipient. Several approaches to target the elimination of cells involved in graft rejection more precisely are currently under investigation. They usually involve the use of antibodies against markers expressed by activated T cells, such as MHC II antigens and the IL2 receptor.

Irrespective of their specificity, monoclonal antibodies and antilymphocyte/thymocyte globulins cannot be used for prolonged periods of time, because of their heterologous nature. Sooner or later, and in spite of their immunosuppressed state, patients receiving these heterologous immunoglobulins will become sensitized to them and will produce antibodies to horse or mouse immunoglobulins. This can result in side-effects such as allergic reactions or serum sickness. But more importantly, the production of these antibodies will result in almost immediate elimination of newly administered antilymphocyte antibodies. Therefore, most groups reserve the use of these agents to the reversal of acute rejection episodes and use chemical immunosuppressants for long-term prevention.

A recent approach that is reported to be very efficient in experimental animals is the use of hybrid molecules of IL2 and the toxic A chain of diphtheria toxin (DT). These hybrid molecules bind through the IL2 moiety and therefore are targeted towards activated lymphocytes. Their toxic effect is mediated by the diphtheria toxin moiety, which is internalized only by the cells binding IL2. Early reports of studies in experimental animals seem to suggest that the administration of IL2-DT conjugates may result in long-term tolerance to grafted organs, which remain viable without the need for long-term immunosuppression. The potential impact of this approach in human transplantation is extraordinary.

C. Total Lymphoid Irradiation

Irradiation of those areas of the body where the lymphoid tissues are concentrated is almost exclusively used to prepare leukemic patients for bone marrow transplantation. Irradiation will combine two potential benefits: the elimination of malignant cells and the ablation of the immune system. The immunosuppressive effect of irradiation seems to be due to the greater radiosensitivity of helper T cells, which will result in a marked predominance of suppressor/cytotoxic T cells among the residual lymphocyte population surviving after irradiation.

D. Immunosuppression Side Effects

Effective long-term immunosuppression is inevitably associated to a state of immunoincompetence. The immunosuppressed patient is susceptible to a wide variety of infections, particularly those caused by infectious agents that are not often seen as pathogens in immunocompetent individuals, such as cytomegalovirus, varicella-herpes virus, *Pneumocystis carinii, Toxoplasma gondii*, etc. Cytomegalovirus infections are particularly ominous, because this virus can further interfere with the host's immune competence and, by infecting the kidney, may trigger rejection in a nonspecific way.

Also, whether a consequence of the oncogenic properties of some immunosuppressive agents or whether a consequence of disturbed immunosurveillance, the incidence of malignancies is significantly increased in transplant patients. In those patients with survival times following transplantation of 10 years or longer, the frequency of skin cancer is a staggering 40%, and an additional 10% develop other types of malignancies, with lymphomas being relatively frequent. Interestingly, lymphomas in transplant patients tend to spread to areas usually spared in nontransplanted patients, such as the brain. The reasons for the predominance of skin cancer and lymphoma among transplant patients are unknown.

IV. THE TRANSFUSION EFFECT

For many years blood transfusions were generally avoided in potential transplant recipients because of the fear of sensitization to HLA, blood group, and other antigens. However, for many years. Opelz, Terasaki and co-workers had claimed that kidney graft survival was longer in patients who had received blood prior to transplantation. The publication of prospective studies confirming this observation in the early 1980s (Fig. 27.2) led to the adoption of a deliberate transfusion policy in most transplantation centers.

The mechanism responsible for this so-called transfusion effect are not yet fully understood. It has been demonstrated that following transfusion there is a depression of cellular immunity indices, which according to some studies seems to become more accentuated and long-lasting with repeated transfusions. The induction of "enhancing" antibodies has also been suggested as an explanation for the transfusion effect. Such antibodies react with antigenic determinants of the grafted tissue without activating complement or inducing cytotoxicity, thereby blocking other potentially cytotoxic antibodies or T cells from binding to the same antigens and prolonging (enhancing) graft survival. Finally, it has also been suggested that the transfusion effect may be mediated by anti-idiotypic antibodies reacting with the T-cell receptors of effector T cells. The interaction of T-cell receptors with anti-idiotypic antibodies may result in inhibition

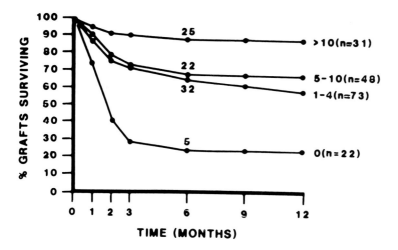

FIGURE 27.2 Actuarial kidney graft survival rates according to the number of transfusions received before transplantation. Numbers of transfusion are indicated at the end of each curve, and numbers of patients are given in parentheses. Numbers of graft survivals for each group at 6 months are as indicated. Number of patients at risk at 6 months are indicated. p (weighted regression analysis) was <0.0001 at 3, 6, and 12 months, indicating that the improvement in graft outcome was dependent upon an increased number of pretransplant transfusions. (Reproduced with permission from Opelz, Graver, and Terasaki. *Lancet* *I*: 1223, 1981.)

of rejection by either physical blocking of subsequent interactions between cytotoxic T cells and grafted tissues or by up-regulating suppressor T cells that will prevent the expansion of helper and cytotoxic T-cell populations. The administration of whole blood, packed cells, or buffy coat is more efficient than the administration of washed red cells in producing the transfusion effect, suggesting the key role of leukocytes in the induction of this phenomenon. Some animal studies show that soluble lymphocyte extracts may produce effects similar to those of whole blood transfusion.

Considerable uncertainty remains about the optimal number of pretransplant transfusions, the advantages of concomitant administration of immunosuppressive drugs, and whether donor blood is preferable to random blood. However, it seems clear that not all transplant candidates benefit from a deliberate transfusion program. Patients younger than 21 years and women without history of pregnancy show minimal increases in graft survival. Also, about 30-40% of patients given pretransplant transfusions develop cytotoxic antibodies to multiple HLA specificities in high titers that in effect delay or preclude transplantation.

This observation led to the suggestion that pretransplant transfusions actually helped separate responsive patients, who develop cytotoxic antibodies and would tend to reject the graft energetically, from nonresponsive individuals, who would be more likely to accept the graft. Most authors, however, believe that this selection cannot totally explain the transfusion effect. In any case, the real possibility that a patient given pretransplant transfusions may develop high titers of cytotoxic antibodies has resulted in the recommendation that the titers of cytotoxic antibodies should be determined after each transfusion and the protocol interrupted as soon as a significant increase in their titer is detected.

Somewhat ironically, it may be that pretransplant transfusion will fall out of favor before a good understanding of their mechanism of action is obtained. Recent data comparing the survival of patients treated with CsA, with and without having undergone pretransplant transfusions, suggests that the 5-year survival of each group is virtually identical. If these studies are confirmed, the rationale for pretransplant transfusion protocols will be significantly weakened.

V. GRAFT-VS.-HOST REACTION

Whenever a patient with a profound immunodeficiency (primary, secondary, or iatrogenic) receives a graft of an organ rich in immunocompetent cells, there is a considerable risk that a graft-vs-host (GVH) reaction may develop. Such reactions are a significant problem in infants and children with primary immunodeficiencies on whom a bone marrow or thymus transplant is performed with the goal of reconstituting the immune system, and in adults receiving a bone marrow transplant. As pointed out earlier, many patients receiving bone marrow transplants have received cytotoxic/immunosuppressive therapy, and their immune system is completely or partially destroyed.

When a graft containing immunocompetent cells is placed into an immunocompetent host, the transplanted cells can recognize as nonself some host antigens. In response to these antigenic differences, the donor T lymphocytes proliferate and differentiate into effector cells that attack recipient cells, producing the signs and symptoms of GVH disease (GVHD). The probability of developing GVHD is greater in the two-month period immediately following transplantation.

The crucial role played by the donor T cells is evidenced by the fact that their elimination from a bone marrow graft avoids GVH reactions. The initial proliferation of donor T cells appears to take place in lymphoid tissues, particularly in the liver and spleen (leading to hepatomegaly and splenomegaly). Later, at the peak of the proliferative reaction, the skin and intestinal walls are heavily infiltrated, leading respectively to skin rash and diarrhea. At that stage, the majority of the proliferating cells are of host origin and include T and B lymphocytes and monocytes/macrophages. The proliferation of host cells is probably a result of the release of nonspecific mitogenic and differentiation factors by activated donor T lymphocytes.

Experimentally, it can be demonstrated that the injection of allogeneic T lymphocytes to an animal a few days before antigenic challenge can substantially increase the levels of antibodies produced (allogenic effect). It appears that during the mutual recognition as nonself of the two allogenic cell populations, helper T cells are activated and release both interleukin 2 and a nonspecific soluble factor (allogenic factor). These two factors in turn promote further proliferation and differentiation of helper T cells, which will be able nonspecifically to enhance the response of B cells antigenically stimulated at the time.

In the case of the GVH reaction, the reaction of donor lymphocytes against host alloantigens may lead to the release of IL2 and allogenic factor(s), which may eventually be responsible for indiscriminate stimulation of recipient T and B lymphocytes as well as for recruitment and activation of host monocytes. In the chronic phases of GVH, the consequences of this general immunoregulation disorder become obvious. The patient may develop, among other complications, autoimmune hemolytic anemia. At the same time, the capacity to mount an effective immune response to a given infectious agent is compromised, and the patients become immunodeficient. Finally, if the GVH reaction is not controllable, the patient with GVH disease starts losing weight and develops terminal cachexia (runt disease). An interesting and as yet unexplained observation is that the incidence of malabsorption and runting associated to GVHD is very low in a germ-free environment. It has been suggested that the normal bacterial flora may trigger the reaction, perhaps by inducing antibodies with cross-reactivity towards gut epithelial cells.

Once a GVH reaction is initiated, its control may be extremely difficult. Cyclosporine A administration has met with some success, both in therapy and in prophylaxis (patients treated with CsA have less frequent and less severe episodes of GVHD). The most efficient approach to the prevention of GVHD is to eliminate T cells from the graft. Obviously, this is not possible when the graft is given to a child with primary immunodeficiency, but it can be effective in cases of bone marrow transplantation to leukemic patients or patients with aplastic anemia. T-cell depletion can be achieved in a variety of ways, including pretreatment of the bone marrow with antilymphocyte/thymocyte immunoglobulin or with monoclonal antibodies reacting with T cells (e.g., anti-CD3). The major problem with this approach is that the transplant of T-cell-depleted bone marrow into immunosuppressed adults results in a persistently profound state of severe immunodeficiency with increased incidence of opportunistic infections. Replacement therapy with intravenous gamma globulin can be of value for the prophylaxis of infections in patients with bone marrow transplants.

SELF-EVALUATION

Questions

Choose the one best answer to the following questions.

27.1 The graft "enhancement" effect refers to
A. Graft rejection inhibition by a high titer of serum antigraft antibodies.
B. Graft rejection acceleration by a high titer of serum antigraft antibodies.
C. Graft rejection acceleration by an accumulation of lymphocytes at the graft site.
D. Graft rejection inhibition by the injection of immunosuppressive agents.
E. Graft rejection inhibition by the injection of soluble transplantation antigens.

27.2 The major complication resulting from the heterologous nature of monoclonal anti-CD3 antibodies used in the treatment of graft rejection is
A. Serum sickness.
B. Profound immunodeficiency.
C. Carcinomas of the skin.
D. Graft-vs.-host reaction.
E. Development of food allergies.

27.3 The beneficial effects of multiple transfusion in graft survival can be attributed to several factors except
A. The exclusion of high responders from transplantation.
B. The production of enhancing antibodies.
C. The production of complement-fixing anti-HLA antibodies.
D. The stimulation of suppressor cells.
E. The induction of tolerance against MHC antigens.

27.4 The major pathogenic factor(s) in hyperacute graft rejection is (are)
A. Preformed cytotoxic antibodies.
B. Predifferentiated cytotoxic T lymphocytes.
C. Natural killer cells.
D. Killer (K) lymphocytes.
E. Anti-Rh antibodies.

27.5 The most frequent malignancies in immunosuppressed patients are
A. Solid carcinomas.
B. Kidney tumors.
C. Hepatomas.
D. Lymphomas.
E. Epithelial tumors.

27.6 The graft-vs.-host reaction is characterized by
   A. Frequent spontaneous remission.
   B. High incidence of epithelial malignancies.
   C. Proliferation of both donor and recipient lymphocytes.
   D. Production of autoantibodies by grafted B lymphocytes.
   E. All of the above.

Each set of questions below consists of a set of lettered headings followed by numbered phrases. For each numbered phrase, choose the one lettered heading that is best. In each group, the lettered heading may be used once, more than once, or not at all. (A) Bone marrow transplant; (B) Kidney transplant; (C) Heart transplant; (D) Thymus transplant; (E) Skin graft.

27.7 CMV infection can play a role in rejection.

27.8 Most frequently associated with GVHD in adults.

27.9 Patient survival time has significantly increased with the use of cyclosporine.

27.10 Graft survival is enhanced by multiple transfusions prior to transplantation.

Answers

27.1 (A) The antibodies responsible for "enhancement" are believed to be noncomplement-fixing, non-ADCC-inducing antibodies that bind to the graft tissue antigenic sites blocking recognition by cytotoxic T cells.

27.2 (A) Although many complications may result from the use of anti-lymphocyte antibodies in the treatment and prevention of rejection episodes due to the profound immunosuppression associated to their use, the complication directly related to the heterologous nature of these antibodies is serum sickness, caused by the production of antimouse immunoglobulin antibodies by the patients receiving this type of therapy.

27.3 (C) Complement-fixing anti-HLA antibodies are likely to be cytotoxic and lead to hyperacute rejection.

27.4 (A)

27.5 (E)

27.6 (C) The autoantibodies frequently detected in GVHD are produced by proliferating host cells, non-specifically stimulated during the reaction.

27.7 (B)

27.8   (A) Thymic transplants are also frequently associated to GVHD but are
           performed in infants with severe combined immunodeficiency or
           thymic aplasia rather than in adults.

27.9   (C)

27.10 (B)

BIBLIOGRAPHY

Bach, J. F. and Sachs, D. H. Transplantation immunology. *New Engl. J. Med.*
    327:489, 1987.

Carpenter, C. B. Immunobiology of transplantation. In *Renal Transplantation*,
    M. R. Garovoy and R. D. Gutmann (Eds.). Churchill Livingstone, New York,
    1986.

Cecka, J. M. The transfusion effect. In *Clinical Transplants* 1987. P. Terasaki
    (Ed.). UCLA Tissue Typing Laboratory, Los Angeles, California, 1987.

Hall, B. M., Tiller, D. J., and Hardie, I., et al. Comparison of three immunosup-
    pressive regimens in cadaver renal transplantation: long-term cyclosporine,
    short-term cyclosporine followed by azathioprine and prednisolone, and
    azathioprine and prednisolone without cyclosporine. *New Engl. J. Med. 318*:
    1499, 1988.

Mickey, M. R. HLA matching effects. In *Clinical Transplants 1987*. P. Terasaki
    (Ed.). UCLA Tissue Typing Laboratory, Los Angeles, California, 1987.

Strom, T. B. Immunosuppressive agents in renal transplantation. *Kidney Inter-*
    national 26:353, 1984.

Strom, T. B. Toward more selective therapies to block graft rejection. *AKF*
    Nephrology Letter 4:13, 1987.

28

Tumor Immunology

HENRY C. STEVENSON and KWONG-Y. TSANG

One of the most intellectually attractive concepts in clinical immunology has been the postulated role of the immune system in antitumor defenses. It is becoming clear that such a postulate may have serious flaws, but nevertheless it has been the major impulse for decades of medical research in this area and in spite of all uncertainties the interest in basic and applied research in cancer immunology continues to be a dominant force in immunology. For the past 100 years, efforts at numerous levels have been mounted in hopes of developing an immunologic cure for cancer. An important step toward the achievement of this goal was accomplished in 1985 when the National Cancer Program officially designated cancer biotherapy as the fourth modality in cancer treatment, after surgery, radiation therapy, and chemotherapy. Unfortunately, we are still faced with many agonizing dilemmas, including an incomplete understanding of the nature of the malignant process and the mechanisms of human-immune-system responses to malignant cells. However, promising inroads into this difficult area have been made and will be summarized in this chapter.

I. WHAT IS CANCER?

Cancer is a term used to encompass a wide range of clinical disease states that involve virtually every tissue type of the body and every stage of differentiation of these tissues. Cancer cells are said to be *malignant* as they demonstrate

513

fewer of their normal cellular functions (become dedifferentiated). As cancer cells become more malignant, they become more "renegade" in nature; they cease participating in the overall mission of supporting the survival of the organism as a whole and begin competing with normal cells for both space and the limited resources that the organism has available.

As shown in Figure 28.1, the malignant cell has a number of distinguishing characteristics. Because it is capable of successfully competing with normal

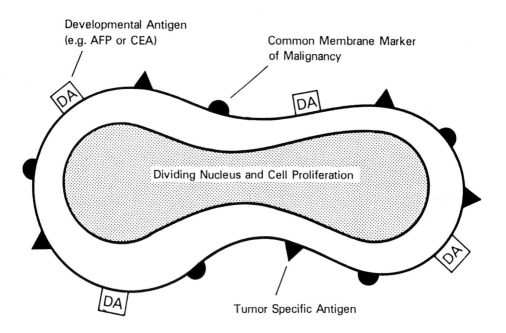

- More dedifferentiated = Less capable of normal cellular functions = More malignant
- Progressive cancer = Malignant cells successfully competing with normal cells for space and resources
- Causes of malignancy include:
    - Defects in proto-oncogene-related cellular machinery (including overproduction of growth factors)
    - Defects in anti-oncogene protection machinery
    - Virus, chemical or radiation injury to above genes

FIGURE 28.1 Schematic representation of the characteristics that distinguish malignant cells from their normal counterparts.

cells, it will tend to proliferate more rapidly than normal cells; in fact, it is frequent to see actual mitoses in cancer specimens obtained from patients. Moreover, the tumor cell may express developmental antigens that are usually seen only in the prenatal period. Examples of these antigens are alpha fetoprotein (AFP) and carcinoembryonic antigen (CEA).

Tumor cells appear to express other types of unique antigens as well. One of these types of antigens are the so-called *tumor-specific antigens*. These are membrane molecules found on tumor cells from the same tissue type; tumor-specific antigens may be uniquely different from one cancer patient to another, even though both patients have the same type of tumor. As will be shown later, tumor-specific antigens are still in the process of being characterized; many controversies exist regarding their exact molecular structure and the timing of their appearance during the malignant process. However, there is some evidence that specific immunologic responses can be mounted to these tumor-specific antigens, as will be discussed below.

Another group of molecules found on malignant cells appear to be common membrane markers of malignancy that are shared on virtually all tumor cell types. These types of common tumor markers also have not been entirely characterized, but there is some evidence that they may be a type of ganglioside (glycolipid). It appears that common tumor markers of malignancy, when expressed, will stimulate nonspecific immune recognition and elimination of cancer cells themselves.

One area of active scientific inquiry focuses on a group of genes, found within normal cells, known as *proto-oncogenes* (such as *myc* and *ras*); many of these genes appear to code for protein products that are an integral part of the normal cellular machinery of all living cells. However, proto-oncogenes also are related to genes found in certain retroviruses that are capable of causing cancer in animal systems. Moreover, slight changes in the genetic structure of proto-oncogenes may cause crucial components of the normal cellular machinery to fail. Such proto-oncogene-related defects may be responsible for the emergence of certain types of cancer. Another mechanism whereby certain defective proto-oncogenes have been associated with cancer has been by their overexpression, including the overproduction of certain normal growth factors that may be associated with the emergence of malignancy.

Another class of genes that have been associated with the development of cancer are the so called *anti-oncogenes*. These are genetic elements found in normal cellular DNA, which when omitted (for example by chromosomal deletion) are associated with the development of cancer. Evidence for anti-oncogene-associated cancers is plentiful; such cancers include retinoblastoma, certain forms of lung cancer, and certain forms of colon cancer. The exact mechanisms whereby anti-oncogenes protect against the emergence of malignancy when they are intact, and the mechanism for the development of malignancy when they are defective, are not clear. It does appear however, that three major types of cellular insults can promote the development of malignancy, by producing defects either in proto-oncogenes or in anti-oncogenes; certain viruses, certain chemicals, and certain types of radiation injury. Examples of virus-associated cancers include cervical cancer (papilloma viruses), Burkitt's lymphoma (Epstein-Barr virus), hepatocellular carcinoma (hepatitis B virus), and certain types of lymphocytic leukemia and lymphoma associated to the human retrovirus HTLV-1 (see Chapter 29). Carcinogenic chemicals include benzene derivatives and a variety of antineoplastic agents that are known to damage DNA, such as nitrogen mustard. Probably all forms of radiation are capable of inducing malignancy, depending on the dose intensity; gamma radiation has been most associated with this phenomenon. The unifying hypothesis regarding these potential causes of cancer focuses on the ability of these agents to interact with and alter the function of the normal host DNA, including proto-oncogenes and anti-oncogenes.

From an immunologic perspective, there are three aspects of cancer immunobiology that have commanded the most attention recently. First is the expression of tumor-specific antigens and common membrane markers of malignancy that might allow the immune system to distinguish malignant cells from normal cell types and arrange for their destruction. Secondly, since the immune system is also a potent source of growth factors (some of which may enhance cancer cell growth), immune-system-mediated tumor promotion may occur. Finally, the emergence of cancer cells within the body may not be a rare or unusual event at all; of the trillions of normal cells found in the body, several hundred per day may be undergoing malignant degeneration in response to the cancer-promoting stimuli cited above.

II. TUMOR ANTIGENS

Tumor cells possess many antigens not found in differentiated cells. These antigens vary in their biologic role, cell location, and specificity. Defining and discussing the terms that are pertinent to these various tumor antigens will help clarify their differences.

A. Classification

1. Tumor-Associated Antigens

The designation tumor-associated antigen (TAA) is often applied to antigens present on tumor cells and undetectable in normal adult cells except under special circumstances. In this group we include embryonic antigens such as carcinoembryonic antigen and alpha fetoprotein.

2. Tumor-Specific Antigens

Tumor-specific antigens (TSA) are antigens that are uniquely present on tumor cells and are qualitatively different from antigens on any normal cell. However, many tumor immunologists are reluctant to use the term tumor-specific because the absolute specificity of these antigens is difficult to prove.

3. Common Membrane Markers of Malignancy

These are poorly characterized glycolipid antigens shared by a variety of tumors. It is likely that NK cells, for example, recognize these types of antigens.

B. Embryonic or Oncofetal Antigens

Tumors sometimes are characteristically associated with cell-surface antigens that are normally expressed only in embryos or in fetuses. These are referred to as embryonic antigens or oncofetal antigens.

1. Alpha Fetoprotein

Alpha fetoprotein (AFP), a glycoprotein with an approximate molecular weight of 70,000 daltons, is found in the fetal sera of all mammalian species; it is synthesized mainly in the yolk sac endoderm and liver parenchymal cells. AFP levels in fetal sera begin to decline in the last months of gestation, and although AFP is still present at birth, it totally disappears within a very short period thereafter. AFP is also produced by certain tumor cells, namely hepatocellular carcinoma and germ-cell teratocarcinoma. Elevated serum AFP levels (i.e., 500-1000 ng/ml) may be utilized as a specific marker for the detection of these tumors (the positive correlation of elevated AFP levels with hepatocellular carcinoma is about 80% in Africa, but only 50% in Europe and the United States). However, some colorectal cancer patients with liver metastases, and some acute hepatitis patients, have been described as showing elevated AFP levels. With the development of highly sensitive immunoassays, AFP can now be detected in normal adult sera, in the sera of acute hepatitis patients, and in the sera of pregnant women. The quantitative determination of low AFP levels has thus far not been proven to be of any significant diagnostic value.

2. Carcinoembryonic Antigen

Carcinoembryonic antigen (CEA) was initially discovered in extracts of human colonic tumors. It is present not only in all colorectal tumors but also in cancers of the pancreas, stomach, breast, lung, and many other neoplasms, as well as in fetal and normal adult colonic mucosa. It can be released in large concentrations by noncancerous, inflammatory lesions of the colon. The presence of CEA in organs other than those of the digestive system (lung and breast) has also been confirmed. CEA is a glycoprotein with an approximate MW of 200,000. Plasma

CEA levels were initially reported to be elevated in 35 out of 36 colorectal cancers and in 3 out of 32 other cancers of the digestive tract. However, subsequent studies have shown not only significantly lower positivity among colorectal cancer patients (i.e., an average of 30-40% significant elevations) but also very much higher positivity rates among patients with nondigestive cancer (approximately 50%). Positivity has also been quite frequently noted in cases of alcoholic cirrhosis, alcoholic pancreatitis, ulcerative colitis, sigmoiditis, peptic ulcer, polyposis of the colon, and heavy smoking. At present, therefore, the quantitation of CEA by radioimmunoassay should not be considered as a diagnostic test. However, utilization of a CEA assay for the follow-up of cancer patients who have already undergone therapy appears to be of much greater value. For example, complete surgical resection of a colorectal tumor is associated with a rapid postoperative decine of serum CEA to a normal value, and no recurrence has been detected among those patients whose CEA values remain normal. A partial decline of CEA value is usually a good indication of incomplete tumor resection and is often associated with a rather rapid regrowth of tumor. More notably, the reappearance of a positive CEA value in patients who had remained negative for a certain period of time is a sensitive and reliable indicator of recurrent tumor growth; positive CEA reappearance consistently precedes clinical detection of recurrence. By constantly monitoring treated patients' plasma CEA levels, chemotherapy or radiotherapy can be initiated at much earlier disease stages, before clinical signs of recurrence are detectable.

C. Diagnostic Applications of Tumor Antigens

A comparatively new approach to the problem of distinguishing normal from tumor cells is through the use of monoclonal antibodies that react with a given type of tumor associated antigen, but fail to react against cells from tumors of different histological types and normal cells from the same species. Many research groups are currently investigating the use of monoclonal antibodies for the early diagnosis of melanoma, colon carcinoma, colorectal carcinoma, breast carcinoma, pancreatic carcinoma, ovarian carcinoma, and other tumors. When used diagnostically, these monoclonal antibodies are labeled with biologically-safe isotopes and injected in patients, to visualize and localize areas of tumor growth.

III. IMMUNOLOGICAL DEFENSE MECHANISMS

Tumor-associated antigens can activate a complete set of specific and nonspecific defense mechanisms, both humoral and cellular. Host antitumor immunity involves a complex series of events that result from the participation of the various "arms" of the immune system. These include T cells, B cells, monocytes/macrophages, NK cells, and a variety of soluble products (biological response modifiers) that regulate the interactions of the different cells involved in the process.

A. T and B Lymphocytes

T lymphocytes play an important dual role, as cytotoxic effector cells and as the central modulating cells that control the antitumor immune response. The major role of B lymphocytes is the production of antitumor antibodies that may induce complement-dependent cytotoxicity of tumor cells or may mediate antibody-dependent cell-mediated cytotoxicity (ADCC) in the presence of killer (K) cells. The effect of antitumor antibodies, however, is not always beneficial. In some cases, the antibodies may not cause cytotoxicity and may block the recognition of antigenic determinants by cytotoxic T cells (blocking antibodies). Also, soluble immune complexes constituted by antitumor antibodies and shedded tumor antigens could be generated, and these are known to suppress cytotoxic-T-cell and NK-cell functions, at least in vitro.

B. Natural Killer (NK) Cells

It has been fairly well established that NK cells play a significant role in the first line of defense against neoplastic cells in experimental animals. Their activity can be augmented in vitro by α interferon, interleukin 2, and adjuvants such as BCG and *C. parvum*.

C. The Monocyte/Macrophage System

The differentiation of cytotoxic macrophages reacting with tumor cells is dependent on the release of T-cell products as a consequence of antigen recognition. Mononuclear phagocytes, NK lymphocytes, and PMN all bear Fcγ receptors and thus can readily interact with and destroy IgG-coated target cells (ADCC). Alternatively, these same three cell types also have the capacity for killing tumor targets in the absence of antibody coating; in the case of NK lymphocytes this is termed natural killing, whereas in the case of mononuclear phagocytes and PMNs, this is called spontaneous killing. These three nonspecific effector cell types appear to recognize a common membrane marker of cancerous cells that appears to be shared by many different types of malignant cells. Local activated T lymphocytes may secrete nonspecific immunoregulatory factors (see below) that are capable of up-regulating the tumor killing function of mononuclear phagocytes, NK lymphocytes, and PMN.

D. Immune Surveillance

The immunologic surveillance theory enunciated by Thomas and Burnet proposes that frequent spontaneous mutations naturally occur in somatic cells, some of which may result in neoplastic transformation. Such transformations are often accompanied by the production of abnormal cell-surface protein antigens, and consequently many neoplastically transformed cells are sufficiently antigenic in the host to cause their elimination by cytotoxic T lymphocytes. In rare instances, weakly immunogenic cells or mutant cells that have lost rather than acquired antigens can escape this defense mechanism and develop into malignant tumors. In individuals whose immune competence is impaired or depressed, whether by genetic factors or by treatment with immunosuppressant drugs or irradiation, even highly immunogenic cells may survive and result in increased incidence of tumors.

Although the concept of immunologic surveillance was widely accepted, recent studies seriously question its validity, and to this day it remains hypothetical. In general, it may be reasonable to assume that there are immunologic mechanisms that can be triggered as defenses against neoplastic outgrowth, and resultant therapeutic attempts that enhance the functions of such immune mechanisms are valid; however, the assumption that malignant neoplastic outgrowths occur only if the tumor is not antigenic, or if the host immune defense capability is somewhat impaired or deregulated, is not supported by most investigators.

E. Escape from Host Immunity

The postulated host defense mechanisms against cancer are obviously ineffective whenever tumor growth occurs. Several mechanisms have been proposed to explain how tumor cells escape or evade immunity and grow unchecked. Of these mechanisms, the most credible are immunoselection and enhancement.

1. Immunoselection

Most tumor cell populations appear to be heterogeneous mixtures of different subclones, some of which may have decreased antigenicity. These poorly antigenic variants may have an advantage under the selective pressure exerted on the tumor cells by the host immunity, and their proliferation will increase the general immunoresistance of the tumor.

2. Enhancement

Immunological enhancement has been observed in animal experiments when animals are immunized with inactivated tumor cells before they are infected with live cells. Thus treatment intended to increase the immune response of the host against the tumor sometimes leads to the opposite result. The enhancement in tumor growth can be mediated by several mechanisms. For example, the production of noncytotoxic antitumor antibodies (blocking antibodies), which bind inconsequently to the antigenic sites of the tumor and prevent the recognition of the same sites by potentially effective cytotoxic T cells, facilitates tumor growth. Alternatively, blocking of the immune response can be mediated by other factors present in the serum of the tumor-bearing animal (blocking factors). Among these factors, free tumor antigen or antigen-antibody complexes deserve special mention. The shedding of free tumor antigen may block the receptors of the cytotoxic cells and induce the formation of immune complexes, which in turn may participate in the stimulation of suppressor cells. Finally, activated leukocytes can also promote tumor growth by releasing growth factors such as interleukin 2 (IL2) and transforming growth factor beta (TGF-β).

IV. CANCER BIOTHERAPY

As shown in Figure 28.2, inhibition or promotion of tumor growth has been subdivided further from a tumor immunology perspective. (1) At the hypothesized earliest level (the single malignant cell), immunosurveillance mechanisms may prevent the emergence of a tumor; (2) leukocyte-derived growth-factor stimulation of cells already committed to malignant transformation could be termed immune-system-related tumorigenesis; (3) in established cancer, tumor inhibition may be induced by therapeutic means (cancer biotherapy); (4) established tumor progression may in certain instances be related to the release of tumor-promoting growth factors by leukocytes.

Cancer biotherapy is currently an established component of cancer therapy. As diagramatically illustrated in Figure 28.3, certain forms of cancer biotherapy research are considered active immunotherapies; these are felt to require an intact patient immune system capable of actively identifying and eliminating malignant cells in response to a biotherapeutic stimulus. Tumor vaccines (see below) are representative of active cancer biotherapies. Passive biotherapies somehow "short-circuit" active immunity; the patient's immune system need not be capable of all tumor recognition/destruction functions; biotherapeutic replacements for certain critical steps are administered to the patient. Adoptive cellular immunotherapy (ACI) and immunotoxins (see below) are representative of passive cancer biotherapies.

From a functional perspective, cancer biotherapy research activity can best be compartmentalized into four groups: (1) tumor vaccines; (2) administration of BRM, biologicals, and/or immunostimulatory chemicals; (3) adoptive cellular immunotherapy (ACI); and (4) affinity column apheresis (ACA).

A. Tumor Vaccines

The vaccination of cancer patients with tumor cell preparations is the earliest form of cancer biotherapy, an attempt to replicate the vaccination strategies

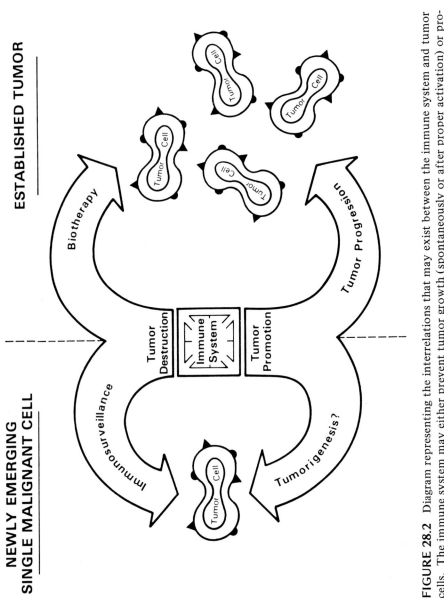

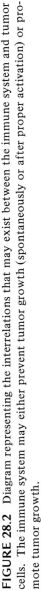

FIGURE 28.2 Diagram representing the interrelations that may exist between the immune system and tumor cells. The immune system may either prevent tumor growth (spontaneously or after proper activation) or promote tumor growth.

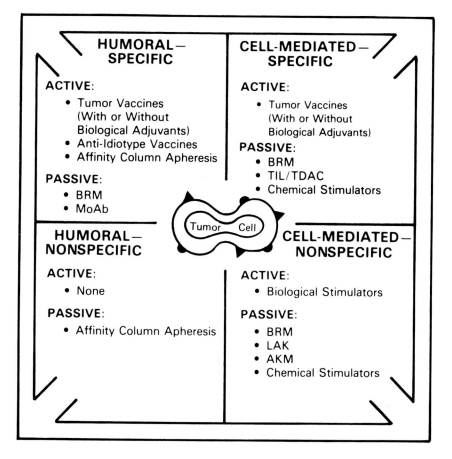

FIGURE 28.3 Schematic representation of the different types of cancer biotherapy.

effective in controlling a variety of infectious diseases. As shown in Figure 28.4, tumor vaccines may be prepared from a patient's own autologous tumor or from similar allogeneic tumor cell lines. These tumor cells may be treated with a variety of enzymatic, chemical, and/or radiation procedures to enhance the expression of tumor antigens and prevent cell division prior to patient reinoculation. Alternatively, a cell-free extract of tumor cell antigen(s) may be prepared and administered back to the patient. Finally, an anti-idiotypic antibody raised against an antitumor antigen monoclonal antibody (thus a "biochemical mirror image" of the original tumor antigen) may be administered in hopes of boosting patient antitumor immunity. A biological adjuvant, such as BCG, may be coad-

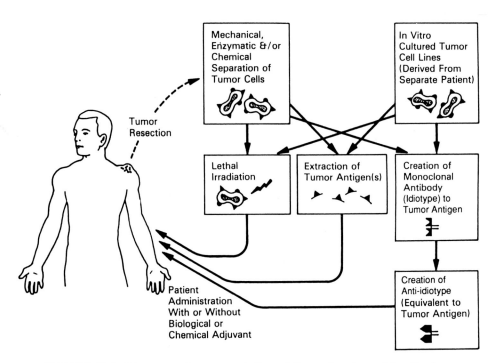

FIGURE 28.4 Diagrammatic representation of the protocols used for the development of tumor vaccines and anti-idiotypic vaccines for use in tumor immunotherapy.

ministered with these vaccines in hopes of enhancing their efficiency. However, it must be noted that anti-idiotypic antibodies can react with the binding site (internal image antibodies) or with nearby regions of the variable region (structural anti-idiotypes). The last type of antibody may block the antigen-antibody reaction (binding-site-related) or not, as diagrammatically illustrated in Figure 28.5. The internal image and binding-site-related antibodies can be used to stimulate humoral immunity towards cellular antigens, but the non-binding-site-related antibodies are inefficient. Therefore, a careful characterization of anti-idiotypic antibodies is required before their use in immunization protocols.

Tumor vaccines are active biotherapies; they require that the patient have intact recognition and elimination immune mechanisms. This basic premise may underlie the lack of universal effectiveness of tumor vaccines to date. Many vaccinated patients demonstrate enhanced cell-mediated immunity upon laboratory testing, and certain tumor vaccines may stimulate a modest immunoglobulin response. However, established tumor burden is generally not affected in

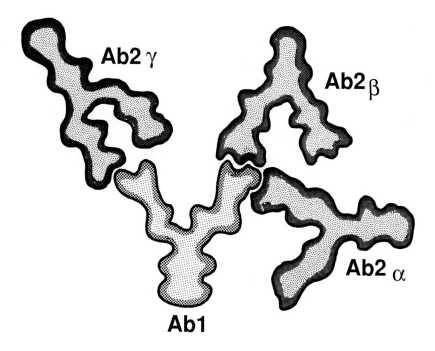

FIGURE 28.5 Schematic representation of the different types of anti-idiotypic antibodies. Anti-idiotypic antibodies can react with the binding site (internal image antibodies) or with nearby regions of the variable region (structural anti-idiotypes).

such patients. Perhaps other required immune system effector mechanisms are defective in certain cancer patients, limiting tumor cell elimination even in the face of antitumor immune response. Alternatively, perhaps the immune response generated by tumor vaccines is not ample enough to control the many distinct cancer cell subpopulations that may emerge during the clinical development of cancer, some of which may express very little or no antigen.

B. Biological Response Modifiers and Immunostimulatory Compounds

The major categories of BRMs that are employed as biotherapies have been cited in Chapter 26; they are generally administered systemically (into the circulatory system) of the cancer patient. Since most BRMs have been successfully produced by genetic engineering techniques, abundant quantities of these agents are available for use in clinical trials; they are substantially pure and free of toxins.

The most striking example of a BRM cancer biotherapy currently employed is the administration of α interferon for hairy cell leukemia. Hairy cell leukemia is a chronically progressive leukemia for which there was no effective therapy prior to 1983. At that time, it was shown that α interferon in modest doses was capable of inducing prolonged durable remissions. In 1987 the Food and Drug Administration approved the use of α interferon for the treatment of hairy cell leukemia. In 1988 α interferon was approved for use also in the treatment of Kaposi's sarcoma in its early stages. Alpha interferon has also been shown to induce remissions in certain types of lymphoma and chronic myelogenous leukemia (CML); certain solid tumors (such as melanoma and renal cell carcinoma) also demonstrate small rates of response to α interferon administration. The mechanism of action of α interferon in patients who do experience remissions is not entirely understood; most of the evidence favors a direct antiproliferative effect of this BRM on the tumor cells rather than an up-regulation of the patient's immune system.

Dozens of other BRMs, other biologicals, and other biologically active chemicals are also undergoing testing. None of these agents (either singly or in combination) has yet been shown to be a panacea for all forms of cancer; in most series, even in "biotherapy responsive" malignancies, response rates are less than 20%. This is perhaps not surprising, given the complexity of the "immune system symphony." The delicate checks and balances required for the successful operation of this system would theoretically preclude duplication by the administration of just a single BRM component. Thus it is possible that our success in the use of single BRMs will be focused on those malignancies that can be directly down-regulated by these agents. Alternatively, we may at some point develop methods for determining precise immunologic defects in the immune system of cancer patients and for administering the appropriate combination of BRMs (at the proper timing and dosage) to reproduce the normal anticancer immunologic symphony.

The most passive form of BRM biotherapy is found when "final effector molecules" are delivered directly to the site of tumor burden. For example, the infusion of IgG or IgM monoclonal antibodies with tumor antigen specificity should permit local complement activation following binding to tumor cells. However, membrane-attack-complex activation has not been found in most cancer patients treated with murine monoclonal antibodies (MoAb), perhaps because most murine MoAb activate human complement poorly. Also, murine hybridomas are antigenic to humans, and this immunogenicity precludes their long term use. With repeated injections of murine monoclonal antibodies, the host will eventually develop antimouse immunoglobulin antibodies; once antimouse antibodies appear in the circulation, any further injections of monoclonal antibodies will result in the rapid formation of immune complexes. The formation of immune complexes has two main consequences; rapid elimination of the monoclonal antibody (with loss of therapeutic efficiency) and development of serum sickness (see Chapter 21). The development of human MoAb with antitumor specificity would solve most of these problems. On one hand, human hybridomas would not be immunogenic. On the other, human hybridomas would be more likely to trigger local complement activation and optimally promote ADCC clearance mechanisms. An interesting alternative is the production of chimeric monoclonal antibodies. These antibodies are produced by immortalized cell lines to which hybrid immunoglobulin genes carry the variable region genes of a murine hybridoma of desired specificity and the constant region genes of human immunoglobulins. The protein product of this hybrid gene has the antigen specificity of the murine antibody and the constant region sequences of a human antibody, thereby being considerably less immunogenic than a murine monoclonal antibody.

An interesting alternative to the therapeutic use of monoclonal antibodies is to use them as targeting devices for other BRMs or toxic compounds. For example, the chemical coupling of LT or TNF-β to a tumor-reactive MoAb could potentially focus these tumor-killing BRM to appropriate loci within the cancer patient. Alternatively, toxic compounds (including radioisotopes, chemotherapeutic agents, or biological toxins) can be chemically coupled to MoAb with preservation of the bioactivity of both. Such monoclonal antibody "immunotoxins" have been used with success in experimental models but have not yet been shown to be reproducibly effective in the cancer patient setting. This could reflect our current inability to focus enough immunotoxin exclusively at the sites of tumor burden to prevent generalized toxicity.

C. Adoptive Cellular Immunotherapy

Adoptive cellular immunotherapy (ACI) was begun in the early 1980s following observations that immune-system subset cells from cancer patients could be upregulated in the laboratory to destroy tumor cells in vitro. Thus various trials began in which patient leukocyte subsets are removed, up-regulated in the laboratory, and then readministered to sites of tumor in the patient. As shown in Figure 28.6, the extraction of T lymphocytes from tumor specimens, and their expansion and activation in vitro in interleukin 2, produces the so-called tumor infiltrating lymphocyte (TIL) or tumor-derived activated cell (TDAC). TIL/TDAC (once generated in the laboratory) can be readministered to the patient, usually with supplementary interleukin 2 to maintain their cytotoxic activity and with cyclophosphamide (presumably to limit the generation of suppressor T lymphocytes).

NK lymphocytes can be removed by apheresis and can also be expanded and activated in vitro with interleukin 2. The resulting lymphokine activated killer

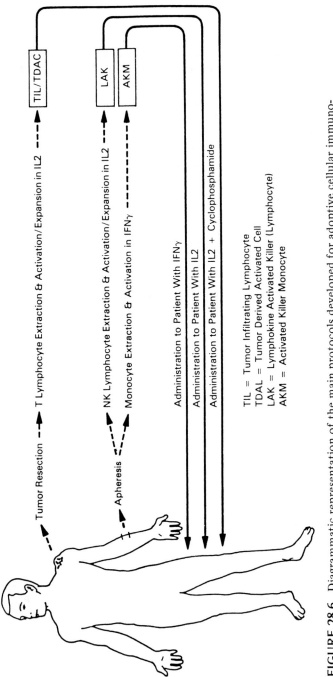

Tumor Resection ---▶ T Lymphocyte Extraction & Activation/Expansion in IL2 ----▶ TIL/TDAC

NK Lymphocyte Extraction & Activation/Expansion in IL2 ---▶ LAK

Monocyte Extraction & Activation in IFNγ ----------▶ AKM

Apheresis

Administration to Patient With IFNγ

Administration to Patient With IL2

Administration to Patient With IL2 + Cyclophosphamide

TIL = Tumor Infiltrating Lymphocyte
TDAL = Tumor Derived Activated Cell
LAK = Lymphokine Activated Killer (Lymphocyte)
AKM = Activated Killer Monocyte

FIGURE 28.6 Diagrammatic representation of the main protocols developed for adoptive cellular immunotherapy.

(LAK) cell can then be readministered to the patient with supplementary interleukin 2 to maintain their cytotoxic activity. Finally, blood monocytes can also
be extracted by apheresis from the cancer patient and activated in vitro to enhanced cytotoxic activity with γ interferon. The resultant activated killer monocyte (AKM) can then be readministered to the patient with supplementary γ interferon to maintain the cytotoxic activity of the infused AKM.

Adoptive cell immunotherapies are truly monumental clinical research ef-
forst. Each ACI trial requires a tremendous effort on the part of clinicians, laboratory personnel, and support personnel. It has been estimated that certain of
these therapies may cost as much as $100,000 per patient. However, the clinical
responses seen in certain ACIs represents the best scientific information to date
that indicates that the immune system can eradicate established tumor. For example, in selected patients with melanoma and renal cell carcinoma, approximately 20% of patients with incurable disease will get responses to LAK cell
therapy; certain patients have had prolonged complete remissions. However,
the time involved, the expense, and the toxicities of certain of these ACIs require that much additional research be done to simplify and improve these forms
of cancer biotherapy.

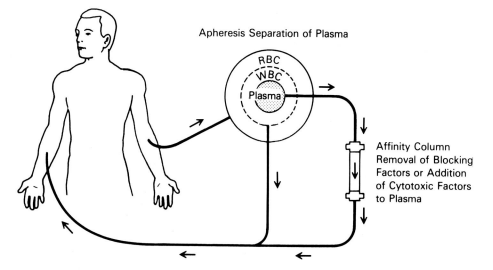

FIGURE 28.7   Schematic representation of the general protocol for the use of
affinity column apheresis in cancer immunotherapy.

D. Affinity Column Apheresis

Affinity column apheresis (ACA) is the final functional grouping of cancer bio-therapy; ACA requires the passage of the plasma of cancer patients over specially formulated affinity columns in order to (1) remove blocking factors of appro-priate immune responses or (2) to activate tumor cytotoxic factors in the plasma (Fig. 28.7). ACA biotherapy originally started with research observations in the 1970s indicating that the plasma of cancer patients contained blocking factors of the immune response. Such blocking factors could include shed tumor anti-gens or antigen-antibody complexes. Many of the ACA cancer therapy trials have focused on passing patient plasma over affinity columns (such as staphyl-ococcus protein A columns) designed to remove immune complexes. The re-sults of ACA trials have been inconsistent to date. In addition, many ACA trials have provided evidence that the passage of patient plasma over affinity columns may also activate cytotoxic factors in the plasma; this observation complicates the task of understanding and scientifically regulating this form of therapy.

V. TUMOR IMMUNOLOGY AND THE FUTURE OF CANCER BIOTHERAPY

Tumor immunology is a necessarily complex area of research investigation, given our incomplete understanding of the nature of the malignancy process and the mechanism of immune responses to malignant cells. However, a variety of can-cer biotherapies (active or passive) have been developed, focusing on specific subcomponents of the cancer patient's immune response. To date, there is clearly no single biotherapy approach effective in all cases of cancer or likely to be so in the near future. Each of the forms of cancer biotherapy reviewed in Figure 28.3 is the subject of continuing long-term scientific investigation.

Overall, the goal of all preclinical tumor immunology research is to charac-terize mechanisms of anticancer immune-system activity with in vitro and ani-mal models. Then each newly developed biotherapy (whether vaccine, BRM, ACI or ACA) should undergo clinical trials to determine its toxicity and effi-cacy rates. If found efficacious, each approved biotherapy will be employed in the general cancer-patient population as quickly as possible; any positive cancer biotherapy result should also stimulate new research to determine its mechanism of action in an attempt to generalize and simplify the treatment. The final goal of tumor immunology research is to develop strategies that will allow us to main-tain enhanced immunosurveillance of normal individuals and thus prevent the emergence of clinical cancer entirely.

SELF-EVALUATION

Questions

Choose the one best answer.

28.1 Activated NK cells
   A. Are called LAK cells when activated in vitro with interleukin 2.
   B. May be up-regulated by α interferon.
   C. May participate in ADCC.
   D. May release NKCF.
   E. All of the above are correct.

28.2 High serum levels of alpha fetoprotein (AFP) are detected in
   A. Pregnant women.
   B. Heavy smokers.
   C. Patients with alcoholic cirrhosis.
   D. Patients with resected cancer of the colon.
   E. Patients with germ-cell teratocarcinoma.

28.3 Which of the following is not considered a passive biotherapy?
   A. In vivo administration of α interferon.
   B. In vivo administration of IL2.
   C. Readministration of activated tumor-infiltrating lymphocytes (TIL).
   D. Readministration of activated killer monocytes (AKM).
   E. Injection of lethally irradiated autologous tumor cells plus BCG.

28.4 Activated mononuclear phagocytes
   A. Are a part of the nonspecific component of cell-mediated immunity.
   B. Kill melanoma cells better than colon cancer cells.
   C. Express antigen-specific receptors.
   D. Cannot be employed in adoptive cellular immunotherapy.
   E. Destroy normal tissues.

28.5 Interleukin 2 has been used immunotherapeutically in protocols involving IL2-mediated expansion of
   A. Helper T lymphocytes.
   B. Antibody-producing plasma cells.
   C. Normal monocytes.
   D. Patient's monocytes.
   E. Tumor infiltrating lymphocytes.

Each set of questions below consists of a set of lettered headings followed by numbered phrases. For each numbered phrase, choose the one lettered heading that is best. In each group, the lettered heading may be used once, more than once, or not at all. (A) Alpha-fetoprotein (AFP); (B) Carcinoembryonic antigen; (C) Both; (D) Neither.

28.6 Pathognomonic when positive.

28.7 Elevated serum levels are found in heavy smokers.

28.8 Useful in the management of patients with cancer.

In Questions 28.9-28.10, match the BRM with the most suitable mechanism for its antitumoral effect. (A) Specific cell-mediated immunity; (B) Specific humoral immunity; (C) Nonspecific cell-mediated immunity; (D) Nonspecific humoral immunity; (E) None of these.

28.9 Toxin-conjugated monoclonal antibodies.

28.10 α interferon.

Answers

28.1 (E)

28.2 (E)

28.3 (E)   Injection of killed tumor cells and BCG is a form of tumor vaccination, whose objective is actively to induce specific antitumor immunity.

28.4 (A)

28.5 (E)   Several different immunotherapy protocols have been tried in which patient's cells have been expanded in vitro and reinfused into the patient, including monocytes (expanded with γ interferon), NK cells, and tumor-infiltrating lymphocytes (these last two types of cells are activated with IL2).

28.6 (D)   Both types of antigens can be increased except with hepatoma or or colon carcinoma; thereafore they are not pathognomonic for a given malignancy.

28.7 (B)

28.8 (C)   Both CEA and alpha fetoprotein levels can be used to monitor progression after surgical excision of a tumor producing either one of of these oncofetal antigens.

28.9 (B)

28.10(E)   The effect of α interferon seems related to an antiproliferative effect rather than to an up-regulation of the immune system.

BIBLIOGRAPHY

Chiao, J. W. (Ed.). *Biological Response Modifiers and Cancer Therapy*. Marcel Dekker, New York, 1988.

Daar, A. S. (Ed.). *Tumor Markers in Clinical Practice*. Blackwell Scientific, Oxford, 1987.

Dilman, R. O. Antibody therapy. In *Principles of Cancer Biotherapy*, R. K. Oldham (Ed.). Raven, New York, 1987.

Hanna, M. G., Hoover, H. C. Peters, L. C., Key, M. E., Haspell, M. V., McCabe, R. P., and Pomato, N. Fundamental and applied aspects of successful active specific immunotherapy of cancer. In *Principles of Cancer Biotherapy*, R. K. Oldham (Ed.). Raven, New York, 1987.

Krolick, K. A. Selective elimination of autoreactive lymphocytes with immunotoxins. *Clin. Immunol. Immunopatholo. 50*:273, 1989.

Oldham, R. K. Immunoconjugates: Drugs and toxins. In *Principles of Cancer Biotherapy*, R. K. Oldham (Ed.). Raven, New York, 1987.

Rosenberg, S. A. A progress report on the treatment of 157 patients with advanced cancer using lymphokine-activated killer cells and interleukin-2 or high-dose interleukin-2 alone. *New Engl. J. Med. 316*:889, 1987.

Stevenson, H. C. and Stevenson, G. W. Adoptive cellular cancer immunotherapy. In *Principles of Cancer Biotherapy*, R. K. Oldham (Ed.). Raven, New York, 1987.

Stevenson, H. C. (Ed.). *Adoptive Cellular Immunotherapy of Cancer*. Marcel Dekker, New York, 1989.

Viale, G. et al. Anti-human tumor antibodies induced in mice and rabbits by "internal image" anti-idiotypic monoclonal immunoglobulins. *J. Immunol. 139*:4250, 1987.

29

Malignancies of the Immune System

GABRIEL VIRELLA and JEAN-MICHEL GOUST

Lymphocytes are frequently affected by neoplastic mutations, perhaps as a consequence of their intense mitotic activity. The malignancies of the immune system are of considerable interest to the immunologist for several reasons. First and foremost, a large amount of our knowledge about the immune system in man has been derived from studies of aberrant situations; for example, the studies on immunoglobulin structure were made possible by the production of large amounts of homogeneous molecules by patients with B-cell malignancies; second, the accurate diagnosis of these situations depends on immunological techniques and on the knowledge of the biological role and characteristics of the normal counterpart to the malignant cell.

We can broadly subdivide the malignancies of the immune system into B-cell and T-cell malignancies. The former are frequently identified by the production of abnormal amounts of homogeneous immunoglobulins (or fragments thereof) by the malignant cells; the latter are usually identified through studies of cell markers. Since the production of homogeneous immunoglobulins may be detected in patients without overt signals of malignancy, the terms *B-cell dyscrasia* and *plasma-cell dyscrasia* are often used to designate all situations in which abnormally homogeneous proteins are detected.

I. B-CELL DYSCRASIAS

A. The Monoclonal Nature of B-Cell Dyscrasias

According to the clonal selection theory of Burnet, immunocompetent cells are organized in families or *clones*. A normal individual has perhaps 10^8 different B-cell clones, each on consisting of a relatively small number of cells producing antibody of a single specificity, able to recognize one or a few closely related antigens. Each B-cell clone produces a homogeneous population of structurally identical antibody molecules reacting with a single antigenic determinant.

Under normal conditions, B-cell clones are stimulated by specific antigens, and the expansion of a stimulated clone is controlled by several feedback mechanisms. In special circumstances, however, a B-cell clone may escape from the normal control mechanisms, proliferate, and produce homogeneous immunoglobulins or fragments thereof (Fig. 29.1). These situations are known as mono-

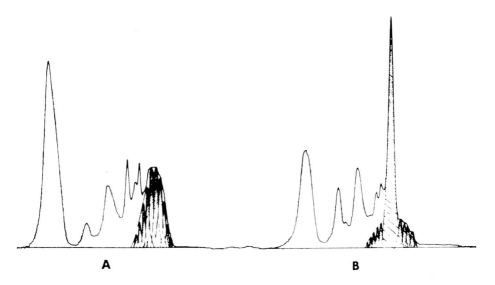

A   B

FIGURE 29.1   The concept of monoclonal gammopathy. In normal sera or in cases of reactive plasmacytosis the gamma globulin fraction is made up of the sum of a large number of different antibodies, each one of them produced by a different plasma cell clone (A); if a B-cell clone escapes normal proliferation control and expands, the product of this clone, made up of millions of structurally identical molecules, will predominate over all other clonal products and appear on the electrophoretic separation as a narrow-based, homogeneous peak in the gamma globulin fraction (B).

clonal gammopathies, plasma cell dyscrasias or B-cell dyscrasias (from the Greek *dyskrasis*, meaning "bad mixture," often used to designate hematological disorders affecting one particular cell line), and the homogeneous immunoglobulin is known as a monoclonal protein or paraprotein. In practical terms, a monoclonal protein is constituted by molecules carrying one single heavy chain class and one single light chain type, or, in some cases, by isolated heavy or light chains of a single type. The escape from feedback control is the result of a neoplastic mutation, but in some cases there is no evidence of malignant growth, so it appears that some mutations may lead to clonal expansion without uncontrolled cell proliferation.

B. Diagnosis of B-Cell Dyscrasias

The diagnosis of a B-cell dyscrasia relies on the demonstration of a monoclonal protein. However, in some instances, B-cell dyscrasias do not result in the secretion of paraproteins. In rare cases of multiple myeloma, for example, the neoplastic mutation alters the synthetic process so profoundly that no paraproteins are produced (nonsecretory myeloma). Similarly, chronic lymphocytic leukemia can be characterized as a B-cell dyscrasia in more than 90% of the cases, but only one-third show paraproteins; the remainder have monoclonal cell-surface immunoglobulins only. B-cell acute lymphocytic leukemias may have as a single marker of their identity a rearrangement of their immunoglobulin heavy chain genes in chromosome 14.

Secreted paraproteins are detected by a combination of methods. Initial screening usually involves the electrophoretic separation of serum and urine from the suspected case (Fig. 29.2). To be sure that urinary proteins are not overlooked because of their low concentration, the urine sample must be concentrated. Electrophoretic studies must usually be supplemented by immunoelectrophoresis or by immunofixation for two reasons: (1) in some cases, paraproteins undetectable electrophoretically may be clearly evident on immunoelectrophoresis or immunofixation studies; (2) more generally, immunochemical studies are essential in order to characterize the paraproteins as containing one of the five possible classes of immunoglobulins, and one of the two possible types of light chains (Fig. 29.3), which is an essential step to confirm the monoclonal nature of a suspected electrophoretic spike. Furthermore, the diagnosis of some specific B-cell dyscrasias, such as light chain disease (a variant of multiple myeloma), Waldenström's macroglobulinemia, or the heavy chain diseases, depends basically on the immunochemical characterization of the paraprotein.

On the other hand, in the majority of cases, the finding of a monoclonal protein does not give a very precise diagnostic indication. For example, the finding of homogeneous free light chains (Bence-Jones protein) in the urine, as the only

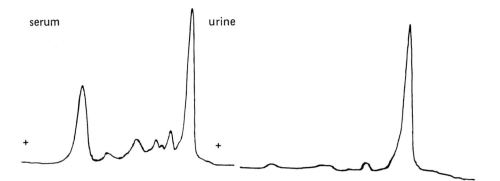

FIGURE 29.2 Electrophoresis of serum and urine proteins from a patient with multiple myeloma. The serum, shown on the left, shows a very sharp peak in the gamma globulin region, with a base narrower than that of albumin, corresponding to an IgG monoclonal component. The urine, shown on the right, shows a sharp fraction in the gamma region with only traces of albumin, meaning that the monoclonal peak is constituted by proteins smaller than albumin, able to cross the glomerular filter. This monoclonal protein in the urine was constituted by free κ type light chains (κ type Bence-Jones protein).

abnormality in a patient, may correspond to one of the following B-cell dyscrasias: (1) light chain disease (a variant of multiple myeloma); (2) chronic lymphocytic leukemia; (3) lymphocytic lymphoma; or (4) "benign" or "idiopathic" monoclonal gammopathy. The precise diagnosis depends on a combination of clinical and laboratory data, as discussed in detail later in this chapter.

C. Physiopathology of B-Cell Dyscrasias

1. Symptoms Resulting from Malignant Cell Proliferation

Symptoms resulting from the malignant proliferation of B-cell clones include (1) enlargement of lymph nodes, spleen, and liver; (2) leukemic invasion of peripheral blood; (3) compressive and obstructive symptoms; and (4) intestinal malabsorption (α chain disease).

Direct compressive and obstructive symptoms can result from a proliferation of plasma cells in soft tissues. Oropharyngeal plasmacytomas often lead to obstructive symptoms. Heavy-chain-producing intestinal lymphomas, when grossly nodular, can lead to intestinal obstruction. On the other hand, compressive symptoms can result from bone destruction, as in cases of multiple myeloma with vertebral body destruction and collapse, resulting in spinal cord compression. Intestinal malabsorption, which is typical of α chain disease, results from

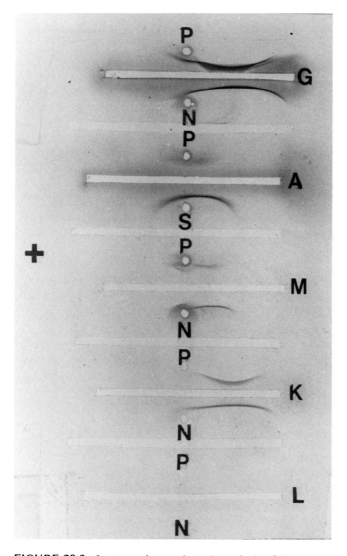

FIGURE 29.3 Immunoelectrophoretic analysis of the serum protein of a patient with multiple myeloma (P), compared to serum from a normal control (N). The following antisera were used: anti-IgG (G), anti-IgA (A), anti-IgM (M), anti-κ chains (K), and anti-λ chains (L). Notice the abnormally homogeneous shape of the precipitation arcs corresponding to the patient's serum when studied with anti-IgG and anti-κ chains, allowing the identification of an IgG κ monoclonal component.

extensive infiltration of the intestinal submucosa by malignant B cells, causing total disruption of the normal submucosal architecture.

2. Symptoms Resulting from General Metabolic Disturbances

These symptoms include (1) bone destruction, hypercalcemia, and renal insufficiency; (2) uremia; and (3) anemia. *Bone destruction* does not result directly from B-cell proliferation but rather from osteoclast hyperactivity secondary to the production of an osteoclast stimulating factor by the malignant B cells and/ or activated T cells. *Renal insufficiency* can result from a diversity of factors, such as hypercalcemia, hyperuricemia, deposition of amyloid substance in the kidney, clogging of glomeruli or tubuli with paraprotein (favored by dehydration), and plasmacytic infiltration of the kidney. *Anemia* (normochronic, normocytic) is frequent and is basically due to decreased production of red cells. A moderate shortening of red-cell survival is also common.

3. Serum Hyperviscosity

The viscosity of serum relative to water increases with protein concentration. IgM and polymeric IgA, because of their high intrinsic viscosity, lead to disproportionate increases of blood viscosity (Fig. 29.4). The hyperviscosity syndrome is a frequent manifestation of Waldenström's macroglobulinemia. However, it is also observed in multiple myeloma patients, mainly in those with IgA paraproteins, and occasionally in IgG myeloma. The symptoms of serum hyperviscosity are related to high protein concentration, expanded plasma volume, and sluggishness of circulation. Table 29.1 lists the main signs and symptoms of the syndrome. Typical fundoscopic changes are shown in Figure 29.5.

4. Symptoms Resulting from the Immunological Activity of the Paraprotein

   a. *Cold Agglutinin Disease.* This is characterized by the presence of a monoclonal antibody (IgM κ in more than 90% of the cases) reacting with the I antigen expressed by the red cells of all adults; it can manifest itself as additional features superimposed on a typical case of Waldenström's macroglobulinemia, with the IgM paraprotein behaving as a cold agglutinin. In other cases, the clinical manifestations are exclusively related to the presence of cold agglutinins, and no evidence of B-cell dyscrasia other than the presence of a monoclonal anti-I antibody can be detected. The clinical manifestations of cold agglutinin disease fall into two categories: (1) cold-induced hemolytic anemia, which is usually mild but in some severe cases can be intense enough to lead to acute renal failure; and (2) cold-induced ischemia, probably due to massive intracapillary agglutination, affecting cold-exposed areas.

   b. *Hyperlipemia.* This can be pronounced in patients with monoclonal gammopathies, and in some cases the monoclonal protein has antibody activity

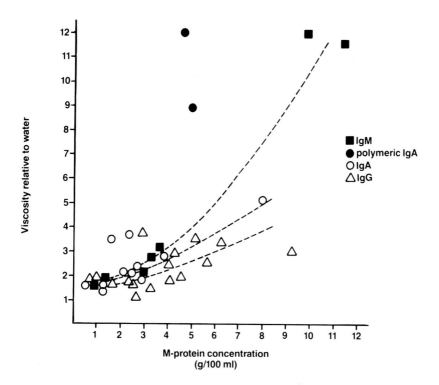

FIGURE 29.4 Plot of relative viscosities versus monoclonal protein concentrations in sera containing IgG, IgA, and IgG monoclonal proteins. The highest relative viscosities were registered with sera containing monoclonal proteins constituted by IgM or polymeric IgA.

to lipoproteins. It has been demontrated that the binding of antibodies to the lipoprotein molecules alters the uptake of intracellular processing of the lipoprotein, resulting in hyperlipemia and increases accumualtion of cholesterol in macrophages.

5. Immunosuppression

One of the classical clinical features of malignant B-cell dyscrasias, particularly of multiple myeloma, is the increased tendency for pyogenic infections. This is paralleled by decreased levels of normal immunoglobulins and decreased antibody production after active immunization. In vitro studies have shown that the number of B cells with surface immunoglobulins is decreased in multiple myeloma, and although the number of antigen-binding cells seems normal, mitogen-induced blast transformation and immunoglobulin synthesis are grossly impaired.

TABLE 29.1   Clinical Manifestations of the Hyperviscosity Syndrome

Ocular
　Variable degrees of vision impairment
　Fundoscopic changes
　　Dilation and tortuosity of retinal veins ("strong-of-sausage" appearance)
　　Retinal hemorrhage and "cotton-wool" exudates
　　Pailledema

Hematologic
　Mucosal bleeding (oral cavity, nose, gastrointestinal tract, urinary tract)
　Prolong bleeding after trauma or surgery

Neurological
　Headaches, somnolence, coma
　Dizziness, vertigo
　Seizures, EEG changes
　Hearing loss

Renal
　Renal insufficiency (acute or chronic) due to
　　(a) clogging of the glomerular vessels with paraprotein and
　　(b) diminished concentrating and diluting abilities

Cardiovascular
　Congestive heart failure secondary to expanded plasma volume

Source: Modified from Bloch, K. J. and Maki, D. G. *Sem. Hematol. 10*;113, 1974.

The depression of the immune response in patients with multiple myeloma appears to be multifactorial. At least two important factors might contribute. In IgG myeloma, the large amounts of circulatory IgG present are likely to have a feedback effect, depressing normal IgG synthesis. A more general mechanism of suppression of the humoral response seems to be mediated by suppressor cells. Phagocytic monocytes (and to a lesser extent T cells) appear to mediate this suppression, which can be demonstrated by cocultures of peripheral mononuclear leukocytes from normal donors and myeloma patients, resulting in impairment of the function of the normal B lymphocytes. Humoral immunosuppression is also observed in mice with experimental plasmacytomas. In contrast to this depression of humoral immunity, both patients and animals with malignant plasmacytomas have normal numbers of T cells and normal cell-mediated immunity, when measured with nonspecific stimulating agents. However, experimental animals are unable to mount an effective immune response against a plasmacytoma. It has been shown that administration of a single, relatively small, dose of cyclophosphamide to mice with plasmacytomas grown to palpable size results in complete tumor remission. The dosage of cytotoxic drug

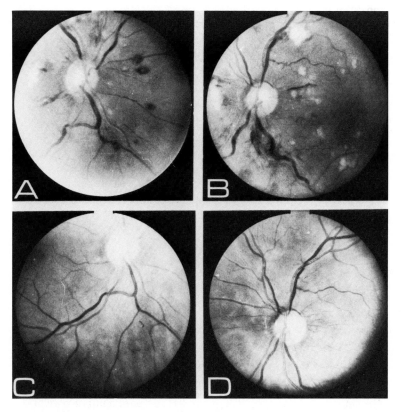

FIGURE 29.5 Fundoscopic examination on a patient with hyperviscosity syndrome. A and B are pictures obtained from the right and left eyes, respectively, at the time of admission. Flame-shaped hemorrhages, "cotton-wool" exudates, and irregular dilation of retinal veins are evident. C and D are pictures obtained from the same eyes after 5 months of therapy, showing total normalization. (From G. Virella et al. Polymerized monoclonal IgA in two patients with myelomatosis and hyperviscosity syndrome. *Brit. J. Haematol 30*:479, 1975.

is not sufficient to destroy the tumor cells, which are obviously present five days after its administration. Administration of cyclophosphamide at the very early stages, when the tumor is still not palpable, is not effective. This result suggests that at the time the tumor has grown to palpable size it has stimulated the immune system, which is kept from rejecting the tumor by an excess of suppressor T cells. This negative balance is offset by cyclophosphamide, believed to affect suppressor cells more easily than effector and helper cells, and the animal is then able to eliminate the tumor by its own immunological means.

In chronic lymphocytic leukemia, in addition to a depression of humoral immunity (milder than that seen in multiple myeloma), there is a depression of T-cell counts and function. Viral and fungal infections, as well as cases of disseminated infection after administration of live attenuated viral vaccines, have been reported in patients with this type of leukemia.

D. Clinical Forms of B-Cell Dyscrasia

1. Multiple Myeloma

The diagnosis of multiple myeloma lies in the following triad; (1) bone lesions, (2) monoclonal protein in serum and/or urine, and (3) bone marrow plasmacytosis. The extent to which these three components are considered in the diagnosis varies from author to author. Basically, typical bone lesions associated with either monoclonal proteins or bone marrow plasmacytosis are diagnostic. Also marked bone marrow plasmacytosis associated with either one of the components of the triad is usually considered diagnostic.

   a. Bone Lesions. The typical features of bone lesions in multiple myeloma are (1) their osteolytic nature (typical lesions appear in the x-ray as punched-out areas without peripheral osteosclerosis) and (2) their multiplicity (multiple punched-out areas appear in the same bone and can be seen in a number of bones in the same patient) (Fig. 29.6). Practically all bones can be affected. In advanced cases, pathological fractures can occur in the long bones, skull, or spinal column. Rarely, a single bone lesion may be detected in one patient; however, such a "solitary bone plasmacytoma" is in fact rarely solitary, and bone marrow aspiration will reveal diffuse plasmacytosis in most cases. Exceptionally, a patient with monoclonal gammopathy and diffuse plasmacytosis can present with no evident bone lesions, or with generalized osteoporosis.

   b. Monoclonal Protein in Serum and/or Urine. In almost all cases of multiple myeloma (98%), a monoclonal protein can be detected by adequate studies. The distribution of monoclonal proteins among the different immunoglobulin classes closely parallels the relative proportions of those immunoglobulins in normal serum: 60-70% of the proteins are typed as IgG, 20-30% as IgA, 1-2% as IgD, and, very rarely, one monoclonal protein can be typed as IgE. A single light chain type is found in these paraproteins. For example, IgG paraproteins can be either κ or λ. The finding of an increased IgG concentration with heterogeneous characteristics, immunochemically demonstrated to result from increased production of both IgG κ and IgG λ molecules, actually excludes the diagnosis of multiple myeloma.

   In the urine, the most frequent finding is the elimination of free light chains, κ or λ (Bence-Jones proteins). These light chains are usually found in addition

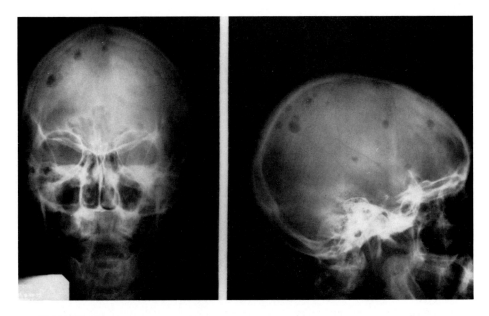

FIGURE 29.6   X-ray of the skull of a patient with multiple myeloma showing typical osteolytic lesions. (Courtesy of Dr. S. Richardson, Division of Hematology, Department of Medicine, Medical University of South Carolina.)

to a monoclonal immunoglobulin detectable in serum, but in about 20-30% of patients with multiple myeloma the only abnormal proteins to be found are the free monoclonal light chains in the urine. Some authors give the designation of *light chain disease* to the form of multiple myeloma in which the only paraprotein consists of free light chains.

Very rarely (in about 2% of cases), no monoclonal paraprotein is detected in the serum or urine of a patient with a typical clinical picture of multiple myeloma. This situation is designated *nonsecretory myeloma.* In many cases, immunofluorescence studies have demonstrated intracellular monoclonal proteins that are not secreted into the extracellular spaces. Nonsecretory plasmacytomas have a very poor prognosis, perhaps indicating that the degree of biochemical disturbance that accompanies the malignant mutation parallels the degree of biological malignancy.

c. Bone Marrow Plasmacytosis.   In multiple myeloma, bone marrow aspirates show increased numbers of plasma cells. In typical cases the plasma cell infiltration is massive, with plasma cells growing in a sheetlike manner. In many instances, however, the only abnormal feature is an increased number of plasma

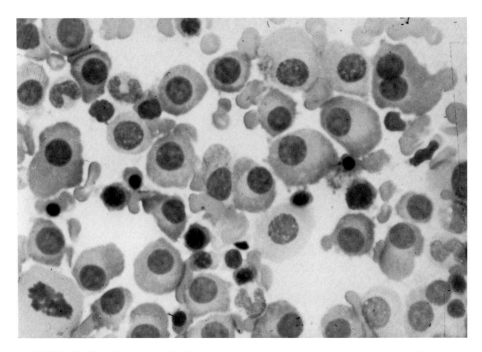

FIGURE 29.7 Plasma cell infiltration of the bone marrow in a patient with multiple myeloma. Note the binucleated plasma cell in the upper right corner of this picture.

cells with more or less mature appearance (Fig. 29.7). Such increases in plasma cell numbers, even when associated with morphological aberrations, are not sufficient to differentiate between malignant and reactive plasma-cell proliferations. The differential diagnosis between malignant and reactive plama-cell proliferations should be based on the immunochemical characteristics of the patient's immunoglobulins. Reactive plasmacytosis is invariably associated with a polyclonal increase of immunoglobulins, while a patient with a malignant B-cell dyscrasia will show either a monoclonal protein or low immunoglobulin levels (if it is a case of nonsecretory myeloma).

    d. Clinical Features. The most frequent clinical symptoms of multiple myeloma are (1) bone pain and "spontaneous" or "pathological" fractures, (2) malaise, headaches, or other symptoms related to hyperviscosity, (3) weakness and anemia, (4) repeated infections, and (5) renal failure.

    The presentation of multiple myeloma can vary considerably. In some cases, anemia is the leading feature and the diagnosis is established when the cause of anemia is investigated. Hemoglobin levels below 7.5 g/dl are usually associated with poor prognosis. Other cases are first seen in a rheumatology outpatient clinic, with "bone pains." Cases with advanced bone destruction may reveal themselves by a fracture after minimal trauma. Symptoms related to hyperviscosity may also lead to hospitalization. Renal failure and repeated infections, which usually occur in advanced stages of the disease, are among the most frequent causes of death but rarely constitute the presenting symptoms. Hyperviscosity-related symptoms can also be life-threatening, but their relief is relatively simple with adequate measures, such as the combination of plasmapheresis and chemotherapy. In contrast, immunosuppression and renal failure may be impossible to treat. The prognosis of a multiple myeloma patient with renal failure, particularly when his blood urea nitrogen exceeds 80 mg/dl, is usually very poor.

   e. Therapy. The basic therapy of multiple myeloma consists of the administration of one of two cytotoxic drugs: melphalan or cytoxan (cyclophosphamide). Different schedules of administration (continuous low dosage of intermittent high dosage) are used by different groups of therapists, and there is no clear evidence in favor of either agent or any of the different therapeutic regimes. Some authors routinely use prednisone in association with the cytotoxic drug, whereas others prefer to use prednisone only in cases with hypercalcemia.

   Besides cytotoxic drugs, other supportive measures are important, such as plasmapheresis (which consists in replacing the patient's plasma by normal plasma or a plasma-replacing solution) in cases with hyperviscosity, hemodialysis or peritoneal dialysis in cases with renal insufficiency, and antibiotic therapy in cases with recurrent infections.

2. Plasma Cell Leukemia

In many cases of multiple myeloma, plasma cells can be seen in low numbers on peripheral blood smears. But some patients have relatively large numbers of plasma cells in the peripheral blood, and in such cases the situation has been designated as *plasma cell leukemia*. Aside from the leukemic aspects, the remaining clinical and laboratory features are indistinguishable from those of multiple myeloma. The prognosis in plasma cell leukemia is generally poor; this may reflect a higher degree of dedifferentiation on the part of malignant plasma cells that lose their normal "homing" patterns.

3. "Benign" or "Idiopathic" Monoclonal Gammopathies

Monoclonal gammopathies can be detected in the serum of clinically asymptomatic individuals or in the serum of patients with a variety of diseases (solid tumors, chronic hepatobiliary disease, different forms of non-B-cell leukemia, rheumatoid arthritis, etc.). Casual relationships between some of these diseases and the monoclonal proteins have been postulated, but this is still a controversial area, since the possibility of coincidence between an "idiopathic" B-cell dyscrasia and any other disease is difficult to rule out.

The designation of benign or idiopathic monoclonal gammopathy is only used when the monoclonal protein is found in an asymptomatic individual or in a patient with a disease totally unrelated to B-lymphocyte or plasma-cell proliferation. The frequency of detection of asymptomatic gammopathies is difficult to establish. Scandinavian authors conducting extensive population studies have given an average figure of about 1%, claiming that this is the most common form of B-cell dyscrasia. The incidence seems to increase in old age, up to about 19% in 90-year-old and older individuals.

The clinical significance of the finding of a "benign monoclonal gammopathy" lies in the need to make a differential diagnosis with malignant B-cell dyscrasia in its early stages. Common sense and careful consideration are essential in handling such cases. For example, in individuals of advanced age it seems preferable to ignore the problem and abstain from any aggressive therapy. In younger patients the problem cannot be so easily ignored, and for years several groups of hematologists have tried to establish criteria for differential diagnosis (Table. 29.2).

It must be stressed, however, that none of these criteria, nor even the association of several of them, is totally discriminatory. A good practical rule is to assume that any monoclonal gammopathy detected unexpectedly during the in-

TABLE 29.2 Laboratory Features That Have Been Proposed for the Differentiation Between Malignant and Idiopathic Monoclonal Gammopathies

Feature	Benign	Malignant
Paraprotein	Complete molecule; little or no Bence-Jones protein	Bence-Jones proteinuria >0.6 g/day
Normal immuno-globulins	Conserved	Depressed
Serum paraprotein	<1 g/100 ml	>1 g/100 ml
Serum albumin	>3 g/100 ml	<3 g/100 ml
Hemoglobin	>7.5 g/100 ml	<7.5 g/100 ml
Serum urea	<80 mg/10 ml	>80 mg/100 ml
Nonspecific proteinuria	Absent	Present
Numbers of B cells in peripheral blood	Normal	Decreased

vestigation of any condition not clearly related to a B-cell dyscrasia, or during screening of a normal population, should be considered as benign until proven otherwise. The best attitude in such cases is to withhold cytotoxic therapy and follow the patients closely, every three to six months, measuring the amount of paraprotein; malignant cases show a progressive increase, whereas in benign cases the levels remain stable. Patients with benign gammopathy have to be observed at least yearly after the first two years of follow-up, since there are documented cases of malignant evolution after benign behavior for five or more years.

4. Waldenström's Macroglobulinemia

Waldenström's macroglobulinemia was the second B-cell dyscrasia to be clinically individualized. First reported by a Swedish clinician, Dr. Jan Waldenström, as a malignancy of lymphoplasmacytoid cells associated with increased levels of serum macroglobulins, it later became better defined when IgM was structurally and antigenically characterized and the existence of a monoclonal IgM protein in the serum was established as the hallmark of this B-cell dyscrasia.

    a. Diagnosis. The two main diagnostic features of Waldenström's macroglobulinemia are (1) the presence of an IgM gammopathy (Fig. 29.8) and (2) the pleomorphic infiltration of the bone marrow with plasma cells, lymphocytes, and lymphoplasmacytic cells.

    b. Clinical Features. The principal clinical features of Waldenström's macroglobulinemia are (1) weakness and anemia, (2) hyperviscosity related symptoms, (3) hepatomegaly, splenomegaly, and lymphadenopathy, and (4) diffuse osteoporosis. Symptoms typical of multiple myeloma, such as bone pain or "spontaneous" fractures, are rare. The immunosuppression is also milder than in multiple myeloma. Hypercalcemia, leukopenia, thrombocytopenia, and azotemia are rarely seen. Renal insufficiency, when present, is usually a manifestation of serum hyperviscosity and can be reversed by plasmapheresis and/or peritoneal dialysis.

    c. Therapy. Waldenström's macroglobulinemia is a disease of old age and frequently follows a benign course. The most common life-threatening complications result from serum hyperviscosity. In such cases, repeated plasmapheresis is often sufficient to keep the patient asymptomatic, avoiding the use of cytotoxic drugs and their side effects. If cytotoxic therapy is thought necessary (due to the severity of the symptoms or the impossibility of keeping the patient on repeated plasmapheresis), chlorambucil (leukeran) is the drug of choice, usually given in a continuous low dosage.

5. The Heavy Chain Diseases

Some B-cell dyscrasias are associated to the exclusive production of heavy chains (or fragments thereof) or to the synthesis of abnormal heavy chains that are not

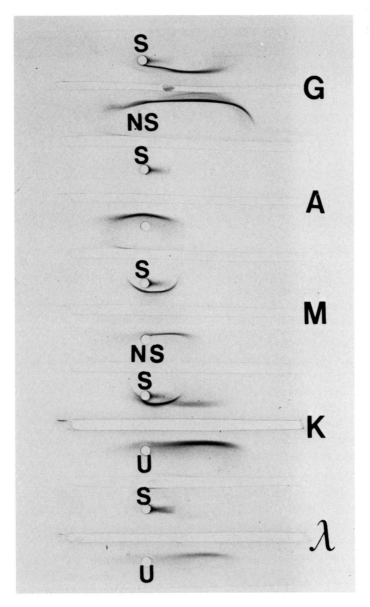

FIGURE 29.8 Immunoelectrophoretic study of the serum of a patient with Waldenström's macroglobulinemia. The patient's serum (S) and the serum of a normal control (NS) were studied with anit-IgG (G), anti-IgA (A), and anti-IgM (M), and the patient's serum (S) and urine (U) were studied with anti κ and anti λ light chain antisera. The paraprotein was typed as IgM-κ.

assembled as complete immunoglobulin molecules and are excreted as free heavy chains. Both types of abnormality can be on the basis of a heavy chain disease. The heavy chain diseases are classified, according to the isotype of the abnormal heavy chain, as γ, α, μ, and δ (one single case of δ chain disease has been reported, and ϵ chain disease has yet to be described).

    a. α Chain Disease. This is the most common and best defined heavy chain disease. It affects patients in all age groups, even children, and is more frequent

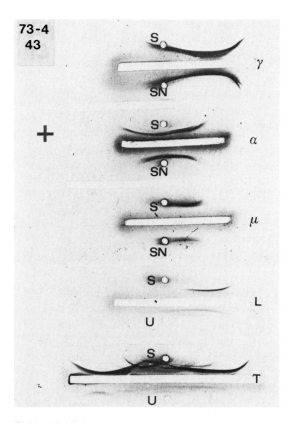

FIGURE 29.9 Immunoelectrophoretic study of a patient with alpha chain disease. The serum (S) and urine (U) from the patient, and a control normal serum (SN), were studied with antisera specific for gamma chains (γ), alpha chains (α), mu chains (μ), total light chains (L), and total serum proteins (T). Notice the anodal prolongation and bowing of the arc obtained with anti-alpha-chain serum, and the lack of correspondence to any abnormality in the precipitin arc obtained with anti-light chains.

in the Mediterranean countries, particularly affecting individuals of Jewish or Arab ancestry. Clinically it is indistinguishable from the so-called Mediterranean-type abdominal lymphoma, characterized by diarrhea and malabsorption unresponsive to gluten withdrawal, with progressive wasting and death. Intestinal x-ray changes suggestive of diffuse infiltration of the small intestine such as thickened mucosal folds, and intestinal biopsy, confirm the diffuse nature of infiltration of the submucosa by reticulolymphocytic cells.

Diagnosis relies on the demonstration of free alpha chains, usually in serum. Routine electrophoresis usually fails to show a monoclonal component, but immunoelectrophoresis shows an abnormal IgA arc with an anodal prolongation that does not react with antisera specific for light chains (Fig. 29.9).

b. γ Chain Disease. This was the first form of heavy chain disease discovered. Clinically it appears as a lymphoma with lymphadenopathy, splenomegaly, and hepatomegaly. Bone-marrow and lymph-node biopsies show lymphoplasmacytic proliferation. The diagnosis, again, is dependent on the immunochemical demonstration of free γ chains in the serum and/or urine.

c. μ Chain Disease. Few cases of μ chain disease have been reported, and clinically it is indistinguishable from chronic lymphocytic leukemia or lymphocytic lymphoma, with marked Bence-Jones proteinuria and small amounts of free μ chains detectable in the serum and sometimes also in the urine.

II. LEUKEMIAS AND LYMPHOMAS

The malignant proliferations of leukocytes can be classified by a variety of criteria. One first important distinction is made between leukemia and lymphoma. *Leukemia* refers to any malignant proliferation of leukocytes in which the abnormal cell population can be easily detected in the peripheral blood and in the bone marrow. In contrast, the term *lymphoma* is used to designate localized malignancies, often forming solid tumors, predominantly affecting the lymph nodes and other lymphoid organs. While lymphomas are always lymphocytic malignancies, leukemias may involve any type of hemopoietic cell, including granulocytes, red cells, and platelets. Finally, leukemias are often classified as acute or chronic based on their clinical evolution and morphologic characteristics, which are closely related. Acute leukemias follow a very rapid progression towards death if left untreated, while chronic leukemias have a more protracted evolution; also, many immature and atypical cells can be seen in the peripheral blood of patients with acute leukemias, while differentiated cells predominate in the peripheral blood of patients with chronic leukemia. However, a leukemic state may evolve from a chronic form to an acute disease, and the type of cell that is proliferating may also change during the course of the disease. For example, transition from a chronic granulocytic stage to an acute and very often fatal lymphoblastic leukemia is characteristic of chronic myelocytic leukemia (CML). Thus an initially relatively benign process can become highly malignant when the transformation strikes a different cell population in the same patient.

In principle, all malignant proliferations of cells identifiable as lymphocytes should be classified as either T- or B-cell malignancies. As discussed in earlier sections of this chapter, the identification of immunoglobulin-producing tumors as B-cell malignancies was relatively easy; currently, with methods allowing not only the sensitive detection of cell markers but also the application of molecular genetics procedures to the study of gene rearrangements, it is possible to classify most leukemias and lymphomas as T or B; and T-cell malignancies can even be subclassified according to the phenotypes of the proliferating cells.

A. Chronic Lymphocytic Leukemia

The first true leukemic process to be identified as a B-cell leukemia, chronic lymphocytic leukemia, has many features in common with Waldenström's macroglobulinemia; it is a disease of old age, often with a relatively benign course. The main difference lies in the rarity of serum monoclonal proteins; most patients are hypogammaglobulinemic, and when monoclonal proteins can be detected they tend to be of the IgM type. Bence-Jones proteins can be detected in the concentrated urine of approximately one-third of the patients. Studies of cell-surface immunoglobulins are positive in about 98% of the patients, most frequently demonstrating a monoclonal IgM. In some cases, cytoplasmic retention of immunoglobulins can also be demonstrated.

Clinical symptoms are often absent or very mild. Malaise, fatigue, or enlargement of the lymphoid tissues felt by the patient are the most frequent presenting complaints. Physical diagnosis shows enlargement of the lymph nodes, spleen, and liver. Viral infections, such as herpes and herpes zoster, and fungal infections are frequent in these patients, pointing to a T-cell deficiency confirmed by the finding of reduced numbers of T cells and reduced responses to T-cell mitogens. The prognosis is determined by the frequency of severe opportunistic infections.

B. Hairy Cell Leukemia

A disease predominantly affecting elderly males, hairy cell leukemia presents with a clinical picture of malaise, fatigue, and frequent infectious episodes. The physical examination usually shows splenomegaly and sometimes generalized lymphadenopathy.

The diagnosis is based on the finding of atypical lymphocytes with numerous finger-like (or hairy) projections from which the disease derives its name. The precise nature of the hairy cells has been extensively debated. These cells have B-cell characteristics (they have membrane immunoglobulins, often with several isotypes, and they synthesize monotypic heavy and light chains), but they also have monocyte/macrophage functions and markers (phagocytic properties, ability to produce and release lysozyme and peroxidase; they contain tartrate-resistant acid phosphatase) and even T-cell features (after mitogenic stimulation, the HCL lymphocytes may form E-rosettes and express the CD2 and CD25 markers).

These contradictory findings are difficult to interpret. It is possible that HCL represents (1) the proliferation of a B-cell precursor that shares monocytic and T-cell markers and functions; (2) a chimera of multiple lineages; (3) a malignant lymphocyte with aberrant gene expression. Without additional data it is impossible to decide which of these possibilities is more likely to reflect accurately the nature of the malignant proliferation in this type of leukemia.

It has been recently reported that α interferon is therapeutically useful (sometimes inducing permanent remissions) in hairy cell leukemia. Apparently this is a consequence of the ability of interferon to down-regulate the proliferating cells, stopping their uncontrolled multiplication.

C. The Acute Leukemias

The term acute lymphoblastic leukemia (ALL) is applied to those acute leukemias in which the malignant cells seen in the peripheral blood are proliferating, immature lymphocytes (lymphoblasts). These leukemias have usually a very poor prognosis. Death usually occurs as a consequence of the massive lymphocytic proliferation in the bone marrow, where the proliferating cells overwhelm and smother the normal hemopoietic cells.

A central idea on which most progress in the treatment of this disease has been based is that the leukemic process results from the proliferation of a single malignant clone. This led to the notion that the cure of the disease depends on the elimination of every single cell from the malignant clone. That goal has been relentlessly pursued with unquestionable success. Twenty years ago the survival of patients with acute lymphoblastic leukemia did not exceed a few weeks; nowadays more than 80% of the patients are cured.

Since ALL are caused by monoclonal proliferations of mutant lymphocytes, the proliferating clone could originate at any point in the differentiation of a hematopoietic stem cell into a mature lymphocyte. It should, therefore, be possible to classify any ALL as either T or B. Also, once "tumor-associated antigens" were defined in several malignancies, it was expected that leukemic cells would also express specific markers. Finally, it was realized that chromosomal abnormalities, initially found in CML, also existed in other types of leukemia; such chromosomal abnormalities are associated with abnormal expression of genes controlling cell growth, which leads to malignant transformation.

1. Classification of Acute Lymphoblastic Leukemias

Early studies of the lineage from which a leukemic cell was derived were based on the identification of B cells by membrane immunoglobulin and of T cells by E-rosetting. This allowed the initial definition of B-cell ALL and T-cell ALL, (Table 29.3), but in the majority of cases of ALL the cells showed neither marker (non-T, non-B ALL). These early observations provided the impetus to search for new ways to reclassify the cases of non-T, non-B ALL as either T-cell or B-cell ALL. With the introduction of monoclonal antibodies directed against T- and B-cell markers, it was determined that up to 95% of these non-T, non-B ALL were in fact B-cell-derived, because the proliferating cells expressed the CD19 and CD20 B-cell markers. The remaining 5% of ALL were of the T-cell type.

2. Prognosis of Different Types of ALL

The most important factor in ALL is the pretreatment blood lymphocyte count (patients with pretreatment lymphocyte counts below 10,000 mm^3 have a better prognosis), but the study of cell markers also has prognostic and thrapeutic implications. Patients with T-cell ALL have lesss than a 20% probability of remaining in remission for more than two years and must be treated as a high risk group; ALL in which the leukemic cells express membrane or cytoplasmic immunoglobulins have even a poorer prognosis and survive less than a year unless very aggressively treated. It thus seems likely that when the acute leukemic transformation occurs at a late stage of B-cell differentiation the resulting leukemic process is extremely difficult to control.

3. T-Cell ALL

Three distinct groups of leukemic processes can be included in the group of T-cell ALL.

   a. T-Cell ALL with Thymic Mass. This type of ALL affects males predominantly over females, and the patients are somewhat older than the children suffering from non-T, non-B ALL. A remarkable feature of this group is the fre-

TABLE 29.3 Classification of ALL According to Classical Membrane-Associated Markers

Patient group	T	B	Non-T, Non-B
Children	20%	1-2%	80%
Adults	10%	2-5%	90%

TABLE 29.4 Classification of T-Cell ALL According to Membrane-Associated Markers Recognized by Monoclonal Antibodies

Patient group	Marker					
	CD5 (Leu 1)	CD2 (T11)	CD3 (T3)	CD4 (T4)	CD8 (T8)	CD1 (T6)
1	+	+	−	−	−	−
2	+	+	−	+[a]	+[a]	+
3	+	+	+	+[b]	+[b]	−

[a]CD4 and CD8 are coexpressed by the malignant cells.
[b]The malignant cells express either CD4 or CD8, but not both.

quent finding of a thymic mass, suggesting that the malignant process arose from this organ. The introduction of monoclonal antibodies that individualize different T-cell subsets allowed a subclassification of T-cell ALL into three groups according to their surface markers (Table 29.4). Not unexpectedly, the membrane markers identified on malignant T cells are often associated in patterns not found among mature, normal T cells.

The first and largest group includes ALL in which the proliferating T cells express the CD5 and CD2 markers. The malignant cell is, therefore, an early T-cell precursor that mutated before the full rearrangement of the T-cell receptor genes, so that the CD3 molecule is not expressed. The second group is constituted by ALL cases in which the proliferating cells have reached a later stage of T-cell differentiation: they express CD3, coexpress both CD4 and CD8 markers, and are also positive for the CD1(T6) marker, indicating an aberrant reversal of a partially differentiated T lymphocyte to an earlier ontogenic stage. The third group is constituted by ALL with proliferating mature T cells, sharing markers (CD4 or CD8, in association with both CD2 and CD3) with the lymphocytes normally found in the peripheral blood and lymphoid organs. It has been suggested that CD8$^+$ T-cell leukemia has a worse prognosis associated to the expansion of suppressor T cells. Because of the relative rarity of T-cell ALL, it has not yet been possible to establish whether any of the subgroups of T-cell ALL has a worse prognosis than that of T-cell ALL in general.

b. T-Cell Leukemia Associated to HTLV-1. This type of T-cell leukemia has a unique goegraphic distribution, closely associated to the first identified human retrovirus (human T-cell lymphotropic virus I or HTLV-1), which is prevalent in Japan and in the Caribbean basin (where the rates of infection reach endemic proportions); the virus has also been reported, although with lower frequency, in the southern United States. The discovery of the link between

HTLV-I and this type of ALL was made possible by the fact that IL2 (TCGF) allows the growth of the leukemic T cells in long term culture. The continuously growing leukemic cells were observed to shed viral particles, which were then isolated and characterized. The proliferative effects of exogenous IL2 on this type of leukemic cell is due to the presence of a gene (*tax* gene) on HTLV-I that induces the permanent expression of IL2 receptors (CD25) in the infected cells. Therefore the overexpression of the CD25 marker separates this type of T-cell leukemia from all others.

The HTLV-I-associated T-cell leukemia develops 10 to 20 years after infection with the virus. This very long latency period and the fact that T-cell ALL is only seen in a fraction of the HTLV-I-infected individuals suggest that malignant transformation does not result exclusively from the viral infection; but the nature of the additional factors leading to leukemic transformation is unknown.

 c. Sézary Syndrome and Mycoses Fungoides. The Sézary syndrome and mycoses fungoides are cutaneous T-cell lymphomas that have also been related to HTLV-I infection. The skin is the original site of malignant cell proliferation in the Sézary syndrome, which is an exfoliative erythroderma with generalized lymphadenopathy and circulating atypical cells with a characteristic multilobulated nucleus (Sézary cells). The phase of cutaneous lymphoma can last many years with little evidence of extracutaneous dissemination. The leukemic evolution is associated with the invasion of the peripheral blood by malignant cells. The malignant cells infiltrating the skin or circulating in the blood are CD4$^+$ and behave functionally as helper T cells when mixed in vitro with T-cell-depleted lymphocytes from a normal donor and antigenically stimulated. This abnormal proliferation of helper/inducer cells may explain the association with autoimmune hemolytic anemia and autoantibody production seen in some patients with Sézary syndrome.

 Mycoses fungoides is clinically similar to the cutaneous phase of the Sézary syndrome, and the infiltrating cells in the skin are also CD4$^+$. No leukemic stage seems to develop in patients afflicted with the disease. However, instead of providing help for in vitro Ig production, the lymphocytes suppress the response of normal allogeneic T and B cells. It has been suggested that the malignant CD4$^+$ cells may in effect be suppressor/inducer T cells.

4. Other Markers of Leukemic Lymphocytes

 a. Enzymes. Since the expression of enzymes of the purine salvage pathway varies during lymphocyte ontogeny, their study in ALL appeared to have obvious interest. The first enzyme studied was adenosine deaminase (ADA). Studies of its expression are important because the enzyme can be used as a basis for specific therapy using 2-deoxycorfomycin, a drug that specifically inhibits ADA and has remarkable therapeutic effects in ADA$^+$ ALL. The second enzyme that attracted the attention of investigators was terminal deoxynucleotidyl transferase (Tdt), which is not expressed by adult lymphocytes but is reexpressed in about 80% of ALL cases; it constitutes a useful marker because its levels fall during remission and increase again before a clinically apparent relapse.

   b.   Common Acute Lymphoblastic Leukemia Antigen (CALLA).   The search for specific tumor markers in leukemia led to the identification of an antigen that was absent from normal peripheral blood lymphocytes but present in the majority of non-T, non-B ALL lymphocytes and was for this reason designated as common acute lymphoblastic leukemia antigen (CALLA). This antigen is almost always expressed in association with a B-cell marker such as the CD19 or CD20 antigens. CALLA positivity identifies patients with a more favorable prognosis. The therapeutic use of monoclonal anti-CALLA antibodies in ALL has been rather disappointing. A sharp decrease in leukemic cell counts is observed after administration of antibody, but this effect is usually of short duration since the CALLA$^+$ lymphocytic population is soon replaced by a CALLA$^-$ population (antigenic modulation) not affected by further administration of antibody. On the other hand, the prolonged administration of anti-CALLA leads to the development of antimouse immunoglobulin antibodies (the monoclonal antibody is of murine origin) that cause rapid elimination of anti-CALLA antibodies from the patient's circulation and may also cause anaphylactic reaction and serum sickness.

   CALLA is also expressed by the lymphoblasts seen during the blastic crisis of patients with CML; these lymphoblasts also express B-cell markers such as the CD20 antigen, establishing their identity as B-cell precursors. When the blast cells seen in the blastic crisis of a patient with CML are CALLA$^+$, TdT$^+$, and CD20$^+$, the crisis responds well to chemotherapy; when none of these markers is expressed survival is limited to a few days. Given the very poor prognosis of the cases with CALLA$^-$ blastic crisis, some groups tried what was initially considered a desperate therapeutic attempt to eradicate the leukemic cells; total body irradiation at sublethal doses followed by bone marrow transplantation. This is now a well accepted protocol for the treatment of forms of ALL associated with poor response to less aggressive therapy. Bone marrow transplantation is associated with a significant risk for developing graft-vs.-host disease; the risk is considerably reduced by (1) using normal bone marrow as closely HLA-matched as possible, (2) depleting T-cell precursors from the bone marrow graft with monoclonal antibodies, and (3) treating the patients with cyclosporin A (see Chapter 26).

5.   Gene Rearrangements in ALL

The treatment of ALL has become progressively more efficient, but it is associated to serious side-effects. Therefore it is necessary to establish beyond questtion the diagnosis of a malignant T- or B-cell proliferation before therapy is initiated. The monoclonal nature of the leukemic process may be difficult to ascertain when the malignant clone does not stand out from within a more polymorphic population of normal and reactive cells (this is particularly true in lymphomas). In these conditions the assessment of rearrangements of the antigen-specific receptor genes of T or B cells is invaluable. With adequate hybridization techniques it is possible to detect a malignant clone with rearranged genome that may constitute only 1-5% of the cell mass examined. The developmental hierarchy of immunoglobulin gene rearrangements during B-cell differentiation is well known. ALL of the B-cell lineage positive for cytoplasmic Ig show a rearranged Cμ gene, but the light chain genes and the T-cell-receptor genes remain in germ-line configuration. In contrast, the immunoglobulin genes remain in their germ-line configuration in leukemic T cells obtained from Sézary syndrome or adult T-cell leukemias. The T-cell receptor, as described in detail in Chapter 10, is constituted by an α/β heterodimer. Each chain is constituted by variable and constant domains under separate genetic control, and the Cβ gene is the first to rearrange as a T cel differentiates. Cells in which *only* the Cβ gene has rarranged do not express the TcR or the CD3 molecule.

6. Chromosomal Abnormalities in Leukemias

a. Chronic Myelogenous Leukemia (CML). This was the first leukemia in which a definite chromosomal abnormality was observed. An abnormal chromosome (Philadelpha or Ph^1 chromosome) is found in 90 to 95% of patients with CML. The presence of the Ph^1 chromosome has prognostic significance: 60% of the patients in whom it is found survive four years after diagnosis as opposed to only 10% of those who do not have this abnormality. The chromosomal abnormality consists of a translocation of the telomeric part of the long arm of chromosome 9 to the telomeric part of the long arm of chromosome 22. The part of chromosome 9 translocated to chromosome 22 contains a proto-oncogene (*c-abl*) that codes for a protein thought to play a very important physiologic role in cell growth and differentiation. During the translocation resulting in the formation of the Ph^1 chromosome, the *c-abl* gene loses its regulatory area; the uncontrolled expression of the gene results in malignant cell proliferation. The fact that the other chromosome involved in the translocation (chromosome 22) carries an actively expressed B-cell-specific gene may explain why the blast cells seen in the crisis are of the B-cell lineage.

b. Burkitt's Lymphoma (BL). Burkitt's lymphoma, endemic in certain areas of Africa and sporadic in the U.S., has been characterized as a B-cell lymphoma expressing monotypic surface IgM. BL cells are characterized by a translocation of the area of chromosome 8, which contains the proto-oncogene *c-myc*, to chromosomes 14, 2, or 22, at a position close to the immunoglobulin heavy or light chains loci. The *c-myc* proto-oncogene is under very tight control and is only transiently expressed during the activation of normal cells. As with the translocation of *c-abl*, the translocation of *c-myc* leaves behind in chromosome 8 areas essential for the control of its expression. Thus the translocated *c-myc* gene becomes constitutively expressed at high levels. BL is epidemiologically linked to infection of the B lymphocytes with the Epstein-Barr virus (EBV). This infection is known to induce a state of active B-cell proliferation that may favor the occurrence of the translocation.

   c.   *T-Cell Acute Lymphocytic Leukemia (T-Cell ALL).* Chromosomal abnormalities involving the T-cell-receptor genes have been observed in at least 40% of the T-cell leukemias. One of the most frequent is a translocation of the area of chromosome 14 which carries the α gene of the T-cell receptor, to the area of chromosome 8 which has the *c-myc* gene. Equally frequent is a translocation of the area of chromosome 7 which contains the β chain of the T-cell receptor, to chromosome 11.

SELF-EVALUATION

Questions

Choose the one best answer.

29.1   HTLV-I induces a T-cell leukemia in which the cells permanently express
   A. The *c-myc* oncogene.
   B. CALLA antigen.
   C. Tdt.
   D. CD5.
   E. CD25.

29.2   In a chronic lymphocytic leukemia,
   A. Most lymphocytes have IgM and/or IgD on their membranes.
   B. Bence-Jones proteinura is detected in less than 5% of patients.
   C. There is no significant compromise of cell-mediated immunity.
   D. Prognosis is worse when the surface immunoglobulin is IgM alone.
   E. The levels of serum immunoglobulins are usually normal.

29.3   All of the following are usually B-cell malignancies except
   A. Chronic lymphocytic leukemia.
   B. Burkitt's lymphoma.
   C. Waldenström's disease.
   D. α chain disease.
   E. Sézary syndrome.

29.4   The finding of Bence-Jones protein in the urine

A. Allows a diagnosis of multiple myeloma.

B. Is proof of the existence of a B-cell dyscrasia.

C. Allows ruling out a diagnosis of benign gammopathy.

D. Has no definite diagnostic implications.

29.5 The finding of a polyclonal increase of serum immunoglobulins

A. Rules out a diagnosis of multiple myeloma.

B. Is characteristic of all heavy chain diseases.

C. Is not compatible with a diagnosis of B-cell dyscrasia.

D. Has been reported in some cases of Waldenström's macroglobulinemia.

E. Is a good prognosis indicator in multiple myeloma.

29.6 The immune depression of B-cell dyscrasias is

A. Equally frequent and intense in all types of B-cell dyscrasia.

B. Believed to be the result of an abnormal helper/suppressor-T-cell ratio.

C. A result of an increased population of suppressor cells including monocytes/macrophages and T cells.

D. A reflection of the general metabolic disturbance that takes place in patients with B-cell malignancies.

E. Predominantly a depression of cell-mediated immunity.

29.7 The distinction between multiple myeloma and reactive plasmacytosis is best made by

A. Finding atypical, multinucleated plasma cells in the bone marrow.

B. Quantitation of serum immunoglobulins.

C. Characterization of the gammopathy as monoclonal or polyclonal by electrophoresis and immunoelectrophoresis.

D. Screening of light chains in the urine.

E. X-ray survey of the skeleton.

29.8 The most reliable criterion for differentiation between benign and malignant B-cell dyscrasias is

A. Age of the patient.

B. Progressive increase of paraprotein levels.

C. Levels of normal immunoglobulins.

D. Presence of Bence-Jones proteinura.

E. Number of B cells in peripheral blood.

29.9 Unexpected in Waldenström's macroglobulinemia would be

A. Increased serum viscosity.

B. Hypercalcemia.

C. Normal or near-normal levels of IgG.

D. Anemia.

E. Mixed cellularity in the bone marrow including plasma cells, lymphocytes, and mast cells.

29.10 A 59-year-old man has been complaining of weakness, repeated pulmonary infections, and "rheumatic" pains for two years. He has been hospitalized because he broke his right humerus falling from a chair. Serum immunoglobulins are

IgG: 600 mg/L   IgA: 450 mg/L   IgM: 200 mg/L

The patient eliminates 2 g of protein daily in the urine.
Most useful for diagnosis will be
A. The heat test for Bence-Jones proteins.
B. Serum electrophoresis and/or immunoelectrophoresis.
C. Urine electrophoresis and/or immunoelectrophoresis.
D. Determination of serum calcium levels.
E. Determination of serum viscosity.

Answers

29.1 (D) In individuals with HTLV-I the leukemic process induces the permanent expression of the IL2 receptor identified by the presence of the CD25 antigen; the cells are otherwise $CD4^+$ T cells for which retroviruses have a special affinity.

29.2 (A) Bence-Jones proteinuria is detected in about one-third of the patients.

29.3 (E) The Sézary syndrome is a malignancy of helper T cells.

29.4 (B) Bence-Jones proteinuria is most often associated with multiple myeloma but can also be seen in patients with other types of B-cell malignancies and even in patients without evidence of malignant B-cell proliferation.

29.5 (A) Although in some cases of lymphocytic lymphoma a malignant, monoclonal, B-cell proliferation may exist in association with a reactive plasmacytosis leading to the simultaneous presence of a monoclonal protein and polyclonal hypergammaglobulinemia, this is not seen in multiple myeloma, in which the immunoglobulins not produced by the proliferating clone are always normal or reduced in levels.

29.6 (C) Depending on the type of B-cell dyscrasia, the suppressor population may be lymphocytic or monocytic.

29.7 (C) Reactive plasmacytosis is associated with polyclonal gammopathy, while multiple myeloma is characterized by a monoclonal gammopathy.

29.8   (B) No other parameter is as reliable.

29.9   (E) Hypercalcemia is usually seen in multiple myeloma, as a conse-
             quence of disseminated osteolysis; in Waldenström's macroglobulin-
             emia there is no appreciable increase of serum calcium, as a rule.

29.10   (C) Since the serum appears not to contain a monoclonal protein (nor-
             mal to low normal levels of IgG, IgA and IgM were assayed), the best
             approach would be to characterize the urinary proteins (Bence-Jones
             protein may be present). The heat test is nonspecific and should not
             be used.

BIBLIOGRAPHY

Forbes, I. J. and Leong, A. S.-Y. *Essential Oncology of the Lymphocyte*
Springer-Verlag, Berlin, 1987.

Fudenberg, H. H. and Virella, G. Waldenström's macroglobulinemia: An inter-
pretive review. In *Cancer Chemotherapy III*, I. Brodsky, S. B. Kahn, and
J. F. Conroy (Eds.). Grune & Stratton, New York, 1978, p. 395.

Fudenberg, H. H. and Virella, G. Multiple myeloma and Waldenström's macroglobulinemia: Unusual presentations. *Sem. Hematol 17*:63, 1980.

Foon, K. A., Gale, R. P., and Todd, R. F. Recent advances in the immunological
classification of leukemia. *Sem. Hematol. 23*:257, 1986.

Gandara, D. R. and Mackenzie, M. R. Differential diagnosis of monoclonal
gammopathy. *Med. Clin. N. Amer. 72*:1155, 1987.

Gordon, J. Molecular aspects of immunoglobulin expression by human B cell
leukemias and lymphomas. *Adv. Cancer Res. 41*:72, 1984.

Kurzrock, R., Gutterman, J. U., and Talpaz, M. The molecular genetics of
Philadelphia chromosome positive leukemias. *New Engl. J. Med. 319*:990,
1988.

Kyle, R. A. and Greipp, P. A. Plasma cell dyscrasias: Current status. *C.R.C.
Crit. Revs. Oncol. Hematol. 8*:197, 1988.

Murphy, S. B. and Gilbert, J. R. (Eds.). *Leukemia Research: Advances in Cell
Biology and Treatment.* Elsevier, New York, 1983. (Includes several chapters on B- and T-cell leukemia.)

Nowell, P. C. and Croce, C. M. Chromosomal approaches to oncogenes and
oncogenesis. *FASEB J 2*:3054, 1988.

Sarin, P. S. and Galli, R. C. Human T-cell leukemia-lymphoma virus (HTLV).
Progr. Hematol. 13:149, 1983.

Toyonaga, B. and Mak, T. W. Genes of the T-cell receptor in normal and malignant cells. *Ann. Rev. Immunol. 5*:585, 1987.

30

Immunodeficiency Diseases

GABRIEL VIRELLA and H. HUGH FUDENBERG

As a rule, a defect in the immune system is suspected when a patient has (1) unusual frequency of infections with common microorganisms, (2) unusually severe infections, (3) infections with usually nonpathogenic organisms, or (4) failure to eradicate infections with antibiotics to which the microorganisms are sensitive.

Three main steps are involved in the investigation of a suspected immuno-deficiency disease:

1. Documentation and characterization of the immunodeficiency state.
2. Exclusion of causes of secondary immunodeficiency.
3. If a diagnosis of primary immunodeficiency disease is indeed made, evaluation of all clinical and laboratory features in order to classify the patient as to the type of immunodeficiency disorder, so as to determine what type of therapy is optimal.

I. CHARACTERIZATION OF AN IMMUNODEFICIENCY STATE

A good history, a careful work-up of the infectious episodes, and a thorough physical examination are of great help in narrowing down the possibilities when evaluating a suspected immunodeficiency. For example, a history of repeated pyogenic infections (tonsillitis, otitis, pneumonia, disseminated impetigo) is suggestive of a B-cell deficiency; a severe mycotic infection, or the development of active infection after administration of a live virus vaccine (Fig. 30.1) suggest a T-cell deficiency; a history of abscess-forming infection with low-grade pathogens (*Staphylococcus epidermidis, Serratia marcescens, Aspergillus* sp.) suggests chronic granulomatous disease. The age and mode of onset are also important to define. The onset of persistent infection of the lungs, diffuse mucosal moniliasis, and chronic diarrhea and wasting, when occurring early in life, are suggestive of severe combined immunodeficiency; the association of neonatal tetany with cardiac malformations, mongoloid facies, and immunodeficiency defines the DiGeorge syndrome, a congenital (but not hereditary) disorder due to the failure of development of the third and fourth pharyngeal clefts, resulting in thymic and parathyroid aplasia or hypoplasia.

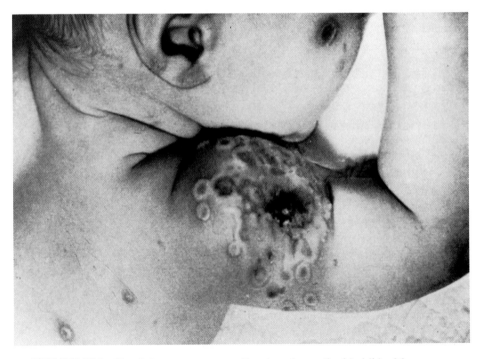

FIGURE 30.1 Vaccinia gangrenosa reaction in a 6-month-old child with combined immunodeficiency. Note the extensive gangrenous and necrotic lesion with satellite poxes around the gangrenous lesion, that eventually spread to the face and buttocks. (Reproduced with permission from Good, R. A. et al., *Progr. Allergy* 6:187, 1962.)

Identification of the etiologic agent(s) responsible for the infectious episode(s) is of great significance, for it not only provides some indication about which arm of the immune system is affected but also indicates whether one is dealing with a broad-spectrum immunodeficiency, in which different microorganisms will be involved in different infectious episodes, or with a selective immunodeficiency, in which all infections are caused by one microorganism or by a group of closely related agents.

Physical examination can also provide useful data. In patients with lack of development of the B-cell system, no peripheral lymph nodes can be felt and the tonsils are atrophic. A patient with chronic granulomatous disease often has scars from previous bone and/or liver abscesses, draining lymphadenitis, and hepatosplenomegaly. Patients with severe, congenital forms of immunodeficiency disease are likely to have growth retardation and, in some cases, other associated congenital abnormalities.

A good family history is very important. Early death of older siblings suffering from repeated infectious episodes is often the only way to document the hereditary character of a congenital immunodeficiency.

II. DIAGNOSTIC STUDIES

Once a patient with suspected immunodeficiency has been identified it is necessary to attempt to confirm the diagnosis. This can be done in many ways that may vary from patient to patient. The main approaches for the diagnosis of deficiencies of humoral and cellular immunity, phagocytic function, and complement have been discussed in earlier chapters. It is necessary to stress at this point that the investigation of an immunodeficiency is a step-by-step procedure in which tests are ordered to confirm clinical impressions or the results of previous tests.

An initial evaluation may involve simple assays such as a white blood cell count with leukocyte differential, immunoglobulin quantitation, isohemagglutinin titers, T- and B-cell counts, an NBT test for phagocytic function, and a CH50 for complement activity. Depending on the results of this initial evaluation and on the clinical impression as to the nature of the immunodeficiency, further tests should be ordered so as to obtain the best possible definition of the nature and degree of immunodeficiency, information essential for rational therapeutic choices.

III. CLASSIFICATION OF THE IMMUNODEFICIENT PATIENT

After completion of a clinical and laboratory study, it becomes important to attempt to classify an immunodeficiency disease by several criteria, because

TABLE 30.1 Criteria for Classification of Immunodeficiency States

By their range
  Broad spectrum
  Restricted (antigen-selective)
By their etiology
  Primary
  Secondary
By the limb of the immune system predominantly affected
  Humoral immune deficiencies
  Cellular immune deficiencies
  Combined immune deficiencies
  Phagocyte dysfunction syndromes
  Complement deficiencies
By the mechanism of transmission
  Genetically transmitted
    X-linked
    Autosomal recessive
    Autosomal dominant
  Sporadic

some important differences in therapeutic approaches depend on this classification (e.g., treatment of primary and secondary immune deficiencies have some common points, but also some important differences). The main criteria currently used to classify immunodeficient patients are shown in Table 30.1.

IV. PRIMARY IMMUNODEFICIENCY DISEASES

An imcomplete classification of the most important clinical forms of primary immunodeficiency diseases is given in Table 30.2. In the following pages, a brief outline of the main features of representative primary immunodeficiency diseases (with the exception of phagocytic deficiencies, which have been discussed in an earlier chapter) is presented.

A. Infantile Agammaglobulinemia (Bruton-Janeway Syndrome)

Infantile agammaglobulinemia is the prototype of "pure" B-cell deficiency. Infectious symptoms usually begin early in infancy (8 months to 3 years); most cases seem to be transmitted by an X-linked mechanism, but in some children the pattern of transmission appears to be autosomal-recessive. It follows that male infants are predominantly affected, but the disorder is also seen in females.

TABLE 30.2 Classification of Broad-Spectrum Immunodeficiency Disease

Humoral immunodeficiencies
    X-linked hypogammaglobulinemia
    Transient hypogammaglobulinemia of infancy
    Common variable unclassifiable immunodeficiency
    X-linked immunodeficiency with hyper-IgM
    Selective IgA deficiency

Cellular (T-cell) immunodeficiencies
    Congenital thymic aplasia (DiGeorge syndrome)

Combined immunodeficiencies
    Severe combined immunodeficiency
    Cellular immunodeficiency with abnormal immunoglobulin synthesis
        (Nezelof's syndrome)
    Immunodeficiency with ataxia-telangiectasia
    Immunodeficiency with eczema and thrombocytopenia (Wiskott-Aldrich
        syndrome)
    Immunodeficiency with thymoma
    Immunodeficiency with short-limbed dwarfism
    Immunodeficiency with lymphotoxins

Phagocytic deficiencies
    Chronic granulomatous disease
    Myeloperoxidase deficiency
    Chediak-Higashi syndrome
    Job's syndrome

Complement deficiencies

Clinically, the most important symptomatology is related to repeated infections caused by common pyogenic organisms (*S. pneumoniae, N. meningitidis, H. influenzae, S. aureus*); these cause pyoderma, purulent conjunctivitis, pharyngitis, otitis media, sinusitis, bronchitis, pneumonia, empyema, purulent arthritis, meningitis, and septicemia. In spite of the severe hypogammaglobulinemia affecting these children, seronegative rheumatoid arthritis develops in about 30-35% of the cases.

These patients have normal peripheral-blood-lymphocyte counts, normal T-cell counts, and normal T-cell function. B lymphocytes, on the contrary, are absent or greatly reduced in the peripheral blood.

Histological examination of a peripheral lymph node draining the site of an antigenic challenge (often difficult to localize) shows lack of germinal centers and secondary follicles. Plasma cells are absent both from peripheral lymphoid tissues and from bone marrow.

This condition is best treated by replacement therapy using gamma globulin (a plasma fraction containing predominantly IgG, obtained from normal healthy donors). The recently introduced intravenous preparations should be preferred, since their effectiveness is comparable to that of the classical intramuscular preparations, but their administration is considerably more comfortable for the patient.

B. Common Variable Unclassified Immunodeficiency ("Acquired" Hypogammaglobulinemia)

This designation includes a large number of cases of primary immunodeficiency, heterogeneous in presentation, with variable ages of onset and patterns of inheritance, whose clinical picture is similar to X-linked agammaglobulinemia but less severe. Sinusitis and bacterial pneumonia are the predominant infections. Intestinal giardiasis is common, and in some patients it can lead to malabsorption.

Lymph node biopsies show morphological changes including necrobiosis of the follicles (also seen in the spleen) and/or reticulum cell hyperplasia (which may lead to lymphadenopathy and splenomegaly).

In contrast to the patients with infantile agammaglobulinemia, those with "acquired hypogammaglobulinemia" have normal or increased numbers of B cells in peripheral blood, but these B cells have defective responses to B-cell mitogens, and no immunoglobulin secretion is seen after adequate stimulation in vitro. The lack of immunoglobulin production can be due to a primary synthetic block in the B cell, to the influence of suppressor factors that can be cellular (suppressor T cells or "suppressor" monocytes) or humoral (some patients' sera can suppress the function of B cells), or to a deficiency in number or function of helper T cells (in some cases caused by antihelper lymphocyte antibodies). In some cases intracellular immunoglobulins may be detected, but they apparently are not normally secreted. T-cell function is usually normal, but it can show a progressive deterioration, particularly in patients who have an associated thymoma.

C. Immunoglobulin A Deficiency

Immunoglobulin A deficiency is the most common immunodeficiency (detected in 1 out of 800 normal Caucasian individuals). In most cases it is asymptomatic, but when combined IgA and IgG2 deficiency exists, the patients have frequent infections with bacteria with polysacharidic capsules (the production of IgG2 antibodies appears to be stimulated predominantly by polysaccharides).

IgA deficiency can also be associated with "autoimmune" disorders (especially pernicious anemia) and with the complex syndrome of lymphoid hyperplasia of the intestine, diarrhea, and malabsorption (Crabbe's syndrome).

Many IgA deficient individuals have antibodies to food proteins, which in most cases appear to be of no consequence, and antibodies to isotypic or allotypic determinants of IgA, which can cause hypersensitivity reactions (which may be fatal) upon transfusion of whole blood and plasma, when these antibodies are present in high titers.

D. Transient Hypogammaglobulinemia of Infancy

As a consequence of a delay in the infant's B cell functional maturation, the hypogammaglobulinemia normally occurring during the second and third months of life, because of progressive catabolism of maternal IgG, may persist until two or three years of age and become more progressively more accentuated (relative to age-matched controls). Peripheral-blood B cells are usually normal in number; in most cases a deficiency of helper T cell function appears to be responsible for the delay in immunoglobulin synthesis.

Supportive therapy with intravenous gamma globulin is indicated; eventually the child will develop his own immunoglobulins and fully recover.

E. Congenital Thymic Aplasia (DiGeorge Syndrome)

The DiGeorge syndrome can be considered as a protoype for a pure T-cell deficiency; it results from defective embryogenesis of the third and fourth pharyngeal clefts at six to eight weeks of fetal life, leading to deficient development of the thymus and parathyroids. This syndrome is not genetically transmitted but probably results from intrauterine infection prior to the eighth week of fetal life.

The main clinical features include neonatal tetany, which results from hypocalcemia secondary to hypoparathyroidism; abnormalities of the heart and large vessels; mental subnormality; and frequent infectious episodes.

The degee of T-cell deficiency is variable; in some cases there are residual T cells and/or partial thymus function (partial DiGeorge syndrome). In these cases, if the patient can be kept alive for a number of years a slow development of immune functions may take place.

The best treatment for the immunodeficiency associated with a complete DiGeorge syndrome is the transplantation of a fetal thymus; if residual T cells can be detected, the administration of immunomodulating agents (e.g., thymosin or transfer factor) may be of benefit and may allow the patient to remain relatively infection-free.

F. Severe Combined Immunodeficiency (Swiss-Type Agammaglobulinemia)

Severe combined immunodeficiency is characterized clinically by persistent infections of the lungs and by mucocutaneous candidiasis, chronic diarrhea, wasting and runting, from the early months of life. Survival beyond the first year of

life is rare. Physical examination shows absence of tonsils, very small or undetectable lymph nodes, signs of pulmonary infection, evidence of poor development, and oral thrush. A thymic shadow is not seen on x-ray of the thorax.

Immunologically, these patients have markedly depressed lymphocyte counts,
in some cases associated with neutropenia. The deficiency in cell-mediated immunity is reflected by negative skin tests, lack of response of cultured lymphocytes to PHA and Con A, and delayed rejection of allogeneic skin allografts.
Immunoglobulins are usually low, but in some cases they can be normal or irregularly affected. B cells and plasma cells can be detected, but antibody responses
are very low to absent.

Therapy for this type of combined immunodeficiency usually involves bone
marrow grafts from HLA-DR matched siblings. The graft is usually successful,
but there is a great risk of the development of graft-vs.-host (GVH) disease. Current attempts at eliminating all cells except stem cells from the graft appear
promising, and the successful grafting of parental haploidentical bone marrow
has been reported.

Graft-vs.-host disease is always a major concern; it can develop not only after
bone marrow or thymic transplants but also after whole fresh blood transfusion
or after infusions of fresh plasma (both whole blood and plasma contain viable
lymphocytes). The reaction is characterized by fever, maculopapular rash involving the volar surfaces, diarrhea, and protein-losing entheropathy, Coombs'
positive hemolytic anemia, thrombocytopenia, and splenomegaly. In full-
blown cases the outcome is generally poor, and death occurs within 10 to 14
days from the onset of symptomatology. The reaction may be prevented in the
case of blood transfusion by using frozen or irradiated red cells.

Many of the children with the autosomal recessive variety of severe combined
immunodeficiency lack adenosine deaminase (ADA) in their lymphocytes, red
cells, and other tissues. The lymphocytes are predominantly affected; the enzyme deficiency causes intracellular accumulation of deoxyadenosine triphosphate, a substance extremely toxic for lymphocytes. Prenatal diagnosis of this
disease is often attempted by culturing amnion cells and determining ADA levels
in the cells. In this special type of combined immunodeficiency, frozen and
irradiated red cells can be administered as a source of ADA, as a palliative therapeutic measure. Gene therapy is also being actively investigated, since if the
normal gene for ADA synthesis could be introduced in T-cell precursors obtained from the patient's bone marrow, and those cells then reinjected, it should
be possible to replace the ADA-deficient lymphocyte population, at least partially, by lymphocytes carrying the ADA gene. The positive cells, by breaking
down deoxyadenosine triphosphate, would prevent their accumulation in cytotoxic levels even in ADA-deficient lymphocytes, and thus preserve the latter
from destruction.

Another group of children with combined immunodeficiency is characterized by profound lymphopenia with lack of expression of class I MHC and β_2 microglobulin on the residual lymphocytes (*bare lymphocyte syndrome*). These findings were considered as confirmatory of the importance of MHC expression for cell differentiation and activation. However, at least one adult asymptomatic patient has been reported who had normal lymphocyte counts associated with lack of expression of MHC I, and normal β_2 microglobulin. This patient complained of sinobronchial disease without any other clinical evidence of immunodeficiency.

G. Immunodeficiency with Ataxia-Telangiectasia

Ataxia-telangiectasia is genetically transmitted following an autosomal recessive pattern of inheritance. The initial symptoms are of progressive cerebellar *ataxia* beginning in early childhood, associated with insidiously developing *telangiectasia* (first appearing as a dilation of the conjunctival vessels). The capillary abnormalities are systemically distributed, and they involve the cerebellum, causing the motor difficulties characteristic of ataxia. In late childhood, recurrent sinobronchial infections begin and lead to bronchiectasia. The immunodeficiency is characterized by associations of thymic hypoplasia, T-cell deficiency, and low immunoglobulin levels, particular of IgA, which is low or absent in 80% of the patients. It is believed that ataxia-telangiectasia is basically a disease of aberrant gene control, in which DNA repair genes could be deficient. The existence of a generalized defect in tissue maturation is suggested by the persistently increased levels of serum alphafetoprotein and carcinoembryonic antigen in many patients with this disease. Defects in DNA repair mechanisms are supported by the high frequency of lymphoreticular malignancies; these, and the rupture of telangiectatic brain vessels, are the most common causes of death, which usually occurs before puberty.

H. Immunodeficiency with Thrombocytopenia and Eczema (Wiskott-Aldrich Syndrome)

The Wiskott-Aldrich syndrome is charactereized by eczema, thrombocytopenia, and frequent infections with onset late in the first year of life. It is a genetically transmitted disease, with an X-linked recessive pattern of inheritance. The immunological disturbances are believed to result from a defect in a subset of monocytes with antigen-presenting function; in its absence both cellular and humoral immune responses are compromised.

The infections that affect patients with the Wiskott-Aldrich syndrome can be caused by all types of microorganisms—viruses, bacteria, fungi, and parasites such as *Pneumocystis carinii*, which suggests the combined nature of the immunodeficiency. Very early in life the lymphoid system appears normal. As the infant grows, lymphopenia develops, evident in the peripheral blood, thymus, and all other lymphoid tissues. This is associated with a variable loss of CMI. Humoral immunity is also affected. IgM tends to be low, and natural antibodies (usually of the IgM class) are lacking. The response to bacterial polysaccharides is deficient. Infection is the most frequent cause of death, but some children develop lymphoreticular malignancies that can have a fatal evolution.

The immunological defects can be corrected by bone marrow transplantation, but given the potential risk of this type of therapy, attempts at immunostimulation with transfer factor have been made, with mixed success; this may reflect differences in the criteria used for the selection of lymphocyte donors for preparation of the dialyzable extracts (donors with high CMI reactions to common microbial antigens should be preferred). Thrombocytopenia usually responds to splenectomy.

I. Antigen-Selective Immune Deficiencies

Antigen-selective immune deficiencies are often undiagnosed, since most of the tests used for general evalution of the immune system are usually within normal limits. Accurate identification of the infective organisms, and investigation of the ability to generate specific immunity to the identified infectious agents, should be undertaken in every case in which a predisposition to infections is not associated with readily detectable immunodeficiency. Two major types of antigen-specific deficiencies have been identified.

1. IgG Subclass Deficiency

IgG subclass deficiency has been detected in patients with repeated infections often involving pneumococcus and meningococcus (bacteria with polysaccharide capsules), normal total immunoglobulin levels, and lack of IgG2 (associated or not to IgA deficiency). In other patients, other subclasses may be affected, and the pattern of infections is not clear. Thereapy with gamma globulin is usually associated with clinical improvement.

2. Chronic Mucocutaneous Candidiasis

Some patients with chronic infection of skin and mucosae with *Candida albicans* have been shown to have a selective CMI deficiency. The humoral response to *C. albicans* is normal, and CMI is also normal when tested with other antigens, but deficient results are obtained in in vivo and in vitro tests of CMI against *C. albicans*. Therapy with dialyzable leukocyte extracts (transfer factor), prepared from the lymphocytes of donors with strong CMI against *C. albicans*, is usually beneficial.

J. Complement Deficiencies

Cases of isolated deficiency of each complement component have been reported. Patients with C3 deficiency have an inability to opsonize antigens, and they suffer from recurrent pyogenic infections, as with agammaglobulinemia, in spite of normal B- and T-cell function.

Recurrent pyogenic infections can also be a problem in patients with C3b inactivator deficiency. One such patient was shown to have C3b and activated factor D in serum, but very little factor B and C3, C3 being catabolized at four times the normal rate. It appears that his alternative pathway was spontaneously activated at all times. By releasing C3a he also suffered from "anaphylactoid" features.

Deficiencies of C4, C6, C7, C8, and C9 have been reported to be associated with increased frequency of infections. Bacteria with polysaccharide-rich capsules (Neisseria meningitis, Streptococcus pneumoniae) are usually involved as pathogens. The infections are far more severe than usually observed in non-complement-deficient individuals.

V. SECONDARY IMMUNODEFICIENCY DISEASES

Many factors influencing the function of the immune system can lead to variable degrees of immunoincompetence. Some of the factors are environmental, others are poorly understood responses to trauma, and still others are side effects of therapeutic intervention. In some cases the primary disease that causes the immunodeficiency is very obvious, while in others a high degree of suspicion is necessary for its detection. As a rule, secondary immune deficiencies occur late in life, but some causes of secondary immunodeficiency may have greater clinical consequences in infancy, so that the distinction cannot be based on age alone.

A. Immunodeficiency Associated with Malnutrition

Severe protein-calorie malnutrition in man causes a depression of cell-mediated immunity of variable expression. Anergy (lack of reactivity in skin tests for cell-mediated immunity), low T-cell counts, depressed lymphocyte reactivity to PHA, and depressed release of MIF have been reported by different groups. Some humoral immune responses may also be affected. Several causes for this deficiency have been suggested, including general metabolic depression, thymic atrophy with low levels of thymic factors, or increase in mononuclear suppressor cells. An important practical point is that children with malnutrition should not be vaccinated with live attenuated vaccines, which are generally contraindicated in immunodeficient patients.

B. Immunodeficiency Associated with Zinc Deficiency

The discovery that cattle with zinc deficiency secondary to genetically determined malabsorption develop lymphoid hypoplasia identical to a rare disease in
man named *acrodermatitis enteropathica*, which is a congenital disease characterized by diarrhea and malabsorption (affecting zinc, among other nutrients),
aroused considerable interest in a possible association between zinc deficiency
and immunodeficiency. Patients with acrodermatitis enteropathica often present with epidermolysis bullosa and generalized candidiasis, associated with combined immunodeficiency that can be corrected with zinc supplementation. Evidence of thymic function impairment in patients with zinc deficiency has been
published, reinforcing the case for such association. However, most causes of
zinc deficiency (low meat consumption, high fiber diet, chronic diarrhea, chronic
kidney insufficiency, etc.) do not appear to lead to a depletion severe enough to
result in immunodeficiency. On the other hand, parenteral alimentation without
zinc could be a significant cause of zinc deficiency that could lead (by itself or
in association to other factors) to secondary immunodeficiency.

C. Immunodeficiency Associated with Vitamin Deficiencies

Several vitamin deficiencies, including deficiencies of pyridoxine, folic acid, vitamin A, pantothenic acid, and vitamin E, are associated with and presumably the
cause of abnormalities of the immune response. Deficiencies of the first three
vitamins are usually associated with cellular immunodeficiency; pantothenic
acid deficiency is usually associated with a depression of the primary and secondary humoral immune responses; vitamin E deficiency is associated with a
combined immunodeficiency. It appears likely that vitamin deficiencies play
also some role in the pathogenesis of protein-calorie malnutrition, to which
they are inevitably associated.

D. Immunodepression Secondary to Protein Loss

1. Protein-Losing Enteropathy

The association between protein-losing enteropathy and immunodeficiency has
been cited as a classic example of secondary immunodeficiency for many years.
Intestinal lymphangiectasia is perhaps the best known cause of protein-losing
enteropathy. In this disorder a combined immunodeficiency state develops,
with general depression of immunoglobulin levels, lymphocytopenia, and depressed cell-mediated immunity, as reflected by cutaneous anergy, prolonged
graft survival, and depressed mitogenic responses to several stimuli. Both immunoglobulins and lymphocytes are lost into the gastrointestinal tract. Intestinal lymphangiectasia can be either a primary or a secondary disorder, e.g.,
secondary to constrictive pericarditis. In cases of intestinal lymphangiectasia

developing as a complication of constrictive pericarditis, pericardectomy can result in progressive recovery with normalization not only of the severe protein imbalance but also of immune functions.

2. Nephrotic Syndrome

The nephrotic syndrome is one of the most frequent causes of secondary hypogammaglobulinemia. It affects primarily IgG since this immunoglobulin is of smaller molecular size than IgM and IgA and therefore can pass more readily through a damaged glomerular filter. However, several authors have pointed out that the magnitude of the urinary loss of IgG is not sufficient to explain the reduction in its serum levels. A loss of the feedback mechanism that usually leads to a compensatory increase of IgG synthesis has been postulated; another possibility is the triggering of suppressor cells or the depression of helper-T-cell function by unknown mechanisms.

E. Immunodeficiency Associated with Uremia

Patients with renal failure and uremia are predisposed to infection. That cell-mediated immunity is affected in uremia was suggested early in the transplantation era, since uremic patients had depressed delayed hypersensitivity and delayed graft rejection. Systematic studies of immune function in uremia have provided evidence for a combined defect of cellular and humoral immunity. Uremic patients have lymphopenia, a low incidence of positive skin test reactions to a battery of common antigens, and low antibody response to the flagellar and somatic antigens of *Salmonella typhi*.

The depression of humoral immunity in uremia is incomplete. Severe depression of all immunoglobulins can be observed in patients treated with hemodialysis and immunosuppressants, but it is impossible to ascribe this effect in uremia per se. In patients with uremic renal failure not receiving immunosuppressive therapy, humoral immune responses appear to be at least partially conserved.

In contrast, the depression of cellular immunity appears more consistent and has been more thoroughly studied. Patients with chronic renal failure have reduced lymphocyte responses to mitogens such as PHA and PPD. Interestingly, the depression is usually more pronounced in patients with urea levels below 200 mg/dl than in those with levels exceeding this value; thus urea alone cannot be responsible for this CMI deficiency.

Plasma or serum from uremic patients has a suppressive effect on the mitogenic responses of normal lymphocytes in vitro. The suppressive activity is present in dialysates of uremic serum containing substances of molecular weight less than 20,000. Methylguanidine and "middle molecules" (molecular weight approximately 1,200) isolated from uremic sera have been shown to suppress the in vitro mitogenesis of normal lymphocytes.

F. Burn-Associated Immunodeficiency

Bacterial infections are a frequent and severe complication in burn patients; they often lead to death. There are several factors that may contribute to the incidence of infections in burn patients, ranging from the presence of open and infected wounds to a general metabolic disequilibrium.

Burn patients have a wide spectrum of immunological abnormalities. Abnormal neutrophil function has been reported, with defective chemotaxis and depressed oxidative metabolism. In great part the neutrophil dysfunction seems to result from exaggerated complement activation (mostly by proteases released in injured tissues). C3b, for example, when present in circulation, is opsonically inactive and inhibits the bactericidal function of neutrophils. A circulating factor that inhibits C3 conversion (therefore preventing proper bacterial opsonization) has also been detected in burn patients.

Other reported abnormalities include (1) an inability to produce a primary humoral response to heterologous erythrocytes (very likely a T-dependent antigen in humans); (2) normal to enhanced secondary immune responses to tetanus toxoid; (3) an impairment of cell-mediated immunity, suggested by a prolongation of skin homograft survival. Confirmatory evidence of a depression of cell-mediated immunity was obtained by in vitro studies showing depressed responses to mitogenic stimuli and depressed mixed lymphocyte culture reactions in patients with burns (Fig. 30.2). This lack of reactivity was associated with severe lymphopenia.

A controversy exists as to the nature of the putative T-cell defect in burn patients. Some authors have reported a circulating immunosuppressive factor in the serum of burn patients and suggested that this activity resides within a lipid-protein complex released by damaged epithelial cells, of molecular weight 10^6 daltons. This factor appears to be relevant to the clinical course of the patient, since its levels are greater in patients with more severe, more extensive, or more complicated burns; its levels show spikes immediately preceding or concomitant with septic episodes. However, it is not quite clear whether infections are the consequence of immunosuppression or vice versa. On the other hand, patients with higher levels of suppressive factor seem to retain skin homografts for longer periods of time.

An alternative explanation for the depression of cell-mediated immune response in burn patients is an increase in suppressor-cell activity. Suppressor T cells are increased in burn patients and thermally injured experimental animals. Both in humans and in animals, increased suppressor T cells are demonstrable 4 to 8 days after thermal injury, preceding severe sepsis by 4 to 5 days. The increased suppressor-cell activity, like the serum suppressive reactivity, is associated with very poor prognosis (66% mortality vs. 0% mortality in those patients with no evidence of suppressor activity). In humans, suppressor activity is re-

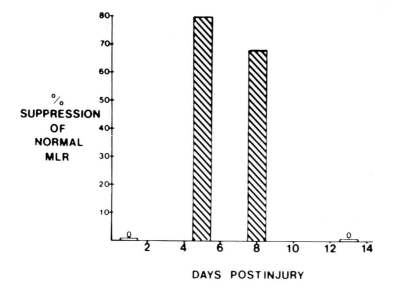

FIGURE 30.2 Development of suppressive activity in the mononuclear cells of burn patients. The effect of adding 1×10^5 mononuclear cells from severely burned patients to triplicate cultures containing 2×10^5 cells from a highly responsive normal individual and 1×10^5 mitomycin-treated normal stimulator cells was assessed. The bars represent the percentage suppression of the normal mixed leukocyte reaction (MLR) when cells from burn patients were studied at various times after injury. (Reproduced with permission from Miller, C. L. and Baker, C. C. *J. Clin. Invest. 66*:202, 1979.)

flected by depressed mitogenic responses to PHA of unfractionated leukocytes, and when lymphocytes from patients showing depressed mitogenic responses were added to mixutres of lymphocytes showing strong mixed lymphocyte reaction, a depression of the MLC was observed. According to other authors, burn patients have activated monocyte/macrophages releasing large amounts of PGE_2, which is known to inhibit T-lymphocyte function.

In conclusion, the immune system is profoundly altered in burn patients, probably as a consequence of multiple factors. All arms of the immune system are affected and although the depression is reversible it unfortunately affects the patient at a time when he most needs the integrity of his antimicrobial defenses. To date, efforts to up-regulate immune functions in burn patients have been inconclusive.

G. X-Ray and Drug-Induced Immune Deficiencies

The use of potentially immunosuppressive drugs in several types of clinical situa-
tins, mainly in patients with homografts and patients with malignancies, autoimmune diseases, or hypersensitivity diseases, has been associated with a progressive increase of infectious complications presumably related to excessive suppression of the normal immune response.

Two main features characterize the infections that appear in immunosuppressed patients: first, they usually involve low-grade pathogens, bacteria, or other
microorganisms not usually associated with clinical disease; second, the extent
and distribution of the infection are unusual, differing from those commonly observed in noncompromised hosts.

The mechanisms of action of most immunosuppressive agents have been characterized in clinical and experimental studies. The main effects of corticosteroids in humans seem to be related to depressed function of neutrophils and
monocytes, as well as depressed effector functions of lymphocytes, such as release of lymphokines and cytotoxicity. It seems likely that this inability of
lymphocytes and monocytes to participate in an adequate immune response
may be the best explanation for the development of cutaneous anergy in cor-
ticosteroid-treated patients.

Most cytotoxic drugs destroy cells more or less nonspecifically, and their
effects on immunocompetent cells depend both on the proliferative state of the
cell and the cell-cycle specificity of the drug. In general, such drugs are effective in suppressing primary immune responses and ineffective in suppressing immunological memory. The same difference in sensitivity between primary and
secondary responses can be observed with irradiation.

H. Surgically Induced Immunodeficiencies

In general, surgical intervention and general anesthesia are associated with transient depression of immune functions, affecting the mitogenic responses of PBL,
cutaneous hypersensitivity, and humoral immune responses. A transient severe
lymphopenia can occur in the immediate postoperative period, and complete
normalization of immune function may take ten days (for mitogenic responses)
to a month (for delayed hypersensitivity reactions and the humoral immune
response). In conventional surgery it is likely that immunosuppression results
predominantly from general anesthesia.

Some surgical interventions have a more direct and long-lasting effect on the
immune respone. Splenectomy is a particularly important cause of immune depression. Splenectomized patients have normal humoral immune responses following injection of soluble antigen, but they are weakly responsive to particulate
antigens. As such, these patients are prone to severe septicemia; the offending

organisms are common pyogenic bacteria such as *Streptococcus pneumoniae* (50% of the cases), *Haemophilus influenzae, Staphylococcus aureus*, group A *Streptococcus*, and *Neisseria meningitidis*. The rate of mortality is high.

These findings can be correlated with the role of the spleen in trapping and clearing cellular antigens and in recruiting immunocytes in the initial phases of the immune responses. Splenectomized patients, especially children, as well as patients with sickle cell anemia who develop splenic atrophy, have depressed serum IgM levels, depressed primary immune responses, delayed macrophage mobilization, and suboptimal levels of opsonins and cytophilic antibodies.

The patients with sickle cell anemia who undergo autosplenectomy usually die of infection (usually involving *S. pneumoniae*) before puberty. The peripheral blood smear in these patients may give indications, through the presence of morphological abnormalities (i.e., inclusion bodies in red cells) suggestive of splenic atrophy. Clinical trials with agents that may prolong normal splenic function are currently underway in several African countries where the disease is prevalent.

I. Immunosuppression Associated with Bacterial Infections

The best characterized example of immunodeficiency associated with bacterial infection is in patients with lepromatous leprosy, whose previously positive skin tests become negative in what is usually described as a state of anergy. These patients also have delayed rejection of skin grafts. In vitro, lymphocyte responses to PHA and to *Mycobacterium leprae* are depressed. In experimental animals, mycobacterial infections can lead to excessive suppressive activity by both lymphocytes and monocytes, but there is no data to suggest that this is also the case in man.

J. Immunosuppression Associated with Parasitic Infections

There is ample evidence obtained in in vitro studies suggesting that patients with schistosomiasis and malaria have depressed lymphocyte reactivity to schistosomal antigens, and in the case of malaria, to many antigens unrelated to the infecting hemoflagellate. In schistosomiasis the defect appears to be explained by an increased population of monocytes able to suppress specifically the antiparasitic response, which may be related to the presence of soluble immune complexes (blocking factors) in the patient's sera. In animal models of malaria there is an activation of suppressor monocytes leading to generalized immunosuppression whose degree is directly correlated to the extent of infection.

In humans, parasitic-associated immunodeficiency appears to be more significant as a parasitic protection mechanism than as a cause of secondary infections.

K. Immunodeficiency Secondary to Viral Infections

The first observation of infection-associated immunodeficiency was published by Von Priquet in 1908 when he described a transitory state of anergy during the acute stage of measles. The application of modern immunological techniques to the study of this immunodeficiency has demonstrated both lymphopenia and a depression of the response of peripheral blood lymphocytes to mitogens and antigens such as PHA and *Candida albicans*. This state of immunosuppression usually lasts no longer than 3-4 weeks and is apparently caused by an increased population of suppressor T cells. The induction of suppressor cells has been demonstrated in vitro in humans and in vivo in experimental animals infected with reovirus type 2 and influenza A2 virus, among others. In humans, rubella vaccination is associated with a depression of T-cell responses to PHA; this appears secondary to an increase in suppressor T cells. Alternative possibilities to explain the immunodeficiency associated to viral infections include direct lymphocytotoxicity of the virus causing lymphopenia, the effects of PGE_2 released from activated monocytes/macrophages, and the production of lymphocytotoxic antibodies. The profound effect of viral infections on the immune response is best exemplified by the acquired immunodeficiency syndrome, as discussed in the next section.

VI. ACQUIRED IMMUNODEFICIENCY SYNDROME (AIDS)

A. Etiology and Definitions

The etiologic agent of AIDS is the human retrovirus HIV, which belongs to the *Lentiviridae* family. This virus is constituted by two identical strands of (+) RNA, a nucleocapside whose major component is protein p24; a second protein coat lies between the nucleocapside and the envelope (p18 is its major constituent); and there is a viral envelope, in which glycoprotein spikes are inserted (gp160). There are two major envelope glycoproteins derived from a common precursor (gp160); the smallest (gp41) is inserted in the cell membrane, and the largest is extracellular (gp120). The numbers (18,24,41,120,160) refer to the molecular weight in kilodaltons of each protein and glycoprotein. The HIV genome includes the usual retroviral genes—*gag* (structural proteins), *pol* (polymerase, in this virus being a reverse transcriptase), and *env* (envelope glycoproteins), plus four regulatory genes of which the *tat* (transactivatory of transcription) gene, which promotes the transcription of viral genomes as well as posttranscriptional events, is the most important.

The designation *acquired immunodeficiency syndrome* (AIDS) is a clinical definition of the full-blown phase of HIV disease and is reserved for patients with specific conditions defined by the Centers for Disease Control. A majority

TABLE 30.3 Infections Most Commonly Diagnosed in Patients with AIDS

Pneumocystis carinii pneumonia

Chronic cryptosporidiosis

Toxoplasmosis

Extraintestinal strongyloidosis

Isosporiasis

Candidiasis (oral is common as a prodromal manifestiona; esophageal, bronchial, and pulmonary are pathognomonic)

Cryptococcosis

Histoplasmosis

Mycobacterial infections (particularly extrapulmonary tuberculosis or infections caused by atypical mycobacteria, such as *M. avium intracellulare*)

Disseminated cytomegalovirus infection

Disseminated herpes simplex infection

Progressive multifocal leukoencephalopathy

Multidermatomal herpes zoster

Recurrent salmonella bacteremia

Invasive nocardiosis

of these patients present with opportunistic infections, caused by a variety of common and uncommon agents, listed in Table 30.3.

In addition, patients with HIV infection and some secondary cancers (Kaposi's sarcoma, non-Hodgkin's lymphoma, or lymphoma of the brain) may also be diagnosed as having AIDS if other criteria are simultaneously fulfilled. Finally, AIDS patients may also present with progressive wasting syndrome and serious dementia. In all cases, the diagnosis of AIDS is possible only in patients in which HIV infections can be documented. This documentation may be serological, when confirmatory tests for anti-HIV antibodies are positive at the time of diagnosis or have been documented to be positive in the past for HIV, or it may involve isolation of viral particles from infected cells, detection of circulating viral antigens, or identification of integrated viral genomic components.

Not all patients with HIV infection have or will develop AIDS, although at present it is believed that the large majority do so. The precise percentage of those that may remain asymptomatic cannot be calculated, since the follow-up of infected people has not been long enough to establish after how long a time an infected patient can be declared free of the risk of developing AIDS. HIV infection can present itself in a variety of ways.

1. Acute Illness Associated with Seroconversion

The clinical picture is similar to infectious mononucleosis or influenza. A maculopapular rash may be present. Seroconversion can also take place in individuals who remain asymptomatic. The average incubation between exposure and onset of symptoms is estimated to be 3 to 6 weeks; seroconversion usually takes place 8 to 12 weeks after exposure. The first antibodies detected at the time of seroconversion react with gp160 followed by antibodies to p24. As a consequence of this delay in seroconversion, there is a "window" period in which the patient is infected, viremic, and probably contagious, but all serological tests for antibody are negative. This problem is likely to be solved when adequate tests for the detection of circulating viral antigens are developed. Early studies have demonstrated antigenemia preceding seroconversion in some patients.

2. Asymptomatic Infection

The patient remains seropositive without symptoms for variable periods of time (up to at least 8 years at this time).

3. Persistent Generalized Lymphadenopathy

There is no other known cause of lymphadenopathy and the patient does not have constitutional symptoms.

4. Persistent Disseminated Lymphadenopathy with Constitutional Symptoms (AIDS-Related Complex, ARC)

The constitutional symptoms include fever, weight loss, chronic diarrhea, oral candidiasis, and chronic mucocutaneous herpes simplex infection.

5. Full-Blown AIDS

B. Epidemiology and Natural History

HIV is transmitted primarily through sexual contact, particularly among homosexual and bisexual males and female partners of infected males, and through contaminated syringes among intravenous drug users. Less frequent modes of transmission include transfusion and related therapies (e.g., plasma fractions used in the treatment of hemophilia) and transplacental infection. Endemic foci for the disease exist in Africa and Haiti, where heterosexual venereal transmission seems to be the predominant mode of transmission.

Once the HIV virus enters the bloodstream, it tends to infect CD4$^+$ (helper) T cells, using the CD4 molecule as receptor. It also infects monocytes, macrophages, and related cells, which also express CD4 on the membrane (at much lower levels than helper T lymphocytes). Phagocytic monocytes may also be infected by ingesting viral-Ab complexes that bind to these cells through their Fc receptors. It is believed that monocytes and macrophages are sources of persistent viral infection. Also, the microglial cells of the CNS (which are of the monocyte/macrophage lineage) seem to be infected in almost every patient.

HIV replication involves *reverse transcription* of the (+)RNA genome into DNA and integration into the host cell genome. In the early stages of the infection, the virus does not seem to cause widespread T-cell depletion, and it appears to replicate at a very low level. Antigenemia is detectable for variable periods of time (most usually 8-12 months) after seroconversion, progressively declining. A second wave of antigen is detected preceding evolution to AIDS (by as many as 14 months). Coinciding with the second wave of antigenemia, there is a decline in antibody levels, particularly to p24. In terminal stages, antigenemia may decline again, perhaps reflecting the total exhaustion of the $CD4^+$ cell population.

It is not clear what determines the evolution towards AIDS, which is associated with progressive $CD4^+$ depletion causing eventual reversion of the normal CD4:CD8 ratio (not specific for AIDS). Viral replication seems to depend on T-cell activation, perhaps by some other infection. It could be that other infections (venereal or not), by activating infected T cells, would trigger HIV replication and cause the progressive depletion of $CD4^+$ cells. When the total number of $CD4^+$ cells falls below $300/mm^3$ the risk for development of clinical AIDS is significantly increased. The causes of T-cell depletion are not well defined; one possible factor is the formation of syntitia of infected T cells; another is the accumulation of unintegrated DNA in the cytoplasm of infected lymphocytes; according to some authors this DNA is actually expressed, accounting for marked viral proliferation and eventual cell death. The immune response against HIV-infected T cells (mediated both by cytotoxic T cells and by ADCC mechanisms) may also contribute to the depletion. However, the state of marked immunodepression associated with full blown AIDS does not appear to be a result of simple T-cell depletion. Most patients have uninfected $CD4^+$ cells in circulation (until the very late stages) even when there is pronounced immunodepression. It is possible that the virus may block the immune response by a variety of means, including the release of gp120, which binds to CD4 and may block the interaction of this molecule with MHC II antigens, therefore preventing the proper stimulation of helper T cells by antigen-presenting cells. Immune complexes involving viral antigens and the corresponding antibodies may also play a role in depressing immune responses. Furthermore, cytotoxic T-cell responses, NK-cell acitivty, and B-cell responses are depressed. Humoral responses to toxoids, for example, are impaired; this may be in part the result of lack of efficient help, but the B-cell system in HIV infection seems to be in a state of permanent polyclonal activation. Serum immunoglobulin levels are often elevated while the activation of B cells in vitro and the response to active immunization are depressed. The lack of active response can be explained on the basis of the deficiency in helper/inducer T cells, while the increased state of B-cell polyclonal activation may be due to a direct mitogenic effect of the virus on the B-cell population. The depression of cytotoxic T-cell activity is not a consequence of infection ($CD8^+$ cells are not infected) but rather a consequence of lack of help.

Most AIDS patients produce antibodies against HIV, at least in the early stages of infection. However, these antibodies may not deter the progress of the virus, for three reasons.

1. The AIDS virus is a very difficult target for the humoral immune response, because it can integrate in the host cell's DNA and remain silent, without transcription or translation, for long periods of time.
2. There are several HIV serotypes, and HIV mutates at a much faster rate than most other viruses. This is because the reverse transcriptase is error-prone (as are all reverse transcriptases, but the one from HIV is more so than any other). For unknown reasons, the mutations affect predominantly the epitopes of gp120 against which neutralizing antibodies are directed. Thus by the time the immune system has produced an antibody that neutralizes HIV with a particular gp120, the virus may mutate to a new structure that evades the immune response.
3. Finally, the virus survives and multiplies in key cell populations of the immune system that normally should be involved in its destruction (T cells and macrophages), presumably depressing their functions.

C. Serological Diagnosis

The initial screening of anti-HIV antibodies is done by an enzyme-linked im-munoassay test (ELISA) using HIV antigens, obtained from infected H-9 cells, adsorbed to a solid phase. Since this is a screening test, its positivity cutoff is set for maximal sensitivity. This is important, for example, when blood is screened in blood banks. The test is still very specific although rarely it may yield false positive results (multiparous females and patients with autoimmune diseases are more likely to have false positive results; this often involves anti-bodies reacting with cellular antigens from the tissue culture where the HIV virus was grown).

If a given individual is positive in an ELISA test, the test should be repeated to rule out a technical problem. If it remains positive it should be confirmed by either the Western blot (immunoblot) test or by indirect immunofluorescence. the Western blot, which is approved by th F.D.A. as the confirmatory test, in-volves separation of viral antigens in an SDS-polyacrylamide gel electrophoresis (which separates them by size), transfer of the separated antigens into a nitro-cellulose membrane, incubation of the "blotted" membrane with the patient's serum, and detection of antigen-antibody complexes with a peroxidase-labeled antihuman immunoglobulin reagent. A Western blot is considered positive if antibodies to p24, p31, and either gp41 or gp160 are simultaneously detected.

D. Therapy and Immunoprophylaxis

The mainstay of therapy at this time is Azidodideoxythymidine (AZT), which is phosphorylated by cellular thymidine kinases and is taken up preferentially by HIV polymerases (while cellular DNA polymerases continue to take up thymidine triphosphate). Upon incorporation of AZT triphosphate into the viral DNA chain, DNA transcription terminates and viral replication is prevented. The drug has serious side effects, but it appears to be beneficial in the patients that tolerate it. Other chain terminators such as $2',3'$-dideoxycytidine (ddC) are being tried and may prove advantageous.

Peptide T, a synthetic peptide analogous to the CD4-binding epitope of gp120, is under investigation. By binding to CD4 it would block viral adsorption. Its efficacy has not been confirmed, and there is concern that it may cause severe immunosuppression by preventing the interaction between MHC II antigens in the antigen-presenting cell and CD4, which seems essential for the effective triggering of helper-T-cell functions.

Recombinant CD4 analogues are being tried with the rationale that their introduction in circulation would block the viral binding sites and inhibit the infection of $CD4^+$ cells. A conjugate of CD4 protein and the toxic chain of ricin toxin has been used with success in experimental conditions, but its clinical efficiency is unknown.

Interferon α seems to inhibit HIV budding and has been approved by the F.D.A. for use in patients with Kaposi's sarcoma.

Other therapeutic measures in patients with HIV infection include the use of immunomodulating agents, such as thymosin, interleukin 2, and isoprinosine, in the hope of restoring the immune functions in AIDS patients or preventing the evolution toward AIDS in patients still asymptomatic or with the ARC; and the use of colony stimulating factors and erythropoietin in conjunction with AZT, as a way of minimizing the adverse effects on erythropoiesis and granulocytopoiesis. Chemotherapy specifically directed against the pathogens affecting AIDS, as in the case of the treatment and prophylaxis of *Pneumocystic carinii* pneumonia with pentamidine, may prolong survival, but the prognosis of patients with symptomatic AIDS remains extremely poor.

Great interest has surrounded the potential development of AIDS vaccines. Four basic types of vaccines are being tried:

1. Killed, genetically deficient viral particles
2. HIV subunits with adjuvants
3. Recombinant viruses containing the HIV *env* gene
4. Anti-idiotype vaccines using monoclonal anti-CD4 antibodies to raise an anti-idiotype that will compete with CD4 for binding to HIV, or vaccines using monoclonal antibodies to gp120 to raise an anti-idiotype resembling the epitope against which neutralizing antibodies are directed and which, in turn, would elicit a third anti-idiotype, this one with neutralizing effects on the viral particle

Killed vaccines have been attacked on the basis of difficulties in obtaining pure virus and of the possibility that the vaccine may contain fragments of viral RNA that, if reverse transcribed and integrated in the wrong position, could induce malignant transformation by activating a cellular proto-oncogene, for example. Recent reports, however, indicate that HIV-infected chimpanzees become apparently HIV-free and resistant to HIV superinfection, and that uninfected chimpanzees receiving the vaccine become only transiently infected when receiving a challenge dose of HIV. The vaccine has also been administered to patients with ARC without serious side effects, but it is not known whether the vaccine confers long-term protection against the development of AIDS.

Vaccines using isolated gp120 or recombinant viral particles induce neutralizing antibodies but fail to protect recipient chimpanzees against HIV challenge infection. In humans, recombinant gp160 and recombinant vaccinia virus vaccines have been tried, but their effectiveness is not clear.

Several other approaches are being tried, ranging from using multiple gp120 proteins in a single vaccine to using peptides representing more conserved regions (such as the CD4-binding domain). It is also believed that an efficient vaccine should stimulate cell-mediated immunity, which may be the only way to eliminate virus-infected cells that apparently can be involved in the transmission of HIV infection. Certain conserved epitopes of gp120 appear more effective in inducing T-cell-mediated immunity, but whether this knowledge can be applied in a practical vaccine is not known.

Besides general questions concerning the efficiency of the vaccine, related to the dormant nature of the infection in many asymptomatic carriers, and with the possibility of inducing enhancing antibodies that may be deleterious rather than protective, two main problems arise in the development of HIV vaccines.

1. The variability of gp120, against which neutralizing antibodies are directed. Different strains of HIV diverge by as much as 20% in the structure of gp120, and antibodies or CMI elicited with one strain do not cross-neutralize other strains. Furthermore, the virus infecting a given individual may undergo mutations, and a single amino acid substitution of a critical epitope of gp120

may render the virus insusceptible to neutralizing antibodies elicited earlier in the disease.

2. The difficulty in testing protection by the vaccine. There are no good animal models (chimpanzees are close, but far from perfect; they are susceptible to HIV infection but do not develop symptoms). Using the vaccine in seronegative individuals of populations at risk meets with a variety of problems such as the need to protect vaccinated subjects against discrimination based on seropositivity (which one hopes to achieve through vaccination), changes in behavior which may reduce the risk of natural infection in vaccinated volunteers, therefore giving a false notion of efficacy of the vaccine, possible adverse effects of the vaccine (antibodies may help to "select" mutant viral strains and may assist viral infection of macrophages), liability of vaccine producers if serious side effects are observed, etc.

SELF-EVALUATION

Questions

Choose the one best answer.

30.1 A large majority of individuals with serum IgA deficiency
  A. Are equally deficient in secretory IgA.
  B. Have an associated autoimmune disease.
  C. Have a partial or total deficiency of secretory component.
  D. Have a marked predisposition for upper respiratory infections.
  E. Have associated, but less pronounced, deficiencies of all major immunoglobulins.

30.2 The pathogenesis of some cases of adult-onset hypogammaglobulinemia may be related to
  A. The administration of live viral vaccines in the first few months of life.
  B. Increase in number and/or activity of suppressor T cells that block B-cell differentiation into antibody secreting cells.
  C. Failure of stem cell differentiation to B lymphocytes in the bone marrow.
  D. Deficient antigen processing and presentation by phagocytic cells.
  E. Total absence of B lymphocytes from lymphoid tissues and peripheral blood.

30.3 A pediatrician asks for an immunological work-up for cellular immunity in a 3-year-old child who has been acutely ill with measles in the past few days. Skin tests with candidid, SK-SD, PPD, and mumps antigen are negative. Lymphocyte transformation with PHA, measured by incorporation of ^{3}H-thymidine, is of 3,000 cpm; with Con A, the mitogenic response similarly measured is of 5,000 cpm. MIF tests using measles antigen and PPD are negative. In your report to the referring physician you will state that

A. The patient has primary cell-mediated immunodeficiency.
B. The patient has no immune abnormality.
C. No conclusion is possible.
D. There is a depression of cell-mediated immunity that could be secondary to the viral infection; the studies should be repeated 4 weeks later.
E. The results are difficult to interpret; blood shoud be collected as soon as possible to repeat in vitro studies.

30.4 The finding of antibodies to p24, p31, and gp160 in the serum of an individual previously found to be repeatedly positive in screening enzymo-immunoassays indicates that
A. The individual has AIDS.
B. The individual is infected with HIV.
C. The results of the screening tests were false positives.
D. The individual's immune system is functioning normally.
E. A second confirmatory test should be run.

30.5 In a normal 3-month-old child you expect to see
A. IgM as the quantitatively predominant serum immunoglobulin.
B. A concentration of IgG close to that of an adult, due to the persistence in circulation of maternally transferred IgG.
C. Generalized hypogammaglobulinemia.
D. Total lack of serum IgA.
E. Significantly lower levels of all immunoglobulin classes relative to normal adults levels.

In Questions 30.6-30.10, match each numbered word or phase with the one lettered heading that is most closely related to it. Each lettered heading may be selected once, more than once, or not at all. (A) Acquired agammaglobulin (common, variable, immunodeficiency); (B) Autosomal recessive form of severe combined immunodeficiency; (C) C6 deficiency; (D) DiGeorge syndrome; (E) Infantile agammaglobulinemia.

30.6 Associated with adenosine deaminase deficiency.

30.7 Defective differentiation of the third and fourth pharyngeal pouches.

30.8 Associated with frequent infections with *Neisseria* sp.

30.9 Absence of lymphocytes with surface immunoglobulin.

30.10 Associated with tetany and cardiac abnormalities.

Answers

30.1 (A)   Only one case of apparent selective deficiency of secretory IgA
(i.e., lack of secretory IgA coexisting with normal levels of serum
IgA) is known, while in all cases of serum IgA deficiency secretory
IgA has also been found to be deficient.

30.2 (B)   In most cases of adult-onset agammaglobulinemia, a variant of common variable immunodeficiency, the patients have normal B-cell
numbers, and one of several immunoregulation abnormalities (including excess of suppressor cells) appears to be responsible for the
deficiency.

30.3 (D)

30.4 (B)   The simultaneous finding of antibodies to p24, p31, and gp160 or its
components (gp120,gp41) in a Western blot is considered as confirmatory of HIV positive serology, and by inference of HIV infection. Positive serology is the rule in patients with symptomatic
AIDS, and it cannot be considered as an indication of a normally
functioning immune system.

30.5 (E)   The immunoglobulin levels of a child cannot be considered normal
or abnormal relative to those of an adult, but they should be compared to those of a reference group of children of the same age. At
3 months of age immunoglobulin levels in normal infants are significantly lower than those of an adult.

30.6 (B)

30.7 (D)   Characteristically, infants with the DiGeorge syndrome have combined aplasia of the thymus and parathyroids, and other congenital
abnormalities of the heart and large vessels.

30.8 (C)   Neisseria infections are frequently seen in patients with deficiency of
the late complement components.

30.9 (E)   In contrast to what is seen in patients with common variable immunodeficiency, infants with infantile agammaglobulinemia have a
marked depression or absence of B cells in the peripheral blood.

30.10(D)

BIBLIOGRAPHY

Chandra R. K. (Ed.). *Primary and Secondary Immunodeficiency Disorders.*
Churchill Livingstone, New York, 1984.

DeVita, V. T., Hellman, S., and Rosenberg, S. A. (Eds.). *AIDS—Etiology, Diagnosis, Treatment, and Prevention*, 2nd Ed. Lippincott, Philadelphia, 1988. (Perhaps the best comprehensive textbook on AIDS published to date.)

Durack, D. T. Infection in compromised hosts. In *Clinical Aspects of Immunology*, 4th Ed. Blackwell Scientific, Oxford, 1982, p. 1713.

Fishinger, P. J. Progress in vaccine development against AIDS. In *AIDS Updates July/August 1989*, De Vita, V. P., Ed. Lippincott, Philadelphia, 1989.

Good, R. A. and Pahwa, R. N. The recognition and management of immunodeficiency disorders. *Pediatric Infec. Dis. J. 7*(suppl), May, 1988.

Hansbrough, J. F., Zapata-Sirvent, R. L., and Peterson, V. M. Immunomodulation following burn injury. *Surg. Clinics N. Amer. 67*:69, 1987.

Hayward, A. Immunodeficiency. In *Clinical Aspects of Immunology*, 4th Ed. Blackwell Scientific, Oxford, 1982, p. 1658.

Kantoff, P. W., Freeman, S. M., and Anderson, W. F. Prospects for gene therapy for immunodeficiency disease. *Ann. Rev. Immunol. 6*:581, 1988.

Rosen, F. S., Cooper, M. D., and Wedgewood, R. J. P. The primary immunodeficiencies. *New Engl. J. Med. 311*:235, 300, 1984.

Rosen, F. S. Defects in cell-mediated immunity. *Clin. Immunol. Immunopath. 41*:1, 1986.

Scientific American. *What Science Knows about AIDS*. October, 1988.

Virella, G. and Fudenberg, H. H. Secondary immunodeficiencies. In *The Pathophysiology of Human Immunologic Disorders*, J. J. Twomey, Ed. Urban & Schwarzenberg, Baltimore-Munich, 1982.

WHO Scientific Group on Immunodeficiency. Primary immunodeficiency disease. *Clin. Immunol. Immunopathol. 28*:950, 1983.

Index

About the Editors

Gabriel Virella is Professor of Basic and Clinical Immunology and Microbiology at the Medical University of South Carolina in Charleston, where he has taught since 1975. His teaching has been clearly recognized by his students who have conferred upon him a total of six teaching excellence awards. Previously, he was a senior researcher in immunochemistry and immunopharmacology at the Gulbenkian Institute of Science in Oeiras, Portugal, and he also held postdoctoral fellowships at the University of Birmingham Medical School and the National Institute for Medical Research, London. The author or coauthor of 176 articles and several book chapters, he is a Fellow of the American Academy of Microbiology, as well as a member of the American Board of Medical Laboratory Immunology, British Society for Immunology, Association of Medical Laboratory Immunologists (charter member), and American Association of Immunologists. He is a section editor of *Clinical Immunology and Immunopathology*, and serves as an editorial board member of *Inmunologia* and *Journal of Clinical Laboratory Analyses*. He served as an editorial board member of *Clinical Immunology and Immunopathology* and of *Clinical and Diagnostic Immunology*. Dr. Virella received the M.D. (1967) and Ph.D. (1974) degrees from the University of Lisbon School of Medicine in Portugal.

Jean-Michel Goust is Professor of Immunology and Associated Professor of Neurology at the Medical University of South Carolina in Charleston, where he has taught since 1975. Prior to this he taught and conducted research in experimental pathology and immunology at Pitié-Salpêtrière Hospital in Paris, France. The coauthor of more than 75 articles and text chapters, Dr. Goust served as an editorial board member of *Clinical Immunology and Immunopathology*. He is a member of the Société Française d'Immunologie, American Federation for Clinical Research, American Association of Immunologists, American Society for Microbiology, Society for Experimental Biology and Medicine, and American Association for the Advancement of Science. Dr. Goust studied at the Lycée St. Louis in Paris and received the M.D. degree (1965) from the Faculty of Medicine, University of Paris.

H. Hugh Fudenberg is Professor of Basic and Clinical Immunology, Microbiology, and Medicine at the Medical University of South Carolina in Charleston. The author or coauthor of more than 810 scientific papers and six books, he was one of the original chief editors of the journal *Clinical Immunology and Immunopathology*, and is an editorial board member of many other journals. He is a Fellow of the American Academy of Microbiology and American Association for the Advancement of Science, as well as a member of the American Association of Immunologists, American Society for Clinical Investigation, American Society of Hematology, and many others. Among his many honors are the Pasteur Medal of the Institut Pasteur in Paris, the Petrov Medal for Distinguished Contributions to Oncologic Research (U.S.S.R.), and honorary doctorates from the University of Kuopio, Finland, Université Claude-Bernard, Lyons, France, the Free Science University (combined science faculties of Bologna, Padua, and Venice), Italy, and several others. Dr. Fudenberg received the A.B. degree (1949) from the University of California, Los Angeles, M.D. degree (1953) from the University of Chicago Medical School, and M.A. degree (1956) in immunochemistry from Boston University.